Pain Management for the Otolaryngologist

Editors

ANNA A. PASHKOVA
PETER F. SVIDER
JEAN ANDERSON ELOY

OTOLARYNGOLOGIC CLINICS OF NORTH AMERICA

www.oto.theclinics.com

Consulting Editor
SUJANA S. CHANDRASEKHAR

October 2020 • Volume 53 • Number 5

ELSEVIER

1600 John F. Kennedy Boulevard ● Suite 1800 ● Philadelphia, Pennsylvania, 19103-2899

http://www.oto.theclinics.com

OTOLARYNGOLOGIC CLINICS OF NORTH AMERICA Volume 53, Number 5
October 2020 ISSN 0030-6665, ISBN-13: 978-0-323-73303-8

Editor: Stacy Eastman
Developmental Editor: Laura Fisher

Otolaryngologic Clinics of North America (ISSN 0030-6665) is published bimonthly by Elsevier, Inc., 360 Park Avenue South, New York, NY 10010-1710. Months of issue are February, April, June, August, October, and December. Business and Editorial Offices: 1600 John F. Kennedy Blvd., Suite 1800, Philadelphia, PA 19103-2899. Customer Service Office: 6277 Sea Harbor Drive, Orlando, FL 32887-4800. Periodicals postage paid at New York, NY and additional mailing offices. Subscription prices are $424.00 per year (US individuals), $947.00 per year (US institutions), $100.00 per year (US & Canadian student/resident), $548.00 per year (Canadian individuals), $1200.00 per year (Canadian institutions), $592.00 per year (international individuals), $1200.00 per year (international institutions), $270.00 per year (international student/resident). Foreign air speed delivery is included in all *Clinics'* subscription prices. All prices are subject to change without notice. **POSTMASTER:** Send address changes to *Otolaryngologic Clinics of North America*, Elsevier Health Sciences Division, Subscription Customer Service, 3251 Riverport Lane, Maryland Heights, MO 63043. **Telephone: 1-800-654-2452 (U.S. and Canada); 314-447-8871 (outside U.S. and Canada). Fax: 314-447-8029. E-mail: journalscustomerservice-usa@elsevier.com (for print support); journalsonlinesupport-usa@elsevier.com (for online support).**

Reprints. For copies of 100 or more of articles in this publication, please contact the Commercial Reprints Department, Elsevier Inc., 360 Park Avenue South, New York, NY 10010-1710. Tel.: 212-633-3874; Fax: 212-633-3820; E-mail: reprints@elsevier.com.

Otolaryngologic Clinics of North America is also published in Spanish by McGraw-Hill Interamericana Editores S.A., P.O. Box 5-237, 06500 Mexico D.F., Mexico.

Otolaryngologic Clinics of North America is covered in *MEDLINE/PubMed (Index Medicus), Current Contents/Clinical Medicine, Excerpta Medica, BIOSIS, Science Citation Index,* and *ISI/BIOMED.*

Contributors

CONSULTING EDITOR

SUJANA S. CHANDRASEKHAR, MD, FACS, FAAOHNS
Past President, American Academy of Otolaryngology–Head and Neck Surgery,
Secretary-Treasurer, American Otological Society, Partner, ENT & Allergy Associates,
LLP, Clinical Professor, Department of Otolaryngology–Head and Neck Surgery, Zucker
School of Medicine at Hofstra/Northwell, Hempstead, New York, USA; Clinical Associate
Professor, Department of Otolaryngology–Head and Neck Surgery, Icahn School of
Medicine at Mount Sinai, New York, New York, USA

EDITORS

ANNA A. PASHKOVA, MD
Assistant Professor, Division of Pain Medicine, Department of Anesthesiology, Columbia
University Irving Medical Center, New York, New York, USA

PETER F. SVIDER, MD
Otolaryngology–Head and Neck Surgery, Bergen Medical Associates, Emerson,
New Jersey, USA; Rhinology, Sinus, and Endoscopic Sinus Surgery, Hackensack
Meridian Health, Hackensack University Medical Center, Hackensack, New Jersey,
USA

JEAN ANDERSON ELOY, MD, FACS, FARS
Professor and Vice Chair, Director, Rhinology and Sinus Surgery, Director, Otolaryngology
Research, Co-Director, Endoscopic Skull Base Surgery Program, Department of
Otolaryngology–Head and Neck Surgery, Center for Skull Base and Pituitary Surgery,
Neurological Institute of New Jersey, Department of Neurological Surgery, Department of
Ophthalmology and Visual Science, Rutgers New Jersey Medical School, Chair and Chief
of Service, Department of Otolaryngology and Facial Plastic Surgery, Saint Barnabas
Medical Center, RWJ Barnabas Health, Newark, New Jersey

JENNIFER A. VILLWOCK, MD
Associate Professor, Department of Otolaryngology–Head and Neck Surgery, Kansas
University, Associate Program Director, The University of Kansas Medical Center, Kansas
City, Kansas, USA

AUTHORS

SAI ALLA, MD
PGY-3 Resident Physician, Department of Anesthesiology, Emory University, Atlanta,
Georgia, USA

CATHERINE BANKS, MD
Department of Otolaryngology–Head and Neck Surgery, Prince of Wales Hospital,
University of New South Wales, Sydney, Australia

MICHAEL A. BLASCO, MD
Department of Otolaryngology–Head and Neck Surgery, Princess Margaret Cancer Centre/University Health Network, University of Toronto, Toronto, Ontario, Canada

MICHAEL BOBIAN, MD
Department of Otolaryngology–Head and Neck Surgery, Medical University of South Carolina, Charleston, South Carolina, USA

ELIZABETH BOSCOE, MD
PGY III Resident Physician, Department of Otolaryngology, University of Colorado School of Medicine, Aurora, Colorado, USA

AMISHAV BRESLER, MD
Department of Otolaryngology, Rutgers University, Newark, New Jersey, USA

CRISTINA CABRERA-MUFFLY, MD
Associate Professor, Department of Otolaryngology, University of Colorado School of Medicine, Aurora, Colorado, USA

LAUREN M. CASS, MD, MPH
Department of Otolaryngology–Head and Neck Surgery, The University of Kansas Medical Center, Kansas City, Kansas, USA

KIMBERLY K. COCA, BS
Department of Otolaryngology–Head and Neck Surgery, The University of Tennessee Health Science Center, Memphis, Tennessee, USA

DAVID S. COHEN, MD
Partner Physician, Department of Head and Neck Surgery, Southern California Permanente Medical Group, Harbor City, California, USA

JOEHASSIN CORDERO, MD
Professor, Department of Otolaryngology–Head and Neck Surgery, Texas Tech University Health Sciences Center, Lubbock, Texas, USA

JOHN D. CRAMER, MD
Department of Otolaryngology–Head and Neck Surgery, Wayne State University School of Medicine, Detroit, USA

VANINDER K. DHILLON, MD
Assistant Professor, Department of Otolaryngology, Johns Hopkins University, Bethesda, Maryland, USA

YUSUF DUNDAR, MD
Assistant Professor, Department of Otolaryngology–Head and Neck Surgery, Texas Tech University Health Sciences Center, Lubbock, Texas, USA

JEAN ANDERSON ELOY, MD, FACS, FARS
Professor and Vice Chair, Director, Rhinology and Sinus Surgery, Director, Otolaryngology Research, Co-Director, Endoscopic Skull Base Surgery Program, Department of Otolaryngology–Head and Neck Surgery, Center for Skull Base and Pituitary Surgery, Neurological Institute of New Jersey, Department of Neurological Surgery, Department of Ophthalmology and Visual Science, Rutgers New Jersey Medical School, Chair and Chief of Service, Department of Otolaryngology and Facial Plastic Surgery, Saint Barnabas Medical Center, RWJ Barnabas Health, Newark, New Jersey, USA

ADAM J. FOLBE, MD
Department of Otolaryngology, William Beaumont Hospital, Royal Oak, Michigan, USA; Barbara Ann Karmanos Cancer Institute, Detroit, Michigan, USA

CARRIE L. FRANCIS, MD
Associate Professor, Department of Otolaryngology–Head and Neck Surgery, Assistant Dean, Office of Student Affairs, The University of Kansas Medical Center, Kansas City, Kansas, USA

EVAN M. GRABOYES, MD, MPH, FACS
Department of Otolaryngology–Head and Neck Surgery, Medical University of South Carolina, Charleston, South Carolina, USA

NATASA GRANCARIC, MD
Assistant Professor, Department of Anesthesiology, Columbia University Irving Medical Center, New York, New York, USA

STACEY T. GRAY, MD
Associate Professor, Department of Otolaryngology–Head and Neck Surgery, Massachusetts Eye and Ear, Harvard Medical School, Boston, Massachusetts, USA

ERICA C. GRISSOM, CRNA
Instructor, Department of Anesthesiology, The University of Tennessee Health Science Center, Memphis, Tennessee, USA

ANNIKA GUPTA, MD
Department of Otolaryngology–Head and Neck Surgery, Medical University of South Carolina, Charleston, South Carolina, USA

WAYNE D. HSUEH, MD
Department of Otolaryngology–Head and Neck Surgery, Rutgers New Jersey Medical School, Newark, New Jersey, USA

QASIM HUSAIN, MD
Assistant Professor, Hackensack Meridian School of Medicine at Seton Hall University, Coastal Ear, Nose, and Throat, Holmdel, New Jersey, USA

BABAK JAHAN-PARWAR, MD
Partner Physician, Department of Head and Neck Surgery, Southern California Permanente Medical Group, Baldwin Park, California, USA

ANDREW P. JOHNSON, MD
Assistant Professor, Department of Otolaryngology, University of Colorado School of Medicine, Aurora, Colorado, USA

RAYMOND KIM, MBChB, PhD
Department of Otolaryngology–Head and Neck Surgery, Stanford University School of Medicine, Stanford, California, USA

WOOJIN LEE, MD
Resident Physician, Department of Anesthesiology, Columbia University Irving Medical Center, New York, New York, USA

HO-SHENG LIN, MD
Department of Otolaryngology–Head and Neck Surgery, Wayne State University, Detroit, Michigan, USA

JORDYN P. LUCAS, MD
Department of Otolaryngology–Head and Neck Surgery, Wayne State University School of Medicine, Detroit, Michigan, USA

ANDREW J. MARODA, MD
Department of Pediatric Otolaryngology, Le Bonheur Children's Hospital, Department of Otolaryngology–Head and Neck Surgery, The University of Tennessee Health Science Center, Memphis, Tennessee, USA

NICOLE MATAR, MD
Department of Anesthesiology, Columbia University Irving Medical Center, New York, New York, USA

JENNIFER D. McLEVY-BAZZANELLA, MD
Assistant Professor, Department of Otolaryngology–Head and Neck Surgery, The University of Tennessee Health Science Center, Memphis, Tennessee, USA

TAHA S. MERAJ, MD
Department of Otolaryngology, Wayne State University, Detroit, Michigan, USA

LINDSAY S. MOORE, MD
Department of Otolaryngology, The University of Alabama at Birmingham, Birmingham, Alabama, USA

DANIEL R. MORRISON, MD
Department of Otolaryngology, The University of Alabama at Birmingham, Birmingham, Alabama, USA

BRANDON K. NGUYEN, MD
Department of Otolaryngology–Head and Neck Surgery, Rutgers New Jersey Medical School, Newark, New Jersey, USA

ANNA A. PASHKOVA, MD
Assistant Professor, Division of Pain Medicine, Department of Anesthesiology, Columbia University Irving Medical Center, New York, New York, USA

ZARA M. PATEL, MD
Associate Professor, Director of Endoscopic Skull Base Surgery, Department of Otolaryngology–Head and Neck Surgery, Stanford University School of Medicine, Stanford, California, USA

MADELINE SCANLON, MD, MPH
Resident Physician, Department of Anesthesiology, Columbia University Irving Medical Center, New York, New York, USA

KEROLOS G. SHENOUDA, MD
Department of Otolaryngology–Head and Neck Surgery, Wayne State University, Detroit, Michigan, USA

ANTHONY M. SHEYN, MD
Associate Professor, Department of Otolaryngology–Head and Neck Surgery, The University of Tennessee Health Science Center, Department of Pediatric Otolaryngology, St. Jude Children's Research Hospital, Department of Pediatric Otolaryngology, Le Bonheur Children's Hospital, Memphis, Tennessee, USA

JOSHUA B. SMITH, MD
Department of Otolaryngology–Head and Neck Surgery, The University of Kansas Medical Center, Kansas City, Kansas, USA

NOMITA SONTY, MPhil, PhD
Associate Professor at CUIMC, Departments of Anesthesiology and Psychiatry, Vagelos College of Physicians and Surgeons, Columbia University, New York, New York, USA

MELISSA STRAUB, MD, MPH
Department of Anesthesiology, Columbia University Medical Center, New York, USA

PETER F. SVIDER, MD
Otolaryngology–Head and Neck Surgery, Bergen Medical Associates, Emerson, New Jersey, USA; Rhinology, Sinus, and Endoscopic Sinus Surgery, Hackensack Meridian Health, Hackensack University Medical Center, Hackensack, New Jersey, USA

KATHERINE TINKEY, MD
PGY-4 Resident Physician, Department of Anesthesiology, Emory University, Atlanta, Georgia, USA

JENNIFER A. VILLWOCK, MD
Associate Professor, Department of Otolaryngology–Head and Neck Surgery, Kansas University, Associate Program Director, The University of Kansas Medical Center, Kansas City, Kansas, USA

ERIKA M. WALSH, MD
Assistant Professor, Department of Otolaryngology, The University of Alabama at Birmingham, Birmingham, Alabama, USA

JONATHAN A. WAXMAN, MD, PhD
Department of Otolaryngology–Head and Neck Surgery, Wayne State University, Detroit, Michigan, USA

JOSHUA W. WOOD, MD
Assistant Professor, Department of Otolaryngology–Head and Neck Surgery, The University of Tennessee Health Science Center, Memphis, Tennessee, USA

NAN XIANG, MD
Assistant Professor in Pain Management, Department of Anesthesiology, Emory University, Atlanta, Georgia, USA

GIANCARLO F. ZULIANI, MD
Clinical Associate Professor, Department of Otolaryngology, Wayne State University, Detroit, Michigan, USA; Zuliani Facial Aesthetics, Bloomfield Hills, Michigan, USA

Contents

Many individuals believe that physicians can be difficult when they become patients, as having "just enough" knowledge or attempting to direct one's personal medical care presents problems particularly when dealing with a dynamic issue such as analgesia. Physicians are used to being advocates for their patients, and when they are the patients themselves, there is a certain degree of transition that changes one's perspective and affects how complex medical issues are addressed. There has been an evolution in management of pain concerns in recent decades with growing recognition of the toll of the opioid epidemic on our society.

Nearly 50,000 US adults experience opioid-overdose deaths annually and 1.7 million experience a substance use disorder from prescription opioids. Hence, understanding analgesia strategies is of utmost importance. A preoperative analgesic plan can consist of a brief conversation between the surgeon, patient, and anesthesiologist in an uncomplicated case or range all the way to an involved, multidisciplinary plan for a chronic pain patient. Over the past several decades, there have been myriad studies examining perioperative analgesic regimens for otolaryngologic procedures, many of which have demonstrated the efficacy of nonopioid analgesics.

The perioperative analgesic plan begins with preoperative planning. The surgeon should be versed in practical approaches for managing analgesia in patients with chronic pain. The first step includes evaluating the patient and conducting a focused pain history. Confirming, documenting, and understanding current outpatient prescriptions is critical. Patients should be screened for medical conditions that preclude the use of certain analgesics, or place them at higher risk of respiratory depression. Providers should coordinate with the patient's outpatient prescribers and pain specialists to ensure a safe and effective analgesic plan. Multimodal analgesia should be implemented to optimize analgesia and decrease opioid requirements.

Local anesthesia is commonly used for head and neck procedures. Many anesthetic agents are available, with differing properties that can alter their durations of action and lengths of time to onset. These agents can be used acutely for laceration repair or as adjuncts to intravenous sedation. Local and regional anesthetic agents can also be used for chronic conditions. Several local anesthetic blocks are available. Local anesthesia has the potential for complications, ranging from issues with injection process, such as a broken needle, to reactions of the anesthetic agent. Some populations are more at risk for certain reactions to anesthesia.

Acute pain management following major head and neck (HN) surgery is complex. Multimodal analgesia (MMA) regimens including acetaminophen, nonsteroidal anti-inflammatory drugs, gabapentinoids, and locoregional anesthetics are safe and effective in this population (including patients undergoing HN free flap surgery). Special considerations for patients undergoing HN free flap surgery include judicious use of steroids and attention to donor site pain. Evidence for specific analgesic regimens following transoral robotic surgery is limited but should include MMA and perioperative dexamethasone. Further study is required to optimize combinations, dosages, and duration of perioperative analgesia medications, opioid and nonopioid, for patients undergoing major HN surgery.

A literature review was conducted regarding the assessment and treatment of postoperative pain following surgery for obstructive sleep apnea (OSA). Given the risks of opioid use by patients with OSA, special attention to opioid risk reduction and avoidance is warranted in this population. The results of this review demonstrate the existence of a body of evidence that supports the use of nonopioid analgesics and nonpharmacologic approaches pain management. Strategies for managing postoperative pain should emphasize the use of local anesthetic infiltration, nonsteroidal antiinflammatory drugs, acetaminophen, topical analgesics, surgical wound cooling, and when necessary, safer opioid medications, such as tramadol and intranasal butorphanol.

This article discusses the algorithms and published practice patterns on perioperative analgesia for thyroid and parathyroid surgery. This includes medications and techniques used for general anesthesia, local anesthesia including nerve block methods, and oral medication used for postoperative pain control. The authors also discuss multimodality pain control and the increased trend to reduce opioid analgesics without inadequate pain control or patient satisfaction.

Brandon K. Nguyen, Peter F. Svider, Wayne D. Hsueh, and Adam J. Folbe

Perioperative analgesic management is multifaceted, and an individualized approach should be taken with each patient. Preoperative discussion of the plan for pain control and the patient's postoperative expectations is a necessary facet for optimal outcomes of analgesia. There is the potential for significant abuse and development of dependence on opioids. Nonopioids, such as nonsteroidal anti-inflammatory drugs, acetaminophen, and gabapentinoids, provide reliable alternatives for analgesic management following sinus and skull-base surgery. There is a paucity of literature regarding perioperative pain regimens for sinus and skull-base surgery, and the authors hope that this review serves as a valuable tool for otolaryngologists.

Daniel R. Morrison, Lindsay S. Moore, and Erika M. Walsh

Otologic surgery involves a broad range of procedures. In general, postoperative pain from most otologic surgeries can be managed with little to no opioids, and surgeons should make a concerted effort to minimize narcotic prescriptions in the midst of the opioid crisis. Many procedures, including transcanal surgeries and even postauricular surgeries, may performed with local anesthetic in selected patients. Multimodal pain regimens, local anesthesia, and alternative approaches have shown promise in minimizing narcotic use, and should be considered. Preoperative counseling to appropriately manage expectations and goals is imperative for patient satisfaction and safety.

Taha S. Meraj, Amishav Bresler, and Giancarlo F. Zuliani

Facial plastic surgery, including septorhinoplasty, aging face procedures, otoplasty, and oculoplastic procedures, has varying levels of evidence for the management of acute pain after surgery. This article discusses the available evidence in these procedures and discusses the authors' recommendations for the treatment of postoperative pain, with a focus on decreasing the reliance on opioid pain medication.

Andrew J. Maroda, Kimberly K. Coca, Jennifer D. McLevy-Bazzanella, Joshua W. Wood, Erica C. Grissom, and Anthony M. Sheyn

This article reviews the evidence regarding current perioperative pain management strategies in pediatric patients undergoing otolaryngologic surgery. Pediatric otolaryngology is a broad field with a wide variety of surgical procedures that each requires careful consideration for optimal perioperative pain management. Adequate pain control is vital to ensuring patient safety and achieving successful postoperative care, but many young children are limited in their capacity to communicate their pain experience. Current literature holds a disproportionate amount of focus on pain management for certain procedures, whereas there is a paucity of evidence-based literature informing most other procedures within the field.

chronic pain. Treatment of chronic pain encompasses analgesic medications; adjuvant pharmacotherapy, including antidepressants and anticonvulsants; interventional techniques; as well as integrative medicine.

Controlled substance agreements between providers and patients represent important strategies for setting expectations for chronic opioid therapy. These agreements generally summarize best opioid prescription practices and destigmatize practice policies such as regular toxicology screenings. These controlled substance agreements also set expectations for discontinuation of therapy if appropriate.

Pain is one of the leading reasons that brings patients into health care facilities; yet, it often is left undertreated. The biopsychosocial model of pain, which recognizes that pain is multidimensional, explains the complexities that affect the pain experience and response to treatment. Inclusion of behavioral and psychological factors in medical and surgical evaluations can facilitate an optimal outcome. When pain no longer is acute but becomes chronic, access to psychotherapeutic interventions becomes necessary to improve course and prognosis. Techniques, such as psycho-education, deep breathing, imagery, and addressing expectations and catastrophic beliefs, can be incorporated into medical and surgical practices.

The diagnosis "sinus headache" has been reclassified as "headache attributed to disorder of the nose or paranasal sinuses" by the International Headache Society, but the term is still commonly used by patients and primary care doctors alike. Rhinologic symptoms and headache disorders are common, and they may coexist without a causative relationship. Patients may undergo unnecessary medical interventions because of inadequate understanding of the classifications and management of various headache disorders. Otolaryngologists frequently treat patients with these complaints, and a systematic approach to the differential diagnosis and utilization of a multidisciplinary approach are critical in providing optimal patient care.

In the last 30 years, pain control in the United States has undergone several evolutions impacting the care of surgical patients. More recently, safe pain control has been a subject of quality improvement efforts by otolaryngologists focusing on minimizing opioid consumption. This article discusses the rising overprescription of opioids, influenced by legislation and governmental agencies, and the steps taken to correct and reform policies to decrease the amount of opioids prescribed. Lastly, specific institutional examples of quality improvement protocols implemented to help decrease opioid consumption and prescription are discussed.

A shortage of otolaryngologists is predicted for the coming decades, primarily because of an aging population and aging workforce. However, many factors affect the agility of the workforce to expand or contract. This article discusses what is known about factors of the current otolaryngology workforce, including trends in residency and fellowship training, diversity of the specialty, its geographic distribution, and the challenges of caring for an aging population. Predicting the shortage and possible solutions through modeling is complex and prone to errors caused by incomplete data and assumptions about otolaryngology's similarity to other specialties of medicine at large.

Otolaryngology has historically lagged behind other specialties with respect to diversity, equity and inclusion (DEI) and remains one of the least diverse specialties as it relates to gender, race and ethnicity. Strategies aimed at increasing DEI include programs designed to provide mentorship, coaching, and sponsorship. Pipeline efforts, inclusivity on committees, bi-directional communication, and equal pay are additional DEI efforts that have been successful in recruiting and retaining those underrepresented in medicine (URiM). Closing the equity gap requires commitment; daily action and measuring progress is required. Finally, use feedback to make refinements as opportunities exist to continually improve DEI efforts.

OTOLARYNGOLOGIC CLINICS OF NORTH AMERICA

SERIES OF RELATED INTEREST

Facial Plastic Surgery Clinics
Available at: https://www.facialplastic.theclinics.com/

THE CLINICS ARE AVAILABLE ONLINE!
Access your subscription at:
www.theclinics.com

Foreword

Changing the Management of Pain in Otolaryngology

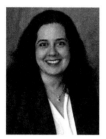

Sujana S. Chandrasekhar, MD, FACS, FAAOHNS
Consulting Editor

Physicians the world over have come to understand the role we have played in contributing to the current opioid epidemic. There are an estimated 2 million patients in the United States who have an opioid use disorder, with approximately 90 deaths occurring every day in the United States from an opioid overdose.[1] However, the roots of this crisis are deeper than a single factor would explain. This issue of *Otolaryngologic Clinics of North America*, guest edited by Drs Eloy, Svider, and Pashkova, takes the reader on a journey to understanding acute and chronic pain, pain psychology, and opportunities for improvement of the quality of care and patient comfort outcomes in Otolaryngology.

Fear of pain is deeply rooted among patients who are about to have surgery. *The Lancet* published a series of articles looking at pain from the surgical perspective. Key statements from the Commentary[2] are as follows: (1) Satisfactory perioperative pain management is crucial; (2) Despite decades of research showing the benefits of various new analgesic strategies, many patients continue to endure severe postoperative pain, and this holds true across all age groups and continents, even after "minor" surgery; and (3) Even as recently as 2016, a study of 799,449 patients in the United States showed that reliance on opioid analgesics remains the mainstay for perioperative pain management,[3] highlighting the ongoing pivotal role of the health care system in this epidemic.

The US epidemic is felt to have 3 phases.[4]) The first phase began in the 1970s with overprescription of opioids for acute pain, and the secondary diversion, misuse and abuse of these legal drugs. It was compounded by the 1990s as chronic pain management needs increased due to greater patient expectations for pain relief and greater survivorship after cancer and complex surgery, among other factors. When effective behavioral therapies, such as cognitive behavioral therapy, were no longer covered adequately by insurers, the pharmaceutical and device industries burgeoned in this

Otolaryngol Clin N Am 53 (2020) xvii–xix
https://doi.org/10.1016/j.otc.2020.07.001
0030-6665/20/© 2020 Published by Elsevier Inc.

sector, and chronic pain became big business by 2000. This, coupled with withdrawal from the market of some nonopioid medications and some unethical kick-back schemes, led to the dramatic rise in rates of overdose and addiction. Phase 2 started around 2010, based on concerns about intertwined opioid analgesic and heroin abuse. Heroin overdose deaths spiked, tripling between 2010 and 2015. This was attributed to an expanded pool of individuals with rising dependency and tolerance, who turned to the cheaper and easier available heroin on the street, as well as the increasing concern among physicians and policymakers regarding opioids. The third phase began in 2013 and continues to today. This phase includes a shocking rise in deaths attributed to illicitly manufactured fentanyl analogs: 540% in the United States between 2013 and 2016. Contrary to the single-blame model that health care overprescription is the gateway to addiction, individuals entering drug treatment nowadays are more likely to report that their first exposure was to heroin and not to a prescribed analgesic.

In 2012, US pharmacies and long-term care facilities dispensed 4.2 billion prescriptions, 289 million (6.8%) of which were opioids. Primary care specialties accounted for nearly half of all dispensed opioid prescriptions. The rate of opioid prescribing was highest for specialists in pain medicine (48.6%); surgery (36.5%); and physical medicine/rehabilitation (35.5%). The rate of opioid prescribing rose during 2007 to 2010 but leveled thereafter as most specialties reduced opioid use. The greatest percentage increase in opioid-prescribing rates during 2007 to 2012 occurred among physical medicine/rehabilitation specialists (+12.0%). The largest percentage drops in opioid-prescribing rates occurred in emergency medicine (−8.9%) and dentistry (−5.7%).[5]

Although otolaryngologists are not the main drivers of the opioid epidemic, we must be cognizant and ensure that we are active participants in managing our patients' acute and chronic pain. This issue of *Otolaryngologic Clinics of North America* covers the issues in actionable detail, and I urge you to read it through. Your patients will thank you.

Sujana S. Chandrasekhar, MD, FACS, FAAOHNS
Consulting Editor, Otolaryngologic Clinics of North America

Past President, American Academy of Otolaryngology–Head and Neck Surgery

Secretary-Treasurer, American Otological Society

Partner, ENT & Allergy Associates LLP
18 East 48th Street, 2nd Floor, New York, NY 10017, USA

Clinical Professor, Department of Otolaryngology–Head and Neck Surgery
Zucker School of Medicine at Hofstra-Northwell, Hempstead, NY, USA

Clinical Associate Professor, Department of Otolaryngology–Head and Neck Surgery
Icahn School of Medicine at Mount Sinai, New York, NY, USA

E-mail address:
ssc@nyotology.com

REFERENCES

1. Schuchat A, Houry D, Guy GP. New data on opioid use and prescribing in the United States. JAMA 2017;318:425–6.
2. Hollman MW, Rathmell JP, Lirk P. Comment: optimal postoperative pain management: redefining the role for opioids. Lancet 2019;393(10180):1483–5.

3. Ladha KS, Patorno E, Huybrechts KF, et al. Variations in the use of perioperative multimodal analgesic therapy. Anesthesiology 2016;124:837–45.
4. Dasgupta N, Beletsky L, Ciccarone D. Opioid crisis: no easy fix to its social and economic determinants. Am J Public Health 2018;108:182–6.
5. Levy B, Paulozzi L, Mack KA, Jones CM. Trends in Opioid Analgesic-Prescribing Rates by Specialty, U.S., 2007-2012. Am J Prev Med 2015 Sept;49(3):409-413.

Preface

Pain Management for the Otolaryngologist

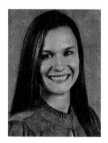 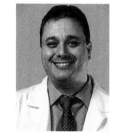 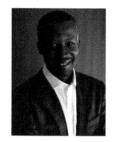

Anna A. Pashkova, MD   Peter F. Svider, MD   Jean Anderson Eloy, MD, FACS, FARS
Editors

There have been extensive paradigm shifts in the management of perioperative analgesia when it comes to surgical patients over the past 3 decades. In the late 1990s, several private and government-based organizations raised recognition of pain as an undertreated "vital sign," a policy that has led to unintended consequences, including the rise of the contemporary opioid epidemic.

An interdisciplinary approach among surgeons, anesthesiologists, pain physicians, and other health care providers has been invaluable in tackling the opioid epidemic, and in this issue of *Otolaryngologic Clinics of North America*, we emphasize our understanding of contemporary strategies for managing pain in the perioperative Otolaryngologic setting. Surgeons must be well versed in appropriate and safe opioid prescription practices, as well as evidence-based nonopioid alternatives and multimodal analgesia. Our hope is that by incorporating evidence-based approaches, the

Otolaryngol Clin N Am 53 (2020) xxi–xxii
https://doi.org/10.1016/j.otc.2020.07.002
0030-6665/20/© 2020 Published by Elsevier Inc.

number of inappropriately prescribed opioids in the perioperative setting decreases while ensuring adequate analgesia for optimal patient management.

Anna A. Pashkova, MD
Division of Pain Medicine
Department of Anesthesiology
Columbia University Medical Center
622 West 168th Street
New York, NY 10032, USA

Peter F. Svider, MD
Otolaryngology–Head and Neck Surgery
Rhinology, Sinus, and Endoscopic Sinus Surgery
Bergen Medical Associates
466 Old Hook Road #1
Emerson, NJ 07630, USA

Jean Anderson Eloy, MD, FACS, FARS
Endoscopic Skull Base Surgery Program
Department of Otolaryngology–
Head and Neck Surgery
Center for Skull Base and Pituitary Surgery
Neurological Institute of New Jersey
Rutgers New Jersey Medical School
Department of Neurological Surgery
90 Bergen Street, DOC 8100
Newark, NJ 07103, USA

E-mail addresses:
ap3762@cumc.columbia.edu (A.A. Pashkova)
psvider@gmail.com (P.F. Svider)
jean.anderson.eloy@gmail.com (J.A. Eloy)

Introduction: Opioid Analgesia: A Patient Perspective

Peter F. Svider, MD[a,b],*

KEYWORDS

- Opioid analgesia • Prescription Opioid • Patient perspective • Physician perspective
- Physician as patient • Pain medication • Opioid crisis

KEY POINTS

- Many individuals believe that physicians can be difficult when they become patients, as having "just enough" knowledge or attempting to direct one's personal medical care presents problems particularly when dealing with a dynamic issue such as analgesia.
- Physicians are used to being advocates for their patients, and when they are the patients themselves, there is a certain degree of transition that changes one's perspective and affects how complex medical issues are addressed.
- There has been an evolution in management of pain concerns in recent decades with growing recognition of the toll of the opioid epidemic on our society.

There is certainly anecdotal evidence supporting the long-held adage that "physicians make the worst patients." Domeyer-Klenske and Rosenbaum identified several different approaches physicians take when treating a colleague, ranging from ignoring the physician-patient's medical background or negotiating care around this background knowledge to allowing physician-patients to drive management.[1] With these considerations in mind, transitioning from being the physician to being the patient does change one's perspective and can provide invaluable strategies for dealing with complex medical issues. A significant portion of medical training involves development of a physician's ability to serve as an advocate for our patients, and these skills are often harnessed excessively when physicians advocate for themselves and/or family members.[2]

When the physician becomes the patient, this can potentially raise problematic issues, such as when physicians try to direct their own care or when the objectivity of the treating physician becomes obscured. The American Medical Association's

Financial Disclosures and Conflicts of Interest: None.
[a] Hackensack University Medical Center, Hackensack, NJ, USA; [b] Bergen Medical Associates, 466 Old Hook Road, Suite 1, Emerson, NJ 07630, USA
* Bergen Medical Associates, 466 Old Hook Road, Suite 1, Emerson, NJ 07630.
E-mail address: psvider@gmail.com

code of ethics explicitly states that "physicians should not treat themselves or members of their immediate families...professional objectivity may be compromised."[3] This represents a particularly dynamic issue when topics such as analgesia come up, as there has been an evolution in familiarity and management of pain concerns in recent decades, with the pendulum swinging from pain as an underrecognized "fifth vital sign" up through widespread recognition of the contemporary opioid epidemic.

As anybody familiar with political discourse nowadays can attest, the opioid "epidemic" has reached critical mass and captured public awareness in recent years. This crisis was initiated around the turn of the century by a variety of organizations trying to shed light on the "underrecognition" of pain control in our health care system. For example, in 2000 JCAHO released standards that maximized awareness of "the right to pain relief." Around this time began a concomitant increase in direct to consumer marketing of painkillers.[4] Consequently, these trends continued, with current economic costs of *prescription opioid misuse* amounting to nearly $80 Billion annually.[5,6] Nearly 50,000 people died from opioid overdoses in the United States in 2017, whereas 1.7 million Americans qualified as having a substance use disorder due to the misuse of prescription opioids.[7] With increasing recognition of these considerations, addressing this crisis from both a supply and demand standpoint has involved a multipronged public health approach, including strategies for reducing access to prescription opioids, minimizing overprescription, diversion, and misuse and doing a better job of educating patients and physicians about the appropriate use of these drugs and available alternatives.[8]

Over the past year, I have had the opportunity to experience our health care system as well as aspects of various analgesia strategies from a patient perspective rather than that of the physician, and this has provided some compelling insights. There is little in the literature or lay press describing physician experiences with opioid analgesia; my hope is stepping back and briefly sharing some of these personal experiences may provide a practical perspective.

After attributing many months of cough, fatigue, and night sweats to other causes, I was diagnosed with lymphoma and started on chemotherapy about 6 weeks after finishing my fellowship and starting practice as an attending. I was doing well on my chemotherapy regimen until experiencing drug-induced pancreatitis, an adverse event specific to one of the induction chemotherapy agents. This pancreatitis itself was initially "mild." Nonetheless, lingering and worsening symptoms along with the development of pseudocysts dragged these sequelae out over many more episodes of pancreatitis lasting months and gave me the unfortunate but eye-opening experience of both acute and chronic analgesic strategies in action. During my first emergency department visit for severe abdominal pain, before seeing a physician an order was written for me to receive 6 mg of intravenous (IV) morphine. For an opioid naïve patient who had never even had any pain medications in their life, having this medication "pushed" very quickly without an explanation of what exactly I was getting was quite an experience; the intentions behind it were good and it ultimately worked very well from an analgesic standpoint, but nothing quite prepares someone for the accompanying "head rush," sensation of passing out, and generalized discomfort that precedes the analgesic effects. Over the remainder of this initial hospitalization along with subsequent ones for lingering and worsening symptoms, I ended up going through a multitude of different phases relating to analgesia, including the following: trying to avoid any pain medicine use at all, trying to minimize intravenous pain medication use, attempting to be comfortable without concern for how much I thought I was using, and in-depth discussions for the most appropriate outpatient regimens to facilitate the use of nonopioid alternatives. Nonetheless, unless one has personally experienced the ebbs and flows of high-dose narcotic usage in both acute and chronic situations, it is impossible to describe the uncertainties and perceptions encountered. During these episodes it was remarkable to learn how my perceptions of narcotic usage (of which I felt I was using a huge amount) diverged with my treatment team's perceptions. In addition to the medical aspects of opioid usage and related health events, there are certainly the psychosocial impacts associated with considering these medications, such as a fear of dependence as well as concerns regarding how continued use could affect one's ability to lead a regular life (ie, working, driving) when not in the hospital. For example, I had worked toward a goal for so long, finally finished residency and fellowship, and 6 weeks into my job as an attending physician when I was starting to see more patients and perform more surgeries, I faced a diagnosis that had a potential to upend all of this. Having an unpredictable schedule, canceling patients frequently, and realizing you have suddenly missed 3 months of work after missing virtually no time the first few weeks of chemotherapy certainly all contribute as a psychosocial stressor. Going through 15 hospitalizations, multiple unexpected surgeries, and countless rounds of chemotherapy all have psychosocial effects, something that can affect analgesic strategies and patient management in general. This stresses the value of adding sections in the present issue such as Pain Psychology: *Practical Approaches for Otolaryngologists*, as the physical aspects of pain may not be the only consideration you are managing.

Although the current issue of *Otolaryngologic Clinics of North America* focuses more on perioperative analgesia, there are several lessons I took away from my personal experiences that I think can be kept in mind and invaluable for anyone managing someone's pain, some of which may be obvious and some of which are not:

- "Evidence-based" practices sometimes go out the window when you are in acute and severe pain, at least from a patient consent and decision-making perspective. This is where it is important for your treating physician to be familiar with evidence-based medicine and quality improvement practices, because in an acute pain crisis, you as a physician are not necessarily having an exhaustive discussion of risks, alternatives, and benefits or discussing outpatient regimens that are appropriate.
- If you find yourself in the situation of being the patient, try not to be your own doctor. This may seem self-evident even beyond us harping on this earlier, but it is actually not too difficult to find yourself placed in this situation. There were multiple times physicians who evaluated me either in the emergency department or elsewhere during these hospitalizations would ask "What do you want to do?" or "How would you like to proceed?" For some of these specific situations, just background knowledge and common sense dictated that they would not have provided these open-ended choices to nonphysicians. Although having the opportunity to participate in decision-making is something that is an important part of the physician patient relationship, being asked these open-ended questions on topics in which patients would normally not be asked for this much input was a bit disconcerting, particularly as this was brought up several times in relation to what should be my pain regimen.
- In situations during my care in which trainees were involved, I could not help but wonder how much formal opioid prescribing education these residents had in their training; I had just been a trainee and realize myself there is a dearth of

formalized opioid prescribing education opportunities. For example, I had just underwent a surgical resection of an infected pancreatic pseudocyst, with my preoperative pain requirements being considerable (2 mg Dilaudid every 2–4 hours); the on-call surgical resident felt they were being proactive in "getting me out of bed" by completely cutting off IV pain medications and replacing with IV Dilaudid with PO oxycodone *after* surgery. This is clearly due to a lack of education and understanding, not a lack of empathy: the resident had no knowledge of opioid conversion ratios and was not aware of the importance of my prior interdisciplinary regimen that the pain team had come up with. This is not to say it is the individual's fault; this ignorance of opioid prescribing education is a systemic issue.

- The urgent and unmet clinical need for stronger education in this regard among trainees has become an issue with a larger overlying societal impact, and recent studies have demonstrated a lack of dedicated training encompassing the appropriate analgesic prescription among surgical trainees.[9] Our hope is that this issue of *Otolaryngologic Clinics* represents an important first step toward addressing this concern.

- Appropriate evidence-based pain management ideally represents an interdisciplinary endeavor, meaning collaboration between physicians and health care providers in several different specialties represents an optimal approach. This point of emphasis cannot be stressed enough, as the present issue is an interdisciplinary venture between otolaryngologists, pain medicine physicians, anesthesiologists, and pain psychologists.

- An abundance of retrospective studies, multiinstitutional trials, and evidence-based systematic reviews and meta-analyses exist regarding pain prescribing practices in surgeries and situations relevant to Otolaryngologists. Many of these have been published over the past 5 years, as there has been increasing recognition of the toll the opioid epidemic has on our society, as well as increased appreciation of how opioids started in the inpatient setting and continued in the outpatient setting (or simply started outpatient after surgery) play a critical role in the misuse and diversion of these medications. These studies cannot be highlighted and emphasized enough, and practical take-home points will be stressed throughout this issue regarding these resources.

REFERENCES

1. Domeyer-Klenske A, Rosenbaum M. When doctor becomes patient: challenges and strategies in caring for physician-patients. Fam Med 2012;44(7):471–7.

2. Luft LM. The essential role of physician as advocate: how and why we pass it on. Can Med Educ J 2017;8(3):e109–16.

3. Fromme EK, Farber NJ, Babbott SF, et al. What do you do when your loved one is ill? The line between physician and family member. Ann Intern Med 2008;149(11): 825–31.

4. Manchikanti L, Helm S 2nd, Fellows B, et al. Opioid epidemic in the United States. Pain Physician 2012;15(3 Suppl):ES9–38.

5. Florence CS, Zhou C, Luo F, et al. The economic burden of prescription opioid overdose, abuse, and dependence in the United States, 2013. Med Care 2016; 54(10):901–6.

6. Pollack HA. So Prescription Opioid Disorders are a $78.5 Billion Problem. Med Care 2016;54(10):899–900.

7. National Institute on Drug Abuse. Opioid Overdose Crisis. 2019. Available at: https://http://www.drugabuse.gov/drugs-abuse/opioids/opioid-overdose-crisis. Accessed November 5, 2019.
8. Clark DJ, Schumacher MA. America's opioid epidemic: supply and demand considerations. Anesth Analg 2017;125(5):1667–74.
9. Yorkgitis BK, Bryant E, Raygor D, et al. Opioid prescribing education in surgical residencies: a program director survey. J Surg Educ 2018;75(3):552–6.

Pain Management for the Otolaryngologist

Overview of Perioperative Analgesia and Introduction to Opioids

Anna A. Pashkova, MD[a,1], Peter F. Svider, MD[b,c,]*,
Jean Anderson Eloy, MD[d,e]

KEYWORDS

- Perioperative analgesia • Pain management • Pain • Sinus surgery
- Head and neck surgery • Pre-operative optimization • Facial plastic surgery
- Non-opioid adjuncts and alternatives

KEY POINTS

- Nearly 50,000 US adults experience opioid-overdose deaths annually and 1.7 million experience a substance use disorder specifically from *prescription* opioids. Surgeons prescribe 36% of opioid medications in the United States.
- Opioids continue to be indicated to treat acute postoperative pain that cannot be expected to be well controlled with other modalities. There is a lack of dedication to prescribing education resources for surgical trainees.
- Excess opioids are prescribed following endoscopic sinus surgery despite the existence of efficacious alternatives.
- Controlled substance agreements set expectations as to the universal precautions providers should practice when prescribing chronic opioids. Standard practices include checking prescription monitoring programs, toxicology screens, and frequent assessment of ongoing risks versus benefits.

OVERVIEW

Educational societies, news media, and the political establishment have extensively reported on the recent upsurge in opioid misuse (**Table 1**). Furthermore, personal

[a] Division of Pain Medicine, Department of Anesthesiology, Columbia University Medical Center; [b] Otolaryngology–Head and Neck Surgery, Bergen Medical Associates, Emerson, NJ, USA; [c] Hackensack Meridian Health, Hackensack University Medical Center, Hackensack, NJ, USA; [d] Department of Otolaryngology–Head and Neck Surgery, Center for Skull Base and Pituitary Surgery, Neurological Institute of New Jersey, Newark, NJ, USA; [e] Department of Neurological Surgery, Rutgers New Jersey Medical School, 90 Bergen Street, Suite 8100 Newark, NJ 07103, USA
[1] Present address: 250 Hempstead Road, Ridgewood, NJ 07450.
* Corresponding author. Bergen Medical Associates, 466 Old Hook Road, Emerson, NJ 07630.
E-mail address: psvider@gmail.com

Otolaryngol Clin N Am 53 (2020) 715–728
https://doi.org/10.1016/j.otc.2020.05.001
0030-6665/20/© 2020 Elsevier Inc. All rights reserved.

Table 1
Select local legislative initiatives targeting narcotic prescription

Max. # of Days[a]	States
14	NV
7	AK, CT, IN, LA, MA, PA, UT, WV
5	AZ, NJ, NC
4	MN
3	FL

[a] Referring to maximum number of days of supply allowed for prescription of initial pain prescription or acute pain prescription for adults.

Data from Prescribing Policies: States Confront Opioid Overdose Epidemic. NCSL 2019. Retrieved from https://www.ncsl.org/research/health/prescribing-policies-states-confront-opioid-overdose-epidemic.aspx.

and societal costs related to the US opioid "epidemic" have become more apparent to the lay public (**Fig. 1**), with multiple local legislative initiatives being passed and several landmark lawsuits making the news. In September 2019, OxyContin manufacturer Purdue Pharma reached a historical tentative settlement for several billion dollars with 23 state attorneys general and 2000 other local governments.[1] As part of the settlement, Purdue did not admit wrongdoing, but, assuming the deal goes through, will declare bankruptcy and reorganize as a company producing medications to fight the opioid epidemic. Proceedings such as these remain fraught with political and ethical considerations on both sides; nonetheless, they have been in the news recently amid the significant increase in opioid-related abuse and deaths in the United States. In 2017 alone, almost 50,000 US adults experienced opioid-overdose deaths (see **Fig. 1**) and 1.7 million experienced a substance use disorder specifically from *prescription* opioids.[2]

Evidence-based medicine plays an increasingly important role in contemporary practice. Notably, surgeons prescribe 36% of opioid medications in the United States.[3] Over the past several decades, there have been myriad studies examining perioperative analgesic regimens for otolaryngologic procedures. Many of these regimens have demonstrated the efficacy of opioid alternatives. Multimodal analgesia should be implemented whenever possible, but for surgeries where postoperative pain cannot be expected to be controlled with analgesic adjuncts, the surgeon must be versed in safe opioid prescription practices. There is a lack of dedicated opioid prescribing education (OPE) resources for otolaryngology and surgical trainees,[4,5] so many of these considerations are generally overlooked (**Table 2**). One of the main points of this issue of *Otolaryngologic Clinics of North America* is to summarize evidence-based cost-effective practices that can be used in many situations. To continue to progress as a specialty, otolaryngologists need to be educated about novel approaches to multimodal analgesia and be familiar with the literature.

Preoperative Optimization

Successful implementation of a perioperative analgesic strategy starts with preoperative planning. Regardless of preexisting comorbidities or analgesic history, there should be an agreed-upon-plan before every elective surgery. This can consist of a brief conversation between the patient, surgeon, and anesthesiologist in an uncomplicated case or range all the way to an involved multidisciplinary plan for a patient with chronic pain (**Box 1**). For patients with chronic pain, it is important to coordinate care with their outpatient provider preoperatively in order to set clear expectations and

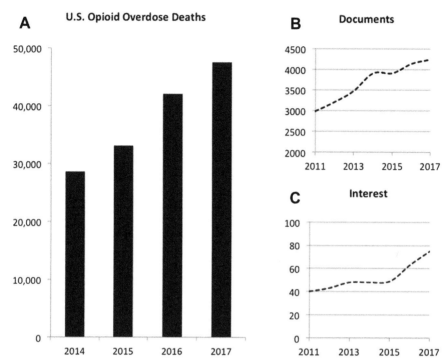

Fig. 1. (*A*) Bar chart: number of US opioid overdose deaths. (*B*) Upper right panel represents number of documents/publications by year on search for perioperative, surgical, surgery, otolaryngology AND analgesia, analgesic, opioid, and pain control. (*C*) Bottom right panel illustrates public interest via Google trends by year (January 1 of each year) for opioids as a class of prescription medications. (*Data from* [A] Drug Overdose Deaths. CDC 2020. Retrieved from https://www.cdc.gov/drugoverdose/data/statedeaths.html; and [B] Document search. Scopus, Elsevier 2020. Retreived from https://www.scopus.com/search/form. uri?display=basic&zone=header&origin=resultslist.)

goals for recovery. Notably, patients with substance use disorders require special attention. Postoperative pain control may be challenging, and discharge planning may be complex if postoperative opioids are indicated. Other issues integral to appropriate preoperative optimization include obtaining adequate nutrition and hydration, minimizing smoking, and providing appropriate deep vein thrombosis prophylaxis.[6,7] As this process is often underappreciated, the authors have dedicated a chapter entitled "Pre-Operative Optimization" in this issue to guide the surgeon in important questions to ask the patient preoperatively, optimization strategies, high-risk patients, and when it is necessary to consult a specialist.

Local Adjuncts

Regional anesthesia and local anesthetics can play a significant role in perioperative analgesia strategy when offered in appropriate circumstances. These agents can be used preoperatively and intraoperatively to minimize the need for postoperative "rescue." Their efficacy has been described for a variety of otolaryngologic surgeries and procedures, including nasal surgeries and thyroid surgery, and are further detailed and illustrated in the Elizabeth Boscoe and colleagues'article, "Local Blocks and Regional Anesthesia in the Head and Neck," in this issue.

Table 2
Select evidence-based recommendations for perioperative analgesia

Reference	Surgery	# Studies/Patients	Highlights
Campbell 2019	Otologic Surgery	23 studies/1842 patients	Acetaminophen + Codeine superior to monotherapies; NSAIDs, a-agonists, and blocks are also viable monotherapies
Nguyen 2019	Septoplasty Rhinoplasty	37 studies	Preponderance of evidence for local anesthetics; NSAIDs decreased VAS scores and postop analgesic use; gabapentin and a-agonists are also evidence-based effective alternatives
Svider 2018	Endoscopic sinus surgery	32 studies/1812 patients	Acetaminophen reduced postoperative opioid requirements, as did NSAIDs (although beware of NSAID intolerance in sinus patients); gabapentin and a-agonists are also postoperative options
Sethi 2018	Endoscopic sinus surgery	155 patients (single-institution)	73.1% reported requiring no opioids; predictors of opioid use included concurrent turbinate reduction or septoplasty
Patel 2018	Rhinoplasty	62 patients (2 institutions)	Patients only used 40% of their hydrocodone/acetaminophen tablets

Abbreviation: NSAID, nonsteroidal antiinflammatory drug.

Perioperative Pain Management

Acute pain management following head and neck surgery represents a significant undertaking and certainly requires a preoperative plan as well as setting clear expectations. Local anesthetics may provide excellent coverage for some smaller head and neck cases, such as patients undergoing thyroid/parathyroid surgery, and there is evidence showing a preponderance of benefit over harm with the use of these

Box 1
Topics to address in order to optimize perioperative care

Analgesia Strategies

Issue
  Is the patient currently on any pain medications?
  Is the patient currently taking any illicit substances? Past use?
    [a] Past pain medications?
    [a] Medication requirements for prior surgeries/procedures
  Is the surgery elective? Inpatient? Outpatient?
    What is the expected level of pain on discussion with the surgeon (ie, is this a small outpatient surgery or a major head and neck resection?)?
  What are the expected morbidities from this surgery?
  Are there any planned regional techniques or local blocks?
    [a] Has a perioperative plan been discussed with the primary care provider?

[a] Particularly important for patients with chronic pain/prior history. Patients should be screened for whether they have chronic pain issues, and if so, there should be discussion with the outpatient provider. Considerations for patients on buprenorphine must occur in advance.

modalities.[8–11] However, depending on the extent of the surgery, some patients undergoing extensive head and neck resections require multidisciplinary care collaboration involving their operating surgeon, anesthesiology, and the pain medicine team. Involving the pain medicine team does not preclude the surgical team's participation in decision-making regarding analgesia, although all subsequent changes and plans should be taken forward together after discussion rather than a unilateral fashion. For physicians taking care of a patient following significant head and neck resection, nonenteral pain management takes on exceeding importance for patients unable to tolerate oral analgesics (see Katherine Tinkey and colleagues' article, "Non-enteral Pain Management," in this issue).

Beyond acute perioperative management following head and neck surgery, the close proximity of numerous critical structures in the head, neck, and skull base that may be affected may necessitate the need for a chronic pain plan. Extensive resection can harbor a wide variety of morbidities that may worsen pain, including those affecting speech, sight, swallowing, and airway patency.[12] Hence, keeping these patients comfortable while offering evidence-based practices can be important in minimizing superfluous subsequent narcotic prescription and decreasing hospitalization stays.[13] This also comes down to understanding the appropriate role of the otolaryngologist regarding interdisciplinary cooperation with pain and palliative physicians. Coming up with a "game plan" encompassing both anticipated immediate perioperative considerations as well as long-term postoperative recovery from an analgesic standpoint may facilitate the patient's suitability for planned adjuvant therapies, especially in patients who are undergoing extensive surgery.[14] In other words, many patients with extensive head and neck cancers may have significant pain before or after chemotherapy/radiotherapy, and all attempts should be made to minimize delays in the administration of adjuvant therapy. This includes ensuring that the patient has adequate pain control.

Obstructive Sleep Apnea and Perioperative Analgesia

Sleep apnea surgery represents a wide range of procedures. These involve inpatient endeavors as complicated as any oncologic surgery (base of tongue surgeries with airway concerns, maxillomandibular skeletal surgery) to more minor undertakings such as uvulopalatopharyngoplasty, nasal airway surgery, and limited palatal techniques. Regardless of surgical complexity, these patients are at greater risk with narcotic exposure due to their underlying obstructive sleep apnea (OSA) and may be more sensitive to the respiratory depressive impacts of opioids. This necessitates a special understanding of opioid alternatives and reinforces the importance of using these alternatives to decrease postoperative discomfort in the care of these patients. Patients with OSA, as previously discussed, benefit from preoperative optimization and have an appropriate anesthesia/analgesia plan; although there are not necessarily myriad studies specific to regimens following sleep surgery, there are evidence-based practices relating to throat surgery and other related techniques. Adverse events attributed to medications including narcotics have been cited in lawsuits related to patients with OSA perioperatively.[15] Appropriate level and duration of monitoring of these patients postoperatively must be ensured, especially for those patients requiring postoperative opioids.

Other Outpatient Perioperative Analgesia Considerations

Although seeking narcotic alternatives and applying appropriate postoperative monitoring is of utmost importance in patients undergoing sleep surgeries, other predominantly outpatient procedures in otolaryngology also warrant a discussion of outpatient analgesic strategies. In an ideal preoperative informed consent process, perioperative quality of life should be discussed as well as long-term considerations; controlling pain in the immediate postoperative period minimizes the number of patients who are afraid of getting these surgeries in the first place. Otologic surgeries and sinus surgeries are generally outpatient and can be seemingly innocuous; however, a significant proportion of opioids prescribed in the United States is by surgeons for outpatient use; hence, there have been multiple papers demonstrating that many of the pills from these prescriptions are unused and in fact may be diverted, intentionally or not.[16] In one analysis of prescription patterns following sinonasal surgery, excess opioids were prescribed 85% of the time; for example, 25.3 tablets were prescribed per each postoperative patient, with a mean value of just 11.8 tablets reportedly being used.[17] Another study looking at opioid utilization following endoscopic sinus surgery also noted that most of the patients prescribed an opioid filled their prescriptions but did not use any opioids postoperatively for pain control.[18]

Perioperative analgesia following facial plastic surgery represents a primarily outpatient undertaking but with several unique considerations. Important differentiating factors include the type of surgery performed and the patient population being managed. There are different strategies and expectations based on whether a patient has underwent a cosmetic, elective procedure versus a reconstructive operation. Hence, setting realistic expectations particularly for aesthetic surgeries will play a significant role in patient satisfaction and the perception of success following a surgery. There may be a real and significant difference in how the elderly man who underwent a reconstruction of a branched-chain amino acid defect perceives their pain and satisfaction as compared with a younger woman undergoing a cosmetic rhinoplasty. Furthermore, psychiatric comorbidities may be far more prevalent in patients undergoing aesthetic procedures, and this can affect how pain is perceived. Considerations unique to pain perception and facial plastic procedures are further detailed in *Acute Pain Management following Facial Plastic Surgery*.

Special Populations

Several noteworthy populations should be considered in the context of providing high-quality evidence-based analgesia. Appropriately optimizing the chronic pain patient has been discussed earlier and also has its own dedicated Natasa Grancaric and colleagues' article, "Postoperative Analgesia in the Chronic Pain Patient," in this issue. Furthermore, although geriatric otolaryngology has been traditionally overlooked,[19,20] there are a whole host of considerations that can affect medication prescription in these patients. Older patients are undergoing surgery, including elective otolaryngologic procedures, in greater numbers than ever before.[21,22] Hence, close monitoring and judicious use of opioid alternatives in this patient population has never been more important, as narcotics have a high propensity to interact with other medications, and this population is characterized by polypharmacy.[23,24] Furthermore, unrecognized interactions with anesthetic agents and the greater potential for derangements of metabolism should prompt caution and really make one give second thought to using opioids in the elderly population until there is greater availability of dedicated high-quality studies exploring this topic.

Children also present a unique challenge, as they may not be able to appropriately communicate their pain in all situations. There are some evidence-based guidelines with regard to the use of nonsteroidal antiinflammatory drugs (NSAIDs), with controversy surrounding whether the use of these agents harbors an increased risk of potentially catastrophic postoperative bleeding. In addition, there is certainly evidence demonstrating the efficacy of narcotics in children, and as many of these opioids are liquid rather than pills they are not necessarily thought of as substances used for misuse and diversion. Nonetheless, there are many surgeons who do not feel comfortable with prescribing narcotics to children, particularly younger ones or those with OSA, and evidence-based recommendations looking at alternatives exist. One analysis of 91 children younger than 10 years demonstrated combination ibuprofen/acetaminophen to provide effective posttonsillectomy analgesia; these patients did better and had fewer concerns compared with a posttonsillectomy morphine group, in which patients experienced a greater number of oxygen desaturation events.[25] Nonetheless, there is not a generalized consensus in the pediatric population, and evidence-based practices are further addressed in the Anthony M. Sheyn and colleagues' article, "Perioperative Analgesia in Pediatric Patients Undergoing Otolaryngologic Surgery," in this issue.

Opioid-Prescribing Education Among Otolaryngologists

Knowledge concerning the opioid "epidemic" is historically novel, as mass marketing of opioids and treatment of pain as a "fifth vital sign" did not show up until the turn of the century. Nonetheless, there have been paradigm shifts in resident education during this time period, including increased pressures regarding requirements that need to be learned in an increasingly limited amount of time. With no requirement for OPE, competing pressures and ignorance of evidence-based alternatives have contributed to the societal problems noted earlier. In one survey of 110 responding surgery program directors, only 22.0% of programs required OPE,[4] and most of these experiences are simply composed of 1 hour of OPE. These considerations, taken in conjunction with a lack of training covering nonopioid adjuncts and alternatives and poor knowledge of dealing with postoperative analgesia in the patient with chronic pain, harken back to the importance of appropriate preoperative optimization. Without specialty-specific educational resources such as those offered in this issue, this lack of familiarity promotes the situation for opioid misprescription, facilitating the opioid epidemic that our society has experienced. The authors hope that the foundational principles provided in the present issue are used to deal with doing their part to address the opioid epidemic.

Controlled Substance Agreements and Other Best Opioid Prescribing Practices

Controlled substance agreements (CSAs) are used for patients who are on chronic opioids and represent a nonlegally binding agreement the provider enters with the patient. These documents set expectations as to the universal precautions prescribing providers should practice. Standard practices include checking prescription monitoring programs and using toxicology screens. Although these are used frequently in nonsurgical settings such as primary care practices and pain medicine clinics, CSAs have invaluable features and can be helpful among patients experiencing chronic pain following surgery. The logistics of implementing CSAs are further discussed in *Controlled Substance Agreements*.

Pain Psychology

A basic understanding of pain psychology is important for providing context into patients with chronic pain or those who require dedicated attention. Surgeons in general have very little exposure to pain psychology despite being the practitioners who are most heavily exposed to pain prescribing practices in an acute setting. This section discusses the role of psychology and nonpharmacologic therapeutics in managing pain, including cognitive behavior therapies and pain-coping strategies. These outcomes can be affected by moods, behaviors, comorbidities, and extent of chronic pain. The surgeon should be familiar with pain psychology in order to recognize when a patient would benefit from referral to a pain psychologist.

Sinus Headache

Sinus headache represents a unique consideration in this issue, in that the definition is not even widely agreed on. Patel and colleagues[26] explored sinus headache in a systematic review of the literature, focusing on standardizing results and definitions. Notably, in the setting of a comprehensive neurologic and ENT evaluation, most of the adults with sinus headaches are ultimately diagnosed with migraines and ideally treated with migraine therapy. Similar findings are noted on focusing on studies involving children and adolescents.[27] This section better organizes the considerations and controversies characterizing "sinus headache" and provides a practical approach for addressing symptomatic complaints.

Quality Improvement

Evolving pain paradigms represent a ripe target for quality improvement via the use of evidence-based practices. Over the past decade, there has been increasing recognition of the importance of quality improvement (QI) in medicine as a strategy for decreasing deleterious outcomes. QI differs from traditional human participant research in that its purpose is to assess an internal system, evaluate an established set of standards, and as a benefit, provide knowledge to directly benefit the process, program, or system. The objective of any QI project is to improve a process and/or system and then ultimately see whether that process can be transferred to another system with comparable standards and results. Several examples of QI in otolaryngology have been applied in recent years. For instance, Du and colleagues[28] implemented a multimodal analgesic protocol for all admitted head and neck patients and used these data to calculate average pain scores and opioid use, comparing results from before after protocol implementation. Implementation of their multimodal analgesia plan reduced opioid use immediately after surgery, demonstrating that such a plan is feasible (although opioid use was not reduced during the entire hospitalization course). Franz and colleagues[29] developed an opioid-sparing protocol following pediatric adenotonsillectomy at the University of Washington, identifying a feasible intraoperative anesthesia protocol that used dexmedetomidine and ketorolac and provided effective analgesia without lengthening recovery or increasing the need for reoperation. Although these studies represent an excellent approach toward tackling problems in an evidence-based manner, otolaryngology remains behind many other surgical disciplines when it comes to a discussion of pursuing QI practices, and further knowledge as to how to improve these trends is mandatory for our specialty to progress.

Introduction to Opioids

Opioids are potent analgesics that continue to be indicated for acute postoperative pain management as part of a multimodal analgesia strategy for surgeries with expected moderate and severe postoperative pain not controlled by other modalities. In addition, opioids are commonly used for cancer-related pain not controlled by other modalities, as well as in the palliative care setting. Nonetheless, opioids have the potential to cause serious adverse events. The otolaryngologist must be well versed in safe opioid prescribing in order to provide safe analgesia to the patient while minimizing side effects.

Opioids work by coupling to G proteins to cause membrane hyperpolarization. They act on the mu, kappa, delta, and sigma receptors.[30] The gold standard of comparing opioids is in the form of oral morphine milligram equivalents (MME). The potency of commonly used opioids are listed in **Table 3**.[30] Opioid conversion is more of an art than a science, and there are interindividual variabilities. Hydrocodone (commonly combined with acetaminophen and branded as Norco and Vicodin) has the same potency as oral morphine. Oxycodone (commonly combined with acetaminophen and branded as Percocet) is approximately 1.5 times more potent than oral morphine. Oral hydromorphone (brand name Dilaudid) is approximately 4 times more potent than oral morphine. Codeine is an inactive prodrug that must be metabolized to morphine by enzyme Cytochrome P460 2D6 (CYP2D6) to produce analgesic effect. Common genetic variability in CYP2D6 may lead to lack of metabolism and no analgesic effect, or more dangerously, ultrarapid metabolism will lead to high morphine levels and potentially lethal overdose.[31] Because of similar concerns with tramadol, the Food and Drug Administration recommends *against* codeine or tramadol use in children younger than 12 years, recommends *against* codeine or tramadol use for posttonsillectomy and adenoidectomy pain, and recommends *against* codeine or tramadol use in children aged 12 to 18 years who are obese, have obstructive sleep apnea, or a weakened respiratory system. Tramadol is approximately 10 times weaker than oral morphine but also has serotonin reuptake inhibitor properties and so has the potential to cause serotonin syndrome when combined with other serotonergic agents.[30,32,33] Transdermal fentanyl may be delivered via fentanyl patch and acts as a long-acting analgesic. Fentanyl patch is administered as mcg/h and is exchanged every 72 hours. Conversion factor for mcg/h to MME over 24 hours range from 2 to 2.4.[30] Thus, a fentanyl patch at 25 mcg/h would be equianalgesic to 50 to 60 mg of oral morphine administered over the span of 24 hours. Analgesic onset time may take 12 hours, longer for maximum concentration, and offset after patch removal is also delayed. As a long-acting opioid, fentanyl patches are contraindicated in opioid naïve patients and contraindicated to treat mild, acute, intermittent, or postoperative pain. Methadone and buprenorphine are long-acting opioids that may be used to treat pain but also may be used to treat opioid use disorder.

To understand a patient's preoperative opioid use or to track the trend in the patient's postoperative opioid consumption, one calculates the patient's MME over 24 hours. This is helpful in several ways. If a patient is on chronic opioids preoperatively, the patient should generally be prescribed at least their preoperative MME in

Table 3
Opioid equianalgesic table

	IV (mg)	PO (mg)
Morphine	10	30
Hydromorphone	1.5	7.5
Oxycodone[a]	-	20
Hydrocodone[b]	-	30
Tramadol	-	300
Codeine	-	4.5[c]

Individual variation and variation in literature exist for opioid equianalgesic conversions.
Abbreviations: IV, intravenous; PO, oral.
[a] Brand name Percocet consists of oxycodone plus acetaminophen.
[b] Brand names Norco and Vicodin consist of hydrocodone plus acetaminophen.
[c] Abnormal metabolism of codeine can result in lower analgesic effects or higher analgesic effects leading to overdose. If converting from one opioid to another, account for incomplete cross-tolerance.

the postoperative period. For surgeries resulting in little to no pain, the patient's preoperative opioid regimen may provide adequate analgesia when combined with postoperative multimodal analgesia. For surgeries resulting in moderate to severe postoperative pain, it is likely that the patient will need their baseline MME plus supplemental opioid in the acute postoperative period. It is therefore important to know the patient's baseline opioid requirement. Postoperatively, a patient's opioid requirement may be tracked as MME to trend whether the patient's opioid requirements are overall decreasing as would be expected as the patient's pain improves while recovering from surgery.

MME is a useful way of thinking and comparing opioid doses. If converting the patient from one opioid to another, "incomplete cross-tolerance" must be taken into account if the patient has been on an opioid long enough to become tolerant to it. Incomplete cross-tolerance is a concept that notes if a patient is on one specific opioid (eg, hydrocodone) or the patient is more tolerant to hydrocodone than other opioids, so a dose reduction of 20% to 50% should be performed to account for the patient's relatively smaller tolerance to the new opioid (eg, oxycodone).[34] From a mathematical standpoint, the equianalgesic dose of hydrocodone, 30 mg, would be oxycodone, 20 mg. Because of incomplete cross-tolerance, prescribing oxycodone, 10 to 15 mg, would be more appropriate and would provide the same analgesia.

Table 4 Opioid side effects	
CNS	Sedation
	Opioid-induced hyperalgesia
	Tolerance
	Assuming $Paco_2$ is maintained stable through artificial ventilation decreases cerebral blood flow, intracranial pressure, cerebral oxygen consumption
	Seizures (tramadol, meperidine)
Cardiovascular	Remifentanil (commonly used in TIVA) may cause bradycardia
	Morphine, hydromorphone, and meperidine cause histamine release
Respiratory	Respiratory depression
	$Paco_2$ increases
	Apneic threshold increases
	Hypoxic ventilatory drive decreases
	Large doses (fentanyl, sufentanil, remifentanil) may cause chest wall rigidity
	Blunt bronchoconstrictive response to airway stimulation
	Histamine release (see cardiovascular) may cause bronchoconstriction
Gastrointestinal	Stimulation of medullary chemoreceptor trigger zone → nausea/vomiting
	Delay gastric emptying time
	Constipation[a]
Genitourinary	Urinary retention
Endocrine	Attenuate stress response to surgery
	Decrease in testosterone, estrogen, cortisol, LH, GnRH

Abbreviations: GI, gastrointestinal; GnRH, gonadotropin-releasing hormone; LH, luteinizing hormone; $Paco_2$, partial pressure of arterial carbon dioxide; TIVA, total intravenous anesthesia.
  [a] Tolerance does not develop to constipation.

Opioids have potential to cause numerous adverse effects (**Tables 4** and **5**).[30,33,35] Cerebral effects include sedation. Opioid-induced hyperalgesia describes a state where patients become more sensitive to painful stimuli. Respiratory depression may occur, and there is higher risk for respiratory depression when opioids are combined with other sedating agents, such as benzodiazepines. Reversal agents, such as intranasal naloxone and subcutaneous naloxone, as well as intravenous naloxone are available. For *chronic* pain, the CDC recommends practitioners consider prescribing

Table 5	
Special considerations for opioids	
Medication	**Consideration**
Morphine	Avoid in patients with significant renal dysfunction. Metabolites morphine-3-glucuronide and morphine-6-glucuronide excreted renally can accumulate in renal dysfunction and lead to overdose
Meperidine	Avoid in patients with significant renal dysfunction due to accumulation of metabolites. Patients with renal dysfunction more prone to toxicity, including seizures. Avoid in patients taking MAOIs due to risk of hemodynamic instability, hyperpyrexia, coma, respiratory arrest, and death.
Tramadol	Has serotonin and norepinephrine reuptake inhibition properties. Caution with other serotonergic agents and MAOIs. Toxicity includes seizures Dose adjustment with renal dysfunction Contraindicated in patients younger than 12 years, patients younger than 18 years following tonsillectomy and/or adenoidectomy, and patients aged 12–18 years who have risk factors that may increase sensitivity to respiratory depression
Codeine	Codeine is a prodrug that must be metabolized by CYP2D6 to morphine for analgesia. Contraindicated in patients younger than 12 years, patients younger than 18 years following tonsillectomy and/or adenoidectomy, and patients aged 12–18 years who have risk factors that may increase sensitivity to respiratory depression
Methadone	Has NMDA antagonism properties Causes QTc prolongation on ECG, exercise caution with QTc prolonging medications Safe in renal dysfunction Long-acting Conversion factor varies based on dose, should only be prescribed by well-versed practiioners
Fentanyl	Available in transdermal formulation (fentanyl patch) Transdermal formulation may take 12+ h for analgesic onset, longer for maximum analgesia Safe in renal dysfunction For opioid tolerant patients only Contraindicated for acute postoperative pain, intermittent pain, mild pain
Remifentanil	Intravenous opioid with fast onset and fast offset Commonly used as part of TIVA May cause bradycardia

Abbreviations: CYP2D6, cytochrome p450 2D6; ECG, electrocardiogram; MAOI, monoamine oxidase inhibitor; NMDA, N-methyl-ᴅ-aspartate; TIVA, total intravenous anesthesia.

home naloxone to patients at increased risk of overdose, including patients with history of overdose, patients with history of substance use disorder, patients concurrently taking benzodiazepines, and patients taking 50 MME daily or higher.[36] Gastrointestinal effects include nausea, vomiting, and delayed gastric emptying time. Patients do not develop tolerance to the constipating effects of opioids, and so patients should be placed on a bowel regimen. Peripheral opioid antagonists, such as methylnaltrexone, promote gastrointestinal motility by blocking peripheral opioid receptors without crossing the blood brain barrier and without reducing effectiveness of opioid analgesia.[35] Opioids may lead to urinary retention. Patients prescribed opioids should be educated regarding potential side effects.

SUMMARY

There has been increasing awareness of the role perioperative prescribing patterns have played in the increase of the opioid epidemic. The rising recognition of the impact that misuse and diversion of opioid prescriptions have played has facilitated a body of literature examining evidence-based alternatives and adjuncts to narcotic prescription in appropriate situations. Opioids are effective for breakthrough pain, but the decision to prescribe them should not be undertaken lightly, as there is myriad evidence supporting efficacious alternatives with regard to patients undergoing otolaryngologic procedures, including acetaminophen, NSAIDs, local anesthetics, and gabapentinoids. Further considerations should be given in order to enhance preoperative optimization regimens in unique populations, including patients with preexisting chronic pain issues, pediatric patients, and the elderly.

REFERENCES

1. Bernstein L, Davis AC, Achenbach J, et al. Purdue Pharma reaches tentative deal in federal, state opioid lawsuits. Washington Post 2019. Available at: https://http://www.washingtonpost.com/health/purdue-pharma-reaches-tentative-settlement-in-federal-lawsuit-and-some-state-litigation/2019/09/11/ce6cb942-d4b8-11e9-9343-40db57cf6abd_story.html. Accessed November 28, 2019.
2. National Institute on Drug Abuse. Opioid overdose crisis. 2019. Available at: https://http://www.drugabuse.gov/drugs-abuse/opioids/opioid-overdose-crisis. Accessed November 5, 2019.
3. Levy B, Paulozzi L, Mack KA, et al. Trends in Opioid Analgesic-Prescribing Rates by Specialty, U.S., 2007-2012. Am J Prev Med 2015;49:409–13.
4. Yorkgitis BK, Bryant E, Raygor D, et al. Opioid prescribing education in surgical residencies: a program director survey. J Surg Educ 2018;75(3):552–6.
5. Lancaster E, Bongiovanni T, Lin J, et al. Residents as Key Effectors of Change in Improving Opioid Prescribing Behavior. J Surg Educ 2019;76:e167–72.
6. Patel KV, Darakhshan AA, Griffin N, et al. Patient optimization for surgery relating to Crohn's disease. Nat Rev Gastroenterol Hepatol 2016;13:707–19.
7. Rizk P, Morris W, Oladeji P, et al. Review of postoperative delirium in geriatric patients undergoing hip surgery. Geriatr Orthop Surg Rehabil 2016;7:100–5.
8. Choi GJ, Kang H, Ahn EJ, et al. Clinical efficacy of intravenous lidocaine for thyroidectomy: a prospective, randomized, double-blind, placebo-controlled trial. World J Surg 2016;40:2941–7.
9. Dumlu EG, Tokac M, Ocal H, et al. Local bupivacaine for postoperative pain management in thyroidectomized patients: A prospective and controlled clinical study. Ulus Cerrahi Derg 2016;32:173–7.

10. Egan RJ, Hopkins JC, Beamish AJ, et al. Randomized clinical trial of intraoperative superficial cervical plexus block versus incisional local anaesthesia in thyroid and parathyroid surgery. Br J Surg 2013;100:1732–8.

11. Ryu JH, Yom CK, Kwon H, et al. A prospective, randomized, controlled trial of the postoperative analgesic effects of spraying 0.25 % levobupivacaine after bilateral axillo-breast approach robotic thyroidectomy. Surg Endosc 2015;29:163–9.

12. Bossi P, Giusti R, Tarsitano A, et al. The point of pain in head and neck cancer. Crit Rev Oncol Hematol 2019;138:51–9.

13. Majumdar S, Das A, Kundu R, et al. Intravenous paracetamol infusion: Superior pain management and earlier discharge from hospital in patients undergoing palliative head-neck cancer surgery. Perspect Clin Res 2014;5:172–7.

14. Mirabile A, Airoldi M, Ripamonti C, et al. Pain management in head and neck cancer patients undergoing chemo-radiotherapy: Clinical practical recommendations. Crit Rev Oncol Hematol 2016;99:100–6.

15. Svider PF, Pashkova AA, Folbe AJ, et al. Obstructive sleep apnea: strategies for minimizing liability and enhancing patient safety. Otolaryngol Head Neck Surg 2013;149:947–53.

16. Reimer J, Wright N, Somaini L, et al. The impact of misuse and diversion of opioid substitution treatment medicines: evidence review and expert consensus. Eur Addict Res 2016;22:99–106.

17. Newberry CI, Casazza GC, Pruitt LC, et al. Prescription patterns and opioid usage in sinonasal surgery. Int Forum Allergy Rhinol 2020;10:381–7.

18. Sethi RKV, Miller AL, Bartholomew RA, et al. Opioid prescription patterns and use among patients undergoing endoscopic sinus surgery. Laryngoscope 2019;129: 1046–52.

19. Eibling D, Kost K. The emerging field of geriatric otolaryngology. Otolaryngol Clin North Am 2018;51:847–52.

20. Mirza N, Lee JY. Geriatric otolaryngology. Otolaryngol Clin North Am 2018;51: xvii–xviii.

21. McIntire JB, McCammon S, Mong ER. Endocrine surgery in the geriatric population. Otolaryngol Clin North Am 2018;51:753–8.

22. Newberry I, Cerrati EW, Thomas JR. Facial plastic surgery in the geriatric population. Otolaryngol Clin North Am 2018;51:789–802.

23. Borsheski R, Johnson QL. Pain management in the geriatric population. Mo Med 2014;111:508–11.

24. Gerlach LB, Olfson M, Kales HC, et al. Opioids and other central nervous system-active polypharmacy in older adults in the United States. J Am Geriatr Soc 2017; 65:2052–6.

25. Kelly LE, Sommer DD, Ramakrishna J, et al. Morphine or Ibuprofen for post-tonsillectomy analgesia: a randomized trial. Pediatrics 2015;135:307–13.

26. Patel ZM, Kennedy DW, Setzen M, et al. Sinus headache": rhinogenic headache or migraine? An evidence-based guide to diagnosis and treatment. Int Forum Allergy Rhinol 2013;3:221–30.

27. Smith BC, George LC, Svider PF, et al. Rhinogenic headache in pediatric and adolescent patients: an evidence-based review. Int Forum Allergy Rhinol 2019; 9:443–51.

28. Du E, Farzal Z, Stephenson E, et al. Multimodal analgesia protocol after head and neck surgery: effect on opioid use and pain control. Otolaryngol Head Neck Surg 2019;161:424–30.

29. Franz AM, Dahl JP, Huang H, et al. The development of an opioid sparing anesthesia protocol for pediatric ambulatory tonsillectomy and adenotonsillectomy surgery-A quality improvement project. Paediatr Anaesth 2019;29:682–9.

30. Centers for Medicaid and Medicare Services. Opioid Oral Morphine Milligram Equivalent (MME) Conversion Factors. Available at: https://http://www.cms.gov/Medicare/Prescription-Drug-Coverage/PrescriptionDrugCovContra/Downloads/Oral-MME-CFs-vFeb-2018.pdf https://wwwcmsgov/Medicare/Prescription-Drug-Coverage/PrescriptionDrugCovContra/Downloads/Oral-MME-CFs-vFeb-2018pdf. Accessed March 1, 2020.

31. Tobias JD, Green TP, Cote CJ, SECTION ON ANESTHESIOLOGY AND PAIN MEDICINE, COMMITTEE ON DRUGS. Codeine: time to say "no". Pediatrics 2016;138 [pii:e20162396].

32. Food and Drug Administration. Codeine and Tramadol Can Cause Breathing Problems for Children. Available at: https://http://www.fda.gov/consumers/consumer-updates/codeine-and-tramadol-can-cause-breathing-problems-children. Accessed March 5, 2020.

33. Baldo BA, Rose MA. The anaesthetist, opioid analgesic drugs, and serotonin toxicity: a mechanistic and clinical review. Br J Anaesth 2020;124:44–62.

34. Smith HS, Peppin JF. Toward a systematic approach to opioid rotation. J Pain Res 2014;7:589–608.

35. Benyamin R, Trescot AM, Datta S. Opioid complications and side effects. Pain Physician 2008;11:S105–20.

36. Centers for Disease Control and Prevention. CDC Guideline for Prescribing Opioids for Chronic Pain — United States, 2016. Available at: https://http://www.cdc.gov/mmwr/volumes/65/rr/rr6501e1.htm. Accessed March 1, 2020.

Preoperative Optimization for Perioperative Analgesia

Nicole Matar, MD, Anna A. Pashkova, MD*

KEYWORDS

- Preoperative optimization • Multimodal analgesia • Acute on chronic pain • Opioids
- Analgesic adjuncts

KEY POINTS

- Preoperative optimization of patients with chronic pain requires a multimodal and collaborative approach.
- Poor pain control is associated with increased morbidity, impaired physical function and quality of life, slowed recovery, prolonged opioid use during and after hospitalization, and increased costs.
- Current outpatient pain regimens and prescriptions should be reviewed and confirmed preoperatively. Methadone and buprenorphine management requires advanced planning.
- Any medical history or patient factors affecting postoperative analgesic choice should be noted.
- A focused social and psychiatric history must be taken with a focus on substance use disorder.

INTRODUCTION

The majority of patients meet their surgical team before entering the operating room. Just like other aspects of medical optimization, patients should undergo preoperative evaluation to optimize postoperative analgesia. This process includes obtaining a thorough pain history, setting expectations, screening for substance use disorders, developing a postoperative analgesia plan, and possibly involving a multidisciplinary team, including anesthesiology, pain medicine, palliative care, psychiatry, and/or addiction specialists. Waiting to consult the pain service team postoperatively misses an opportunity for valuable planning.

Inadequate postoperative pain control is undesirable, but inadequate pain control is cited in more than 80% of postoperative patients.[1] Pain control directly correlates with patient satisfaction. Poor pain control is associated with increased morbidity, impaired physical function and quality of life, slowed recovery, prolonged opioid use during and

Department of Anesthesiology, Columbia University Medical Center, 622 West 168th Street, PH 5-505, New York, NY 10032, USA
* Corresponding author.
E-mail address: apashkova@gmail.com

Otolaryngol Clin N Am 53 (2020) 729–737
https://doi.org/10.1016/j.otc.2020.05.002
0030-6665/20/© 2020 Elsevier Inc. All rights reserved.

after hospitalization, and increased cost of care. Postoperative pain may also lead to prolonged pain or chronic pain conditions.[1] Although a multitude of factors contribute to inadequate postoperative pain control, limited physician understanding of strategies for pain prevention and control is a contributing factor.[2] Preoperative pain is a risk factor for poorly controlled postoperative pain, and so appropriate analgesia for patients with chronic pain conditions requires additional planning.[1]

The distinction between acute and chronic pain is essential to providing appropriate postoperative analgesia. Acute pain is self-limited, provoked by a particular disease or injury, and generally associated with a sympathetic nervous system activation. Chronic pain, in contrast, should be thought of as a disease state. Chronic pain extends beyond the normal healing time of an associated disease or injury.[3] The prevalence of chronic pain is high with up to a quarter of the adult American population with chronic pain.[4] The treatment of acute pain focuses on addressing the underlying cause. Chronic pain, however, requires a different approach aimed at both the physical and the psychosocial state of a patient. Studies have found that patients with various chronic pain conditions may tend to be more sensitive to injury than others.[4] Additionally, patients with chronic pain may be more physically deconditioned than other patients in similar situations. Thus, those with chronic pain undergoing surgery require special care with respect to postoperative pain management. The perioperative period creates a state of acute on chronic pain for many patients, resulting in an increased complexity of treatment for practitioners.

A focused pain history should be part of the preoperative assessment to create an appropriate perioperative pain management plan (**Box 1**). Key aspects should include any history of chronic or acute pain conditions, the location of the patient's pain, and the patient's preoperative pain score. A thorough list of medications should be obtained. The surgeon should be aware of any opioid medications that the patient is taking, and because many medications are written on as as-needed basis ("PRN"), make note of the total daily dose the patient is actually taking. Adjuvant pain medications and doses must be covered. Patients on multiple sedating medications are at higher risk for respiratory depression and death when combined with opioids.[5] Patients should be screened for medical comorbidities, such as obstructive sleep apnea (OSA), that confer a higher risk of postoperative respiratory depression. A psychosocial history should be obtained. Patients with a history of substance use disorder require special consideration if postoperative opioids are indicated, and patients on buprenorphine require advanced planning.

Patients may be on prescription opioids for acute or chronic pain. For patients on opioids for chronic pain, it is important to note the dose and the total amount the patient takes daily. The standard of comparing different opioids is converting the total daily dose to milligrams of oral morphine milligram equivalents (**Table 1**). Postoperatively, the patient should receive opioids to cover their baseline opioid requirement. For surgeries requiring postoperative opioids, higher opioid requirements will be likely. If it is necessary to switch the patient from their home opioid to a different opioid postoperatively, the managing physician should be versed in opioid conversion and take into account incomplete cross-tolerance. Incomplete cross-tolerance means that an opioid-tolerant patient will be most tolerant to the specific opioids they are chronically taking and slightly less tolerant to other opioids. As such, a dose decrease of 25% to 50% should occur when switching between different opioids.[6] Fentanyl is available in a transdermal formulation via patch. Initiation and discontinuation should take into account onset time and offset time.

The home opioid dose may be confirmed via communication with outpatient physicians, pharmacies, or prescription drug monitoring systems. Patients on chronic

---

Box 1
Preoperative assessment

Pain medication history
- Does that patient have any contraindications to NSAIDs?
  - Kidney dysfunction
  - History of gastrointestinal bleed, peptic ulcers, or gastritis
  - Increased risk of bleeding
  - Coronary artery disease
  - Stroke
- Does the patient have any contraindications to acetaminophen?
  - For patients with stable liver dysfunction, the maximum recommended dose of acetaminophen is 2000 mg/d[24]
- Does the patient have any contraindications to gabapentinoids?
  - Must be renally dosed
  - Common side effects include dizziness and sedation
- Does the patient have an increased risk of opioid-induced respiratory depression?
  - Concurrent use of sedating medications (opioids, benzodiazepines, gabapentinoids)
  - OSA or positive STOP-Bang questionnaire
  - Respiratory condition
  - Cardiac condition
- Does the patient have any exacerbating or aggravating factors?
  - Anxiety
  - Sleep deprivation
  - Poor nutrition

Home medications
- Is the patient on chronic pain medications?
- What is the total dose of home opioid medications?
- Who is the outpatient prescribing provider?
- What is the dose of nonopioid pain medications?

Allergies or history of intolerances to pain medications

Social history
- Does the patient have a history of substance use disorder?
- Is the patient on medication-assisted treatment with methadone or buprenorphine?

---

opioids often have a controlled substance agreement with the prescriber that outlines that the patient should not receive opioid prescriptions from any other physicians, and so the patient should notify their opioid provider before any elective surgery. Methadone and buprenorphine are long-acting opioids that can be prescribed for chronic pain or substance use disorder, and are discussed elsewhere in this article.

Practitioners should be aware that patients on chronic opioids often have a tolerance to opioid medications, which consists of a rightward shift of the dose–response curve to opioids. As a result, patients require increasing amounts of the medication to maintain the same pharmacologic effect.[7] Those patients who have developed tolerance are generally less responsive to standard protocols for postoperative pain control. Chapman and colleagues[4] examined postoperative pain in surgical patients over the span of 6 days and found that those with chronic pain conditions prescribed opioids at baseline had a significantly greater difficulty with their postoperative pain control when compared with surgical patients without chronic pain conditions. The initial pain levels were higher and a decrease in postoperative pain was not found on average over a 6-day window. The study did not explain the cause behind the persistence of postoperative pain in patients with chronic pain. However, the concept of opioid-induced hyperalgesia has been discussed and studied by other researchers. The phrase is used to express the concept that

Table 1
Opioid equianalgesia table

| | Equianalgesic Dose | | Conversion Factor | |
	Parenteral (mg)	Oral (mg)	Parenteral Opioid to MME	Oral Opioid to MME
Drug				
Morphine	10	30	3	1
Hydromorphone	1.5	7.5	20	4
Oxycodone	—	20	—	1.5
Hydrocodone	—	30	—	1

Methadone conversion varies by dose. Fentanyl conversion rate of 2.4 is based on micrograms per hour of transdermal patch. Example: A patient on fentanyl patch 25 μg/h is on a dose equivalent to approximately 60 mg oral morphine equivalents over 24 h. If converting between opioids, reduce dose by 25%-50% to account for incomplete cross tolerance. Example of conversion: A patient taking oxycodone 10 mg four times daily preoperatively is taking a total of 40 mg oxycodone daily. This is the equivalent of 60 mg oral morphine over 24 h. Accounting for incomplete cross-tolerance, the patient may be prescribed a total of 30 to 45 mg oral morphine in divided doses over 24 h with equianalgesic effect. This accounts for the patient's baseline opioid requirement, and supplemental analgesia may be needed postoperatively. Doses listed in this table are for comparison purposes only and do not constitute recommended doses.
Abbreviations: MG, milligrams; MME, oral morphine milligram equivalents.
Data from CDC: Calculating Total Daily Dose of Opioids for Safer Dosage. https://www.cdc.gov/drugoverdose/pdf/calculating_total_daily_dose-a.pdf.

chronic opioid users have lower pain thresholds and exaggerated pain levels after acute injuries. Previous studies have demonstrated that animals chronically exposed to morphine have enhanced proinflammatory cytokine levels postoperatively.[4] It has been postulated that patients with chronic pain enter a state of hypersensitivity in their central nervous systems owing to the impaired function in endogenous opioid analgesic systems.[4]

Patients on opioids for chronic noncancer pain scheduled for elective procedures may benefit from opioid tapering preoperatively. Preoperative opioid tapering to the lowest tolerated dose may mitigate opioid tolerance and opioid-induced hyperalgesia, resulting in improved postoperative analgesia. There are data that patients on high-dose opioids have worse outcomes.[2] Hospitalized patients with opioid use have higher rates of hypoxemia, ileus, nausea, pruritis, and cognitive impairment, as well as an increased length of stay, which may also contribute to the higher cost of care.[8] Opioid tapering requires time and advanced planning, which may act as a barrier preoperatively. Another potential barrier is a patient's willingness to taper.[8] However, studies support that opioid tapering for chronic pain leads to unchanged or improved pain scores and better function.[9,10] The reason for tapering should be explained to the patient. The duration of a taper varies based on a patient's need and the complexity of the initial opioid regimen. For those patients who have been taking opioids for weeks to months, the Centers for Disease Control and Prevention recommend a decrease of 10% per week as a reasonable starting point.[11] Abrupt discontinuation of opioids should be avoided. There is not enough data to support preoperative opioid tapering for all patients, and so the surgeon should contact the patient's outpatient opioid prescriber to discuss whether a preoperative taper would be helpful and appropriate. The opioid prescriber can then implement an individualized taper for the patient. The surgeon should also coordinate a tentative postoperative opioid and analgesic plan with the outpatient opioid prescriber. This strategy may help to set expectations for postoperative analgesia with the patient.

Adjuvant chronic pain medications should most often be continued if no contraindications arise. It is important to take into consideration which medications can be administered via additional routes, because select surgeries may preclude patients from taking pills orally in the immediate postoperative period. Nonsteroidal anti-inflammatory drugs (NSAIDs) may be held based on anticipated intraoperative or postoperative blood loss. The management of aspirin prescribed as anticoagulation for a chronic medical condition should be coordinated with the patient's outpatient prescriber. Fluctuations in a patient's renal function may occur in the perioperative period. Practitioners must be cognizant of which medications need to be adjusted for variable renal function (**Box 2**). In the postoperative period, patients often have an increased risk of respiratory depression and apnea with sedating medications. The surgeon should make note of whether a patient is on multiple sedating medications, such as opioids, benzodiazepines, and gabapentinoids, because this will increase the patient's risk of respiratory depression.[5] Opioid overdose mortality is increased 4-fold with concurrent use of opioids and benzodiazepines.[12]

Patients should be screened for conditions that increase risk of postoperative respiratory depression. A meta-analysis by Gupta and colleagues[5] noted that the incidence of postoperative opioid-induced respiratory depression is approximately 0.5%. Patients with preexisting cardiac disease, pulmonary disease, and OSA are at higher risk for respiratory complications.[5] Patients should be screened for OSA and, if necessary, referred to a sleep medicine specialist. The STOP-Bang questionnaire is a common screening tool used for OSA. One study showed a 3.75-fold increased risk of perioperative complications with an STOP-Bang score of 3 or higher.[13] In a study on OSA-related malpractice, 22% of claims alleged that inappropriate medication administration resulted in respiratory depression.[14] Because the majority of opioid-induced respiratory depression events occur within 24 hours of surgery, patients should be counseled on continuous positive airway pressure use postoperatively. If within hospital protocol, patients should be instructed to bring their home continuous positive airway pressure for use in the postanesthesia care unit and for sleep postoperatively. A multimodal analgesia plan should be implemented to minimize sedating medications postoperatively. A meta-analysis by Gupta and colleagues[5] noted that patients who had respiratory events received a higher 24-hour morphine equivalent dose (average of 24.7 mg vs 18.9 mg). Put in perspective, 25 mg of oral morphine is approximately the equivalent of 5 tablets of hydrocodone

---

Box 2
Medication considerations for patients with renal insufficiency

- NSAIDs[a] – avoid use
- Gabapentin – renally dose
- Pregabalin – renally dose
- Tramadol – renally dose
- Morphine – avoid in severe renal dysfunction
- Meperidine – avoid use
- Duloxetine – avoid use if creatine clearance is less than 30 mL/min

Care should be made when prescribing the following medications in the setting of renal injury or failure. Discontinuation or dosing adjustment may be recommended.[a] Coordination of aspirin continuation should be discussed with outpatient provider.

5 mg administered over the span of 1 day. Patients who are at increased risk of postoperative respiratory depression may require longer periods or an increased level of monitoring. Approximately 20% of claims regarding OSA alleged inappropriate monitoring of the patient.[14] The surgery should be booked at an appropriate location for monitoring duration and care.

In the extended postoperative period, patients often have exacerbating factors that contribute to a worse subjective sensation of pain. Special attention should be given to the anxiety, sleep deprivation, and poor nutrition that may arise in the postoperative period.[15]

Patients with a history of substance use disorder require advanced planning. Methadone or buprenorphine are long-acting opioids that are often used as part of medication-assisted treatment to prevent relapse of substance abuse. It is important to note that some patients take methadone or buprenorphine for pain with no history of addiction, and so the indication for these medications is important to clarify. Methadone for substance use disorder is often acquired at a methadone clinic, which will not show up on prescription drug monitoring programs. In this case, the patient's dose should be confirmed with the methadone clinic preoperatively. If a patient recalls a dose lower than what is prescribed, their opioids may be underdosed postoperatively, which may lead to inadequate pain control. If a patient reports a dose higher than prescribed and this higher dose is administered, they are at risk for respiratory depression and opioid overdose. In general, the patient's methadone should be continued preoperatively.

Buprenorphine (commonly combined with naloxone as buprenorphine–naloxone) is a partial agonist of the opioid mu receptor and an antagonist at the opioid kappa and delta receptors. The naloxone is inactive when taken orally, but acts as an opioid antagonist in case the buprenorphine–naloxone is injected intravenously in an abuse attempt. Buprenorphine binds tightly to the opioid receptor and competitively displaces traditional opioids from the opioid receptor. Through this mechanism, the pharmacokinetic properties of buprenorphine interfere with the effectiveness of postoperative opioids. Owing to the long half-life of buprenorphine (20–70 hours reported), it is important to contact the buprenorphine provider to establish a perioperative plan.[16] Different formulations of buprenorphine have different pharmacokinetic properties. For procedures with expected minimal to no pain, it is generally recommended that patients continue taking their buprenorphine without a change in dose and with an avoidance of supplemental opioids. For those procedures expected to result in moderate to severe pain, consideration should be given to weaning off buprenorphine preoperatively. Patients who have discontinued buprenorphine may require tolerant doses of opioids in the perioperative period. If it is discovered that a patient is taking buprenorphine on the day of surgery, and moderate to severe postoperative pain is expected requiring opioids, consideration should be given to postponing an elective procedure. Anderson and colleagues[17] suggests a dose-dependent timeline for the discontinuation of buprenorphine (**Box 3**). The discontinuation of buprenorphine puts the patient at risk for substance abuse relapse, and so should be done only at the discretion of the buprenorphine provider. Other studies recommend continuation of buprenorphine and the use of higher dose opioids postoperatively.[17] In such cases, admission to the intensive care unit may be required for respiratory monitoring. Hospital guidelines should be followed regarding buprenorphine recommendations. Regardless of the decision of continuation or discontinuation of buprenorphine, multimodal analgesia should play a prominent role in the perioperative analgesia plan. The inclusion of NSAIDs, acetaminophen, local anesthetics, and membrane stabilizers will contribute to an overall decrease

---

Box 3
Preoperative buprenorphine discontinuation

- 0–4 mg – discontinue 24 hours before surgery

- >4–8 mg – discontinue 48 hours before surgery

- >8–12 mg – discontinue 72 hours before surgery

Suggested discontinuation time for buprenorphine based on totally daily preoperative dose prior to surgeries with anticipated moderate to severe pain requiring postoperative opioids. Decision to continue or discontinue buprenorphine preoperatively must be coordinated with outpatient prescriber.

Data from T. Anthony Anderson, Aurora N. A. Quaye, E. Nalan Ward, et. al; To Stop or Not, That Is the Question: Acute Pain Management for the Patient on Chronic Buprenorphine. Anesthesiology 2017;126(6):1180-1186. doi: https://doi.org/10.1097/ALN.0000000000001633.

---

in opioid requirements for postoperative patients. Regional techniques should be used when possible.[17]

For patients on methadone or buprenorphine for substance use disorder, a discharge plan should be implemented. Although the surgeon may continue these home medications while the patient is an inpatient, a DEA-X license is required for initiation or outpatient prescription of these medications. Thus, the patient should not be discharged home with a prescription. Instead, coordination and appropriate follow-up with the patient's outpatient provider must be established. Patients with a history of substance use disorder are at higher risk for opioid overdose.[18]

After a focused pain history is obtained, patients should be counseled on expectations regarding postoperative pain management. Patient satisfaction may be increased with a preoperative discussion of pain management expectations. Expectations of pain levels too high or unrealistic expectations of zero pain may be detrimental.[19]

For those patients with implanted pain devices such as intrathecal pump or spinal cord stimulators, it is necessary to formulate a plan for continuation/discontinuation with the patient's chronic pain provider. Intrathecal drug delivery systems, for example, should be continued during the operative period if possible.[20] If there may be consideration of MRI, the compatibility of the device should be confirmed.

For the uncomplicated patient, enhanced recovery after surgery guidelines exist for select surgeries, and may guide the surgeon in developing an analgesic plan. Enhanced recovery after surgery guidelines have been shown to decrease complications, costs, and opioid use postoperatively.[21,22] For the more complex patient, the surgeon should coordinate with the patient's outpatient pain provider. The anesthesiologist will also be instrumental in preoperative, intraoperative, and postoperative strategies to optimize pain control.

Intraoperative analgesia strategies often are managed by the anesthesiologist. However, it is important to ensure a multidisciplinary discussion as to the course of action. Regional anesthetic techniques should be considered and discussed between the surgical and anesthesia teams. Depending on hospital protocol, either the surgical team or anesthesiology team may order analgesics in the preoperative area to aid with postoperative analgesia. Common premedications include NSAIDs, acetaminophen, and gabapentinoids. Home medication reconciliation should be performed so the patient does not receive redundant medications (eg, preoperative gabapentin for a patient taking pregabalin). Preoperative acetaminophen and NSAIDs have been shown to reduce postoperative opioid consumption for a number of different surgeries.[23]

Preoperative gabapentin has been shown to be effective in decreasing acute pain by blocking the development of hyperalgesia and decreasing central sensitization.[24] For those patients with chronic pain, a number of intraoperative strategies have been found to have benefits that extend into the postoperative period. Dosing long-acting opioids intraoperatively and adjuvant medication infusions, such as ketamine or lidocaine, can offer a multimodal plan for postoperative pain relief.[25]

SUMMARY

Preoperative optimization of patients with chronic pain requires a multimodal and collaborative approach. Providers must assess individuals on a case-by-case basis. This approach includes a focused assessment of current outpatient pain regimens and prescriptions, any past medical history that may create contraindications to additional prescriptions, any pertinent psychiatric and social history with a focus on substance use disorder, and a general assessment of pain. The provider must be cognizant of medical conditions, such as OSA, respiratory disease, and cardiac disease, that will put the patient at higher risk for postoperative opioid induced respiratory depression. Special care must be paid to those patients on long-term outpatient opioid prescriptions, especially buprenorphine and methadone. Multimodal analgesia should be used to aid postoperative analgesia and minimize the amount of opioid required for postoperative care. For patients with chronic pain, providers should reach out to the patient's outpatient prescribers and pain specialists to ensure a safe and effective analgesic plan.

REFERENCES

1. Gan TJ. Poorly controlled postoperative pain: prevalence, consequences, and prevention. J Pain Res 2017;10:2287–98.
2. Pivec R, Issa K, Naziri Q, et al. Opioid use prior to total hip arthroplasty leads to worse clinical outcomes. Int Orthop 2014;38(6):1159–65.
3. Grichnik KP, Ferrante FM. The difference between acute and chronic pain. Mt Sinai J Med 1991;58(3):217–20.
4. Richard Chapman C, Donaldson G, Davis J, et al. Postoperative pain patterns in chronic pain patients: a pilot study. Pain Med 2009;10(3):481–7.
5. Gupta K, Nagappa M, Prasad A, et al. Risk factors for opioid-induced respiratory depression in surgical patients: a systematic review and meta-analyses. BMJ Open 2018;8(12):e024086.
6. Smith HS, Peppin JF. Toward a systematic approach to opioid rotation. J Pain Res 2014;7:589–608.
7. Mitra S, Sinatra RS. Perioperative management of acute pain in the opioid-dependent patient. Anesthesiology 2004;101(1):212–27.
8. Blum JM, Biel SS, Hilliard PE, et al. Preoperative ultra-rapid opiate detoxification for the treatment of post-operative surgical pain. Med Hypotheses 2015;84(6):529–31.
9. Fishbain DA, Pulikal A. Does opioid tapering in chronic pain patients result in improved pain or same pain vs increased pain at taper completion? a structured evidence-based systematic review. Pain Med 2019;20(11):2179–97.
10. Berna C, Kulich RJ, Rathmell JP. Tapering long-term opioid therapy in chronic noncancer pain: evidence and recommendations for everyday practice. Mayo Clin Proc 2015;90(6):828–42.

11. CDC Pocket Guide. Tapering opioids for chronic pain. Available at: https://www.cdc.gov/drugoverdose/pdf/clinical_pocket_guide_tapering-a.pdf.   Accessed December 12, 2019.

12. Park TW, Saitz R, Ganoczy D, et al. Benzodiazepine prescribing patterns and deaths from drug overdose among US veterans receiving opioid analgesics: case-cohort study. BMJ 2015;350:h2698.

13. Nagappa M, Liao P, Wong J, et al. Validation of the STOP-Bang questionnaire as a screening tool for obstructive sleep apnea among different populations: a systematic review and meta-analysis. PLoS One 2015;10:e0143697.

14. Svider PF, Pashkova AA, Folbe AJ, et al. Obstructive sleep apnea: strategies for minimizing liability and enhancing patient safety. Otolaryngol Head Neck Surg 2013;149(6):947–53.

15. Borsook D, George E, Barry K, et al. Anesthesia and perioperative stress: consequences on neural networks and postoperative behaviors. Prog Neurobiol 2010;92(4):601–12.

16. Urman RD, Jonan A, Kaye AD. Buprenorphine formulations: clinical best practice strategies recommendations for perioperative management of patients undergoing surgical or interventional pain procedures. Pain Physician 2018;21:E1–12.

17. Anderson TA, Quaye ANA, Nalan Ward E, et al. To stop or not, that is the question: acute pain management for the patient on chronic buprenorphine. Anesthesiology 2017;126(6):1180–6.

18. Dowell D, Haegerich TM, Chou R. CDC guideline for prescribing opioids for chronic pain – United States, 2016. MMWR Recomm Rep 2016;65(No. RR-1):1–49.

19. Geurts JW, Willems PC, Lockwood C, et al. Patient expectations for management of chronic non-cancer pain: a systematic review. Health Expect 2017;20(6):1201–17.

20. Grider JS, Brown RE, Colclough GE. Perioperative management of patients with an intrathecal drug delivery system for chronic pain. Anesth Analg 2008;107:1393–6.

21. Haase GM. Embracing early recovery after surgery (ERAS) protocols: is it time for otolaryngology to join the parade? Am J Otolaryngol 2018;39(5):652–3.

22. Nelson G, Kiyang LN, Crumley ET, et al. Implementation of Enhanced Recovery After Surgery (ERAS) Across a Provincial Healthcare System: the ERAS Alberta Colorectal Surgery experience. World J Surg 2016;40:1092.

23. Kochhar A, Banday J, Ahmad Z, et al. Pregabalin in monitored anesthesia care for ear-nose-throat surgery. Anesth Essays Res 2017;11(2):350–3.

24. Qiu R, Perrino AC Jr, Zurich H, et al. Effect of preoperative gabapentin and acetaminophen on opioid consumption in video-assisted thoracoscopic surgery: a retrospective study. Rom J Anaesth Intensive Care 2018;25(1):43–8.

25. Murphy GS, Szokol JW, Avram MJ, et al. Intraoperative methadone for the prevention of postoperative pain: a randomized, double-blinded clinical trial in cardiac surgical patients. Anesthesiology 2015;122(5):1112–22.

Local Blocks and Regional Anesthesia in the Head and Neck

Andrew P. Johnson, MD*, Elizabeth Boscoe, MD, Cristina Cabrera-Muffly, MD

KEYWORDS

- Local anesthesia • Pain control • Otolaryngology • Education

KEY POINTS

- There are a wide variety of local anesthetic agents with several different properties, such as onset time and length of action.
- Local and regional anesthetic techniques are often used for laceration repair or in addition to intravenous sedation, but some can be used for chronic pain situations, such as trigeminal neuralgia, migraines, and chronic cough, or in addition to topical anesthesia for intubation procedures.
- Although local and regional anesthesia is often safe, there are several complications that are possible, ranging from issues with the injection (eg, a broken needle or nerve injury) to reactions to the anesthetic agent (eg, allergic reaction, systemic toxicity). These possible reactions are even more important in certain patient populations.

INTRODUCTION

Local anesthesia refers to the application of an anesthetic with the intention to induce the loss of sensation in a particular part of the body, as opposed to general anesthesia where the anesthetic is applied systemically, resulting in loss of consciousness. Otolaryngologists perform a variety of procedures under both general anesthesia and local anesthesia. Because surgeons often inject the local anesthetic, it behooves them to understand the pharmacology of common drugs that they may be using. It is also important to have a firm grasp of facial anatomy so that local anesthetic can be precisely applied and to ensure the desired effect of anesthesia is achieved. This article provides an overview of the pharmacology of local anesthetics (**Table 1**) as well as a brief overview of sensory facial neural anatomy.

Department of Otolaryngology, University of Colorado School of Medicine, 12631 East 17th Avenue, MS: B205, Aurora, CO 80045, USA
* Corresponding author.
E-mail address: andrew.p.johnson@cuanschutz.edu

Otolaryngol Clin N Am 53 (2020) 739–751
https://doi.org/10.1016/j.otc.2020.05.004
0030-6665/20/© 2020 Elsevier Inc. All rights reserved.

Table 1
Description and qualities of various local anesthetic agents in otolaryngology

Drug	Classification	Onset	Half-Life (h)	Duration (with Epinephrine)	Lipid Solubility	pKa	Maximum Dose, (with Epinephrine) (mg/kg)	Application
Cocaine	Ester	Rapid	1	5–90 min	++	8.6	3	Topical for use in nasal procedures
Benzocaine	Ester	Rapid	—	5–10 min	—	2.5	—	Topical
Tetracaine	Ester	Rapid	—	120–180 min	++++	8.2	1–3 (1.5)	—
Lidocaine	Amide	Rapid	1.6	120 min (240 min)	++	7.8	4.5 (7)	Local infiltration, IV, intrathecal
Bupivacaine	Amide	Intermediate	3.5	4 h (8–12 h)	++++	8.1	2 (3)	—
Ropivacaine	Amide	Intermediate	1.9	3 h (6 h)	++++	8.1	2–3	—
Prilocaine	Amide	Intermediate	1.6	90 min (360 min)	++	7.8	5 (7.5)	Topical (component of Emla cream)

Data from Refs.[2,32–35]

Mechanism of Action

Local anesthetics inhibit the neuronal pain signal of peripheral nerve endings. Local anesthetic molecules reversibly bind to sodium channels, resulting in their inactivation and cessation of nerve signal propagation by blocking cell depolarization.[1] The fewer sodium channels present, the more easily a nerve signal can be blocked, so the smaller the diameter, the more sensitive a nerve is to local anesthesia. Therefore, smaller nerve fibers are generally easier to anesthetize because they require smaller volumes of local anesthetic for complete nerve signal blockade. In general, the sensitivities of differing nerve fibers from most sensitive to least are as follows: rapid-firing autonomic nerves, followed by sensory nerve fibers, then motor nerve fibers. Within sensory nerve fibers, pain fibers are the most sensitive, followed by pressure, and then proprioception signals.[2]

Classification

Local anesthetics can be classified by their chemical components into 2 groups: amides and esters. All local anesthetics are made up of an aromatic lipophilic ring attached to a hydrophilic tertiary amine by an intermediate chain. The intermediate chain is either an amide or an ester, which plays an important role in the chemical properties of the compound. It also plays a role in the metabolism of the drug, with amides being metabolized in the liver and esters metabolized in the plasma.[2] Simply put, a local anesthetic can be easily recognized as belonging to one chemical group versus the other by the name of the compound. Amides have 2 ls in their names, whereas esters have only 1.[3]

Lipid Solubility

This property is closely related to potency of the local anesthetic (although is not the entire picture). The more potent an agent, the more lipid soluble it likely is. Because nerve cell membranes are primarily composed of lipids, the more lipid soluble an agent is, the easier it can enter the cell membrane. However, other properties, such as vasodilation, can play a role in a drug's potency. Furthermore, agents that are highly lipid soluble can be easily sequestered in nearby lipid tissues, which can result in a longer duration of action but a lower potency.[4]

Protein Binding

This property determines the duration of action of a compound. The higher affinity for protein binding, the longer duration of action y/because of a firmer bond to the sodium channels. However, like potency, duration of action is also affected by the solubility of an agent as well as vasodilation or vasoconstriction.[2]

Diffusibility

This property is related to the speed of action of the local anesthetic, with faster-onset medications being diffused more quickly through tissues.[3]

Ionization

Most local anesthetics are weak bases and therefore exist partly in an ionized state at physiologic pH.[4] The nonionized state (or uncharged form) is the form able to cross the cell membrane. The amount of nonionized local anesthetic that exists in a solution is based on the pH of the environment and the pKa of the compound. The higher the pKa, the more ionized form exists. Therefore, the lower the pKa, the faster the onset of action of the drug. For anesthetics with a larger pKa, the onset of action can be increased by using a higher concentration of the drug.[4] In addition, as the pH of the solution decreases, the equilibrium shifts toward the ionized form of the compound and this decreases the onset of action of the drug. This process explains why it can be difficult to anesthetize an infected area, because the pH is often decreased in infection.[2]

Vasoconstriction

With the exception of cocaine, all local anesthetics have vasodilatory properties to a degree, with lidocaine having the greatest vasodilatory properties of the local anesthetics.[4] Vasodilation is caused by the direct relaxation of the peripheral arteriolar smooth muscle fibers.[3] Vasoconstrictive agents, such as epinephrine, are often added to local anesthetics to increase the duration of action of the drug by delaying absorption and metabolism.[2]

Facial anatomy

The sensory innervation of the face predominantly comes from the trigeminal nerve (cranial nerve V) and its 3 main branches: the ophthalmic nerve (V1), the maxillary nerve (V2), and the mandibular nerve (V3). In general, sensory innervation to the upper third of the face is performed by branches of V1, the middle third of the face by branches of V2, and the lower third by branches of V3. Sensory innervation of the auricle stems from multiple cranial nerves, including the mandibular branch of trigeminal, as well as facial, glossopharyngeal, and cervical spinal nerves. Sensory innervation of the neck comes from the cervical plexus (ventral rami from C1–C4)[5] as well as the vagal nerve (cranial nerve X), specifically the superior laryngeal nerve branch. Some specific terminal nerve branches and their functions are discussed next.

Facial Anatomy

Nerve anatomy of the upper third of the face[5–8]
- Branches of V1
  - Ophthalmic: cutaneous nose, supraorbital region, forehead
  - Supraorbital: upper eye lid, forehead, scalp (to lambdoid suture)
  - Supratrochlear: conjunctiva, upper eye lid, glabella and midline forehead, anterior scalp
  - Infratrochlear: bridge of nose, medial aspect of eyelid below brow
  - Nasociliary: frontal sinus, anterior and posterior ethmoid sinuses, sphenoid sinus, anterior nasal septum, lateral nasal wall, skin of nasal tip, cornea, iris, ciliary body

Nerve anatomy of the middle third of the face
- Branches of V2
  - Zygomaticofacial: skin overlying cheek
  - Zygomaticotemporal: skin over side of lateral forehead and temples
  - Infraorbital: lower eyelid, lateral nares, upper lip
  - Nasopalatine: anterior portion of hard palate behind incisors
  - Greater and lesser palatine: hard and soft palate, lateral nasal wall
  - Superior alveolar: maxillary teeth, nasal floor, gums
  - Sphenopalatine: orbit, nose, buccal mucosa, palate, paranasal sinuses

Nerve anatomy of the lower third of the face
- Branches of V3
  - Buccal: cheek and oral mucosa and gingiva
  - Glossopharyngeal: posterior tongue and pharynx
  - Inferior alveolar: mandibular teeth
  - Lingual: anterior two-thirds of tongue

   ○ Mental: cutaneous chin, lower lip, and side of mandible
   ○ Auriculotemporal: outer ear and temporal region
Nerve anatomy of the auricle
   ○ Auriculotemporal (branch of V3): superior pinna and temporal region
   ○ Facial: ear canal, ear drum, conchal bowl
   ○ Greater auricular (from C2–C3): inferior and posterior pinna, mastoid process, and parotid gland
   ○ Lesser occipital (from C2): posterior medial surface of ear and back of neck
Nerve anatomy of the neck
   ○ Greater occipital (from C2): posterior neck
   ○ Superior laryngeal (branch of vagus): sensation of larynx above vocal cords and supraglottic mucosa
   ○ Supraclavicular (from C3–C4): anterolateral shoulder and clavicle
   ○ Transverse cervical (from C2–C3): neck around sternocleidomastoid muscle

LOCAL ANESTHETIC BLOCKS

There are a wide variety of local anesthetic blocks available. This article provides information on some that are more often used and ones that can used for more chronic conditions, such as glossopharyngeal and trigeminal neuralgia, neurogenic cough, or migraines. These anesthetic blocks have been divided based on their anatomic locations.

Upper Third of the Face

Supraorbital/supratrochlear block
Anatomy The supraorbital and supratrochlear nerves are terminal branches of the frontal nerve, which is a branch of the ophthalmic nerve (V1). The supraorbital nerve exits the skull at the supraorbital notch located at the midpupillary line. The supratrochlear nerve is on average 1.05 cm medial to the supraorbital nerve at its exit point from the supraorbital foramen.[9]

Nerve function Sensation to most of the forehead, with the supratrochlear providing more medial coverage and components of medial nasal dorsum and upper medial eyelid.

   Reasons for regional block:
- Laceration repair
- Adjunct to surgery involving the upper third of the face in the setting of intravenous (IV) sedation
- Postoperative pain control
- Migraines and chronic headaches[10]

How to Injection is usually completed with either lidocaine or bupivacaine, with bupivacaine providing longer-lasting results. A 27-gauge needle is commonly used. In order to complete this nerve block, the supraorbital notch is palpated at the midpupillary line. The injection is carried in a lateral to medial direction, and a small amount of anesthetic (1–3 mL) is applied in a plane deep to the muscle. Ensure that there is no blood return before injection and that the foramen has not been entered. In order to apply adequate anesthesia to the supratrochlear nerve, injection must be carried medially to provide anesthesia to the nerve.

Zygomaticotemporal nerve block
Anatomy The zygomatic nerve is a terminal branch of the maxillary division of the trigeminal nerve (V2). The zygomatic nerve has 2 branches, the zygomaticotemporal and

the zygomaticofacial. The zygomaticotemporal nerve exits the cranium along the lateral orbital rim and is usually anywhere from the level of the lateral canthus to 1 cm inferior.

Nerve function Sensation to small area of the lateral forehead, anterior to hair line and above the zygoma.

Reasons for regional block:
- Used in conjunction with supraorbital nerve block for complete forehead anesthesia
- Laceration repair
- Adjunct to surgery in setting of IV sedation

How to The important aspect in this injection is to access the area behind the lateral orbital rim. In order to accomplish this, start by palpating the zygomaticofrontal suture. Slide the forefinger of the noninjecting hand into the depression just posterior and inferior to the suture. From here, use a 27-gauge 38-mm (1.5 inch) needle and place the needle just posterior to the finger. Slide the needle anteriorly to the area just behind the concave surface of the lateral orbital rim. Inject 1 to 3 mL of local anesthetic into this area.

Midthird of the Face

Dorsal nasal nerve block

Anatomy The dorsal, or external, nasal nerve is a branch of the anterior ethmoidal nerve. The anterior ethmoidal nerve is a division of the ophthalmic nerve (V1). The external nasal nerve ends up exiting the skull base at the junction between the bony and cartilaginous junction of the nose.

Nerve function Sensation to nasal dorsum, nasal alae, and nasal vestibule.

Reasons for regional block:
- Postoperative pain after nasal surgery[11]
- External nasal neuralgia[12]
- Adjunct for nasal surgery

How to A 27-gauge needle is used to inject the bony cartilaginous junction in the sub–superficial musculoaponeurotic system plane. The injection should be lateral to the midline (~5 mm). Approximately 1 to 2 mL of local anesthetic can be used.

Infraorbital nerve block

Anatomy The infraorbital nerve is a terminal branch of the maxillary nerve (V2). This nerve exits the skull at the infraorbital foramen. The foramen is approximately 0.5 to 1.0 cm below the midpupillary line.

Nerve function Sensation to midface, including cheek, upper lips, and lower eyelid.

Reasons for regional block:
- Reduce emergence agitation following nasal surgery[13]
- Laceration repair of the midface
- Adjunct to surgery in setting of IV sedation
- Possible pain reduction following cleft lip repair[14]
- Treat refractory trigeminal neuralgia isolated to the midface[15]

How to There are 2 approaches available. The first is through an intraoral approach. Through this approach, 1 hand palpates the inferior orbital rim and retracts the cheek, which should expose the gingivobuccal sulcus adjacent to the second premolar. A 27-gauge needle is inserted just lateral into the buccal mucosa from the gingivobuccal sulcus and is then carried to approximately 0.5 to 1.0 cm below the infraorbital rim at the midpupillary line. Inject approximately 3 to 5 mL of anesthetic in this area. Care must be taken to prevent anesthetic from entering into the orbit. The other approach is through an external approach. The infraorbital foramen is identified below the inferior orbital rim at the midpupillary line. A 27-gauge needle is used to inject through the skin to the area of the infraorbital rim, and is carried below the muscle. There must be no intraluminal injection because the facial artery is in close proximity.

LOWER THIRD FACIAL BLOCKS
Mental Nerve Block

Anatomy
The mental nerve is the terminal branch of the mandibular division of the trigeminal nerve (V3). This nerve exits the mental foramen between the first and second premolars, roughly 1 cm below the gum line. This nerve should sit in the midpupillary line and be in the same plane as the supraorbital notch and the infraorbital foramen.

Nerve function
Sensation to the lower lip and chin.

Reasons for regional block:
- Laceration repair
- Lower lip procedures
- Treat trigeminal neuralgia isolated to the lower lip[15]

How to
This block is completed intraorally. The lower lip of the side of the injection is retracted, making the mucosa taut at the gingivobuccal sulcus. The first and second mandibular premolars are identified. A 27-gauge needle is inserted approximately 1 cm below the gum line at a 45° angle until bony contact is made. Once this is reached, withdraw the needle slightly and inject approximately 2 to 3 mL of local anesthetic.

NECK REGIONAL BLOCKS
Glossopharyngeal Nerve Block

Anatomy
The glossopharyngeal nerve originates from the medulla and exits the skull base at the jugular foramen. This nerve then descends with the vagus nerve posterior and medial to the styloid process in the parapharyngeal space. Numerous branches exist after the glossopharyngeal nerve has exited the skull base.

Nerve function
Provides motor, special sensory, and sensory information. From a sensory standpoint, it provides somatic information along pharyngeal walls, base of tongue, anterior surface of epiglottis, ear, and tympanic membrane.

Reasons for regional block:
- Treat glossopharyngeal neuralgia[16]
- Reduce posttonsillectomy pain[17]
- Adjunct during upper esophageal or awake airway procedures[18]
- Eagle syndrome[19]

How to

There are both external and intraoral approaches. There are several different ways to approach the external injections, but most use ultrasonography guidance to identify the large blood vessels in the area. The details of the procedure are too in depth for the overall goal of this article, but suffice to say that the injections come with great risk. These risks include bleeding (secondary to location adjacent to the internal jugular vein and carotid) as well as the risk of anesthesia to the vagus nerve (leading to progressive hoarseness, and, if completed bilaterally, bilateral cord paralysis). Intraoral approaches focus more on blocking distal branches of the glossopharyngeal nerve and not necessarily targeting the main trunk. Often, steroids can be used in addition to local anesthetic to provide symptom improvement. From an intraoral standpoint, there are 2 primary techniques. In the anterior tonsillar pillar approach, the tongue is retracted away from the anterior tonsillar pillar. The palatoglossal fold is identified at the base where it transitions to the tongue. From here, a spinal needle is used and 1 to 2 mL of anesthetic is applied roughly 0.5 cm deep in this area.[20,21] The posterior tonsillar pillar approach is similar but targets an injection through the posterior pillar at the base of tongue. This approach is tougher because the tongue has to be retracted further and gagging often occurs.

Superior Laryngeal Nerve Block

Anatomy

The vagus nerve exits the skull base at the jugular foramen and runs the course of the neck in the carotid space. There are several branches of the vagus nerve, including the superior laryngeal and inferior laryngeal nerves. The superior laryngeal nerve splits into 2 components: an external and internal branch. The internal branch of the superior laryngeal nerve enters the larynx through the thyrohyoid membrane.

Nerve function

The internal branch of the superior laryngeal nerve provides sensory information from the larynx. The external branch provides motor control to the cricothyroid muscle.

Reasons for regional block:
- Treatment of neurogenic cough[22,23]
- Adjunct during awake fiberoptic intubation and laryngeal procedures[24–27]

How to

There are several techniques in completing the superior laryngeal nerve block. Ultrasonography can be used to aid in identification of the thyroid cartilage and the hyoid bone, especially in patients with difficult external neck anatomy. This technique can be completed with the patient supine or sitting upright. Usually a combination of local anesthetic and steroid is used. One hand grasps the larynx and displaces the hyoid to the side of the injection. The space between the thyroid cartilage and hyoid bone represents the thyrohyoid membrane. The greater cornu and superior tubercle of the thyroid cartilage can indicate roughly the location of the internal branch. The carotid can be used as a posterior border. The injection can be completed from an anterior to posterior direction, which is thought to provide the most coverage. However, approaching posteriorly allows greater security, knowing that the carotid is posterior to the injection point. The use of a 27-gauge needle and approximately 1 to 2 mL of topical anesthetic mixed with steroid is sufficient. Bilateral injections can be done for fiberoptic intubations, but, for cough in the outpatient setting, unilateral injections should be completed. A trigger point can be palpated and can be used for injection location.[23]

POTENTIAL COMPLICATIONS OF LOCAL AND REGIONAL BLOCKS

Administration of local anesthesia is generally safe and effective, but there are several potential complications associated with the use of local anesthetics.

Overdose

It is imperative to calculate maximum dosages of various local anesthetics to prevent overdose, especially in pediatric patients, because dosages are calculated in milligrams per kilogram. A list of commonly used local anesthetics with their associated maximum dosages is provided in **Table 2**. The addition of epinephrine increases the maximum dose allowable for most local anesthetics. Symptoms associated with an overdose are the same as those seen in systemic toxicity, which is discussed in further detail later.

Intravascular Injection

Even when low doses of local anesthetics are used, injection intravascularly can lead to rapid onset of systemic toxicity. When injecting local anesthetics, the syringe should be drawn back after the needle is inserted to confirm it is not located intravascularly. During negative aspiration, the presence of a flash of blood should prompt repositioning instead of injection. In situations where the anatomy is difficult or there are large vessels in close proximity to the injection site, ultrasonography guidance may be helpful to confirm location of the needle.

Allergic Reactions

Allergic reactions to local anesthetics are very rare, especially with amides, in which the presentation of an allergic reaction should prompt consideration of an overdose or intravascular injection.[28] Esters are more allergenic because of their para-aminobenzoic acid (PABA) structure. Patients with a PABA allergy or atypical pseudo-cholinesterase activity are at higher risk. Tetracaine, specifically, has been shown to have a higher incidence of allergic reactions.

In some cases, patients are allergic to the preservative in local anesthetics, such as methylparaben in amides (which is similar to PABA), or sodium bisulfite, which is commonly found in epinephrine.[28] In addition, when local anesthesia is administered in the setting of latex glove use, consider a potential latex allergy instead. True allergic reactions are either type I or type IV hypersensitivity, with type IV being more common. In patients with a suspected allergy, patch testing can be performed to confirm the diagnosis.

Table 2	
Maximum doses for local anesthetic agents	
Anesthetic	**Maximum Dose (mg/kg)**
Lidocaine	5
Lidocaine with epinephrine	7
Mepivacaine	4.4
Mepivacaine with epinephrine	6.6
Articaine	7
Bupivacaine	1.3
Prilocaine	2.7

Symptoms associated with allergic reaction to local anesthetics include itching, edema, hives, nasal congestion and rhinorrhea, wheezing, shortness of breath, and headache. Severe allergic reactions can lead to toxic eruptions, bronchospasm, and anaphylaxis. For mild reactions, treatment consists of an oral antihistamine and/or hydrocortisone cream. In more severe cases, the use of an epinephrine pen, oxygen supplementation, and urgent transfer to a monitored setting is recommended.

Broken Needle

Rarely, during injection of local anesthetic, the needle breaks off into the tissue. To avoid this complication, avoid using a short needle and burying it to the hub when injecting.[28] In addition, avoiding bending the needle before injection decreases the potential for breakage. Needles that break off should be removed if possible, because, over time, they can migrate and cause damage to vessels or other structures.

Nerve Injury

When local anesthesia is administered close to a named nerve, there is potential for nerve injury. The mechanism for injury can be related to direct trauma from the needle, epineural hemorrhage, or to a neurotoxic effect from the anesthesia. Nerve injury can lead to persistent numbness, burning, or motor deficits.

Methemoglobinemia

Hemoglobin is a protein in the blood that contains ferrous iron. Ferrous iron is adept at releasing oxygen into the tissues as the blood circulates. In cases of oxidative stress, the heme group of the hemoglobin molecule is oxidized to the ferric state, converting hemoglobin to methemoglobin. Because methemoglobin molecules have a limited ability to release bound oxygen to tissues, high levels of methemoglobin in the blood lead to hypoxia. Hypoxia is manifested by a chocolate-brown appearance of arterial blood, in contrast with its typical bright-red hue. Patients being monitored with pulse oximetry show a discrepancy between saturation level and a measured arterial oxygen partial pressure.[29]

Certain local anesthetics can prompt oxidation of the heme group to create methemoglobin. Most cases in the literature involve benzocaine, but prilocaine, lidocaine, and tetracaine have also been implicated.[29] Patients with congenital methemoglobinemia, caused by NADH deficiency, are at higher risk for exacerbation with concurrent use of local anesthetics. In addition, the use of local anesthetics in the setting of other oxidative drugs can prompt methemoglobin production. Methemoglobinemia can cause seizures, respiratory compromise, shock, and coma. In severe cases, hypoxic encephalopathy, myocardial infarction, and even death can occur. Treatment involves the use of methylene blue infusion, which converts to leukomethylene blue, a reducing agent that converts methemoglobin to deoxyhemoglobin.[29] Admission and observation in a monitored setting is recommended, because, in some cases, a rebound effect occurs 4 to 12 hours after the initial successful methylene blue infusion. Patients with glucose-6-phosphate dehydrogenase deficiency typically cannot convert methylene blue to leukomethylene blue, so ascorbic acid is recommended instead.

Systemic Toxicity

Systemic toxicity related to local anesthetics is estimated to occur in 2.5 per 10,000 blockades.[30] The 2 organ systems typically affected by toxicity are the cardiac system and central nervous system (CNS). Risk factors include large doses, rapid absorption, and intravenous injection. There is an inverse relationship between toxicity and speed of injection, with faster injections decreasing the blood level threshold for symptoms.[31]

In cases of systemic toxicity, patients should be admitted to a monitored setting. Resuscitation and monitoring should last until the local anesthetic is completely metabolized.

CNS toxicity typically manifests first, because doses needed to cause CNS symptoms are lower than doses needed to cause cardiac symptoms. Local anesthetics block inhibitory pathways in the cerebral cortex, causing unopposed excitatory activity,[31] which manifests as dizziness, trouble concentrating, confusion, tinnitus, and circumoral numbness. Severe reactions can progress to seizures and respiratory arrest. In patients taking other CNS-suppressing drugs, the excitatory phase may be silent, progressing directly to seizures and respiratory depression. Treatment of CNS toxicity includes securing the airway; providing supplemental oxygen; and the use of benzodiazepines, barbiturates, or propofol to decrease excitatory neurologic activity and seizure risk.[31]

Cardiac toxicity occurs when local anesthetics bind to sodium. Because cardiac cells rely on sodium-initiated depolarization, local anesthetics can affect conduction and contraction, leading to arrhythmias and decreased cardiac output.[30] Small amounts of local anesthetics create vasoconstriction and increased sympathetic activity, which cause a small increase in cardiac output, heart rate, and blood pressure. As toxicity occurs, peripheral vasodilation occurs, leading to hypotension and decreased cardiac output. Profound hypotension, arrhythmias, and cardiac arrest can follow. Treatment options for cardiac toxicity include vasopressin for hypotension and amiodarone for arrhythmias. Intravenous intralipid can absorb circulating local anesthetic and help decrease cardiovascular effects. Use caution with epinephrine, because it can exacerbate arrhythmias. Cardiopulmonary bypass may be used in the most severe situations.

Special Populations

- Cardiac transplant patients: because the heart is denervated, these patients can be more sensitive to epinephrine.[28]
- β-Blockers, amiodarone, and digoxin: there is an increased risk of arrhythmia with the use of bupivacaine in patients on these medications.
- Sulfonamides, chloroquine, dapsone, phenobarbital, and metoclopramide: these medications increase the risk of methemoglobinemia when used in conjunction with local anesthetics.
- Pregnancy: mepivacaine, bupivacaine, and articaine are considered pregnancy category C.[28]
- Porphyria: avoid the use of local anesthetics during a porphyric crisis. It is difficult to differentiate between neurologic sequelae of porphyria and the anesthetic.

SUMMARY

There are a wide variety of local anesthetic agents available. The selection of which to use depends largely on the goal of the regional anesthetic as well as any potential patient comorbidities. Various local anesthetic blocks are described in this article. Although they are often used for laceration repair or local procedures, some can be used for more chronic conditions (eg, neurogenic cough, migraines, or even trigeminal neuralgia). They can often be used as an adjunct to surgical procedures as well (either providing additional benefit in conjunction with IV medications or to aid fiberoptic intubations). Although the use of local anesthetics is generally safe, it is important to be mindful of potential complications and certain patient populations that may be at high risk for certain local anesthetics.

DISCLOSURE

The authors have nothing to disclose.

REFERENCES

1. Thiagarajan B. Local anesthesia of nose and nasal cavity- a review. Global Journal of Otolaryngology 2017;4(4):001–3.
2. Becker DE, Reed KL. Local anesthetics: review of pharmacological considerations. Anesth Prog 2012;59(2):90–103.
3. McLeod IK. Local anesthetics. Medscape 2019. Available at: https://emedicine.medscape.com/article/873879-overview. Accessed October 15, 2019.
4. Eappen S, Datta S. Pharmacology of local anesthetics. Seminars in Anesthesia, Perioperative Medicine and Pain 1998;17(1):10–7.
5. Burnett G, Demaria S, Levine AI. Regional anesthesia and acute pain management. Otolaryngol Clin North Am 2019. https://doi.org/10.1016/j.otc.2019.08.013.
6. Moskovitz JB, Sabatino F. Regional nerve blocks of the face. Emerg Med Clin North Am 2013;31(2):517–27.
7. Szymanski A, Geiger Z. Anatomy, head and neck, ear. In: StatPearls. Treasure Island (FL): StatPearls Publishing; 2019. Available at: https://www.ncbi.nlm.nih.gov/books/NBK470359/. Accessed June 17, 2020.
8. Waxenbaum JA, Bordoni B. Anatomy, head and neck, cervical nerves. In: StatPearls. Treasure Island (FL): StatPearls Publishing; 2019. Available at: https://www.ncbi.nlm.nih.gov/books/NBK538136/. Accessed June 17, 2020.
9. Konofaos P, Soto-Miranda MA, Halen JV, et al. Supratrochlear and supraorbital nerves. Ophthalmic Plast Reconstr Surg 2013;29(5):403–8.
10. Miller S, Lagrata S, Matharu M. Multiple cranial nerve blocks for the transitional treatment of chronic headaches. Cephalalgia 2019;39(12):1488–99.
11. Ibrahim M, Elnabtity AM, Keera A. Efficacy of external nasal nerve block following nasal surgery. Anaesthesist 2018;67(3):188–97.
12. García-Moreno H, Aledo-Serrano Á, Gimeno-Hernández J, et al. External nasal neuralgia: a neuropathic pain within the territory of the external nasal nerve. Headache 2015;55(9):1259–62.
13. Choi H, Jung SH, Hong JM, et al. Effects of bilateral infraorbital and infratrochlear nerve block on emergence agitation after septorhinoplasty: a randomized controlled trial. J Clin Med 2019;8(6):769.
14. Feriani G, Hatanaka E, Torloni MR, et al. Infraorbital nerve block for postoperative pain following cleft lip repair in children. Cochrane Database Syst Rev 2016. https://doi.org/10.1002/14651858.cd011131.pub2.
15. Perloff MD, Chung JS. Urgent care peripheral nerve blocks for refractory trigeminal neuralgia. Am J Emerg Med 2018;36(11):2058–60.
16. Liu Q, Zhong Q, Tang G, et al. Ultrasound-guided glossopharyngeal nerve block via the styloid process for glossopharyngeal neuralgia: a retrospective study. J Pain Res 2019;12:2503–10.
17. Ahmed SA, Omara AF. The effect of glossopharyngeal nerve block on post-tonsillectomy pain of children; randomized controlled trial. Anesth Pain Med 2019;9(2):e90854.
18. Ortega Ramírez M, Linares Segovia B, García Cuevas MA, et al. Glossopharyngeal nerve block versus lidocaine spray to improve tolerance in upper gastrointestinal endoscopy. Gastroenterol Res Pract 2013;2013(2013):4.
19. Maher T, Shankar H. Ultrasound-guided peristyloid steroid injection for eagle syndrome. Pain Pract 2017;17(4):554–7.

20. Saliba DL, Mccutchen TA, Laxton MJ, et al. Reliable block of the gag reflex in one minute or less. J Clin Anesth 2009;21(6):463.
21. Isbir CA. Treatment of a patient with glossopharyngeal neuralgia by the anterior tonsillar pillar method. Case Rep Neurol 2011;3(1):27–31.
22. Dhillon VK. Superior laryngeal nerve block for neurogenic cough: A case series. Laryngoscope Investig Otolaryngol 2019;4(4):410–3.
23. Simpson CB, Tibbetts KM, Loochtan MJ, et al. Treatment of chronic neurogenic cough with in-office superior laryngeal nerve block. Laryngoscope 2018;128(8): 1898–903.
24. Ramkumar R, Arora S, Bhatia N, et al. Ultrasound guided superior laryngeal nerve block as an adjuvant to generalanesthesia during endoscopic laryngeal surgery: A prospective, randomized, double-blind trial. Am J Otolaryngol 2019; 40(1):30–5.
25. Mathur PR, Jain N, Kumar A, et al. Comparison between lignocaine nebulization and airway nerve block for awake fiberoptic bronchoscopy-guided nasotracheal intubation: a single-blind randomized prospective study. Korean J Anesthesiol 2018;71(2):120–6.
26. Chatrath V, Sharan R, Jain P, et al. The efficacy of combined regional nerve blocks in awake orotracheal fiberoptic intubation. Anesth Essays Res 2016; 10(2):255.
27. Sawka A, Tang R, Vaghadia H. Sonographically guided superior laryngeal nerve block during awake fiberoptic intubation. A A Case Rep 2015;4(8):107–10.
28. Ogle OE, Mahjoubi G. Local anesthesia: agents, techniques, and complications. Dent Clin North Am 2012;56(1):133–48.
29. Guay J. Methemoglobinemia related to local anesthetics: a summary of 242 episodes. Anesth Analg 2009;108(3):837–45.
30. Dickerson DM, Apfelbaum JL. Local anesthetic systemic toxicity. Aesthet Surg J 2014;34(7):1111–9.
31. Dewaele S, Santos AC. Toxicity of local anesthetics. In: Hadzic A, editor. Peripheral nerve blocks and anatomy for ultrasound-guided regional anesthesia. 2nd edition. New York: McGraw-Hill; 2012.
32. Mumba JM, Kabambi FK, Ngaka CT. Pharmacology of local anaesthetics and commonly used recipes in clinical practice. In: Erbay RH, editor. Current topics in anesthesiology. IntechOpen; 2017. Available at: https://www.intechopen.com/books/current-topics-in-anesthesiology/pharmacology-of-local-anaesthetics-and-commonly-used-recipes-in-clinical-practice.
33. El-Boghdadly K, Pawa A, Chin KJ. Local anesthetic systemic toxicity: current perspectives. Local Reg Anesth 2018;11:35–44.
34. Rosenberg PH, Veering BT, Urmey WF. Maximum recommended doses of local anesthetics: a multifactorial concept. Reg Anesth Pain Med 2004;29(6):564–75.
35. Heavner JE. Local anesthetics. Curr Opin Anaesthesiol 2007;20(4):336–42.

Acute Pain Management Following Head and Neck Surgery

Michael Bobian, MD, Annika Gupta, MD,
Evan M. Graboyes, MD, MPH, FACS*

KEYWORDS

- Pain • Head and neck cancer • Free flap • Free tissue transfer • Opioid • ERAS
- Analgesia • Multimodal analgesia

KEY POINTS

- Pain management for patients with head and neck cancer is complex; opioids are uniquely hazardous due to altered upper airway anatomy and physiology.
- Several nonopioid analgesics exist for pain management of patients undergoing major head and neck surgery, including nonsteroidal anti-inflammatory drugs, acetaminophen, anticonvulsants, corticosteroids, and locoregional anesthetics.
- In addition to the safe use of multimodal analgesia (MMA), special considerations for patients undergoing head and neck free flap surgery include judicious use of steroids, and attention to donor site pain.
- Evidence for specific analgesic regimens following transoral robotic surgery is limited but should include MMA and perioperative dexamethasone if not contraindicated.

INTRODUCTION

Head and neck cancer (HNC) is diagnosed in 65,000 patients annually in the United States.[1] More than 80% of all patients with HNC experience pain before treatment and more than 40% receive opioids before treatment.[2] Despite advances in radiation and chemotherapy, surgical resection and reconstruction remains a critical component of multidisciplinary HNC management. Aside from the obvious associations with patient comfort and satisfaction, adequate pain control in patients with HNC is critically important because it is associated with microvascular free flap viability[3] and long-term psychosocial well-being.[4]

Although opioid pain medications have been the cornerstone of acute pain management for patients undergoing HNC surgery, there is renewed interest in identifying opioid-sparing analgesic for a number of reasons.[5] First, for patients with HNC

Department of Otolaryngology–Head and Neck Surgery, Medical University of South Carolina, 135 Rutledge Avenue, MSC 550, Charleston, SC 29425, USA
* Corresponding author.
E-mail address: graboyes@musc.edu

Otolaryngol Clin N Am 53 (2020) 753–764
https://doi.org/10.1016/j.otc.2020.05.005
0030-6665/20/© 2020 Elsevier Inc. All rights reserved.

undergoing significant alterations in their upper airway anatomy and physiology, adverse effects of opioids (eg, nausea, vomiting, respiratory depression) can be uniquely hazardous. Second, there is continued emerging evidence that multimodal analgesia (MMA) featuring opioid-sparing regimens is more effective than narcotic analgesia alone.[6,7] Finally, the concern of long-term opioid dependence is particularly significant among patients with HNC, as they are at elevated risk for short-term and long-term opioid dependence compared with the general population.[2] For patients older than 65 years who underwent primary surgical resection for any site HNC, 18% of opioid-naïve patients and 50% for patients using opioids preoperatively developed persistent postoperative opioid use (new opioid prescriptions 90–180 days postoperatively.)[8] Hand in hand with the growing attention to opioid-sparing analgesia has been the explosion of articles developing dsease-specific and procedure-specifc Enhanced Recovery After Surgery (ERAS) protocols.[9]

To help the head and neck surgeon stay abreast of ongoing controversies in managing acute postoperative pain for patients undergoing major head and neck surgery, this article (1) reviews the classes of nonopioid analgesics used for acute pain management following head and neck surgery (**Table 1**); (2) critically analyzes the evidence underlying MMA in this patient population; and (3) describes procedure-specific analgesia recommendations for unique head and neck surgical procedures.

NONOPIOID ANALGESICS
Acetaminophen

Acetaminophen has long been a safe alternative and/or adjunct in managing acute postoperative pain in patients with HNC. In a recent retrospective investigation of patients undergoing major head and neck surgery, the combination of intravenous (IV) acetaminophen with morphine patient-controlled analgesia (PCA) resulted in similar pain relief, as measured by PCA attempts and pain score, with 40% and 30% less total postoperative narcotic use in the first 8 and 24 hours, respectively, compared with standard morphine PCA.[10] Hepatic complications of appropriately dosed acetaminophen are rare. Nevertheless, liver function assessment should be considered in appropriate, high-risk patients before scheduled administration due to the prevalence of alcohol use among patients with HNC.[11] Overall, because it is an efficacious and safe medication, scheduled administration of acetaminophen should be considered following almost all major head and neck surgeries.[6,7,10,12]

Nonsteroidal Anti-Inflammatory Drugs

Nonsteroidal anti-inflammatory drugs (NSAIDs) inhibit prostaglandin production over prolonged time periods, leading to decreased local inflammation. NSAIDs include nonselective cyclooxygenase (COX) inhibitors such as ibuprofen and ketorolac, and selective COX-2 inhibitors such as celecoxib. COX-2 inhibitors provides excellent pain control but have a lower risk of platelet dysfunction and gastrointestinal complications.[13]

A major barrier to widespread use of NSAIDs is concern for postoperative hemorrhage, which can be acutely fatal when occurring in the neck or upper airway. However, a recent retrospective cohort study showed that a regimen including scheduled celecoxib 200 mg twice per day for a minimum of 5 days and ketorolac pro re nata (PRN) for up to 3 days was not associated with an increased risk of bleeding in patients with HNC undergoing free flap reconstruction.[6] A retrospective cohort study of postoperative ketorolac in patients undergoing major head and neck surgeries also found no increased risk of bleeding and favorable free flap outcomes.[14]

Table 1
Recommended dosing and considerations of opioid-sparing analgesic medications

Analgesic Class	Analgesic Name	Dosing	Special Considerations
Acetaminophen	Acetaminophen or paracetamol	Preop • 650 mg – 1000 mg once Intraop • 1000 mg IV once Postop • 650 mg Q 6 h–950 mg Q 8 h	Up to 4 g per 24 h Consider hepatic dosing in patients with reduced liver function
NSAIDs	Celecoxib	Preop • 200 mg once Postop • 200 mg BID	Continue for 5 d post-discharge Consider renal dosing or omission in patients with CKD or decreased GFR
	Ketorolac	Postop Ketorolac 15 mg–30 mg IV Q 6 h PRN[a]	For up to 3 d maximum Consider renal dosing or omission in patients with CKD or decreased GFR
Anticonvulsants	Gabapentin	Preop • 1000 mg–1200 mg once Postop • 100 mg–900 mg TID as tolerated	Up-titration based on side effects Consider renal dosing or omission in patients with CKD or decreased GFR
	Pregabalin	Preop • 100 mg once Postop • 50 mg–300 mg BID as tolerated	Up-titration based on side effects Consider renal dosing or omission in patients with CKD or decreased GFR
Corticosteroids	Dexamethasone	Intraop • 10 mg IV once[b] Postop • 8 mg IV Q 8 h up to 4 d[b]	Consider dose or duration reduction in patients with diabetes mellitus

Abbreviations: BID, twice a day; CKD, chronic kidney disease; GFR, glomerular filtration rate; Intraop, intraoperative; IV, intravenous; NSAID, nonsteroidal anti-inflammatory drug; postop, postoperative; preop, preoperative; PRN, pro re nata; Q, every; TID, 3 times a day.
  [a] Consider 15 mg dose for patient appearing frail or elderly.
  [b] For TORS patients.

It is also important to note that NSAIDs have other long-established risks, including renal dysfunction. As such, the use of ketorolac should be limited to 72 hours.[15] Although the renal complications due to NSAID use are rare in healthy individuals, patients with HNC have additional risk factors including hypovolemia and prior kidney injury from nephrotoxic chemotherapy agents.

Anticonvulsants

Anticonvulsants are defined by their ability to suppress seizures, although several of them are known to also modulate pain pathways. The routine control of neuropathic and postoperative pain remains limited to gabapentinoids, which include gabapentin and pregabalin.[16]

A double-blinded, randomized controlled trial (RCT) comparing gabapentin 300 mg twice daily with placebo in 110 patients undergoing large head and neck mucosal operations showed that gabapentin use resulted in decreased pain during rest, coughing, and swallowing, as well as less nausea and vomiting.[17] In a retrospective study of patients with HNC, the median dose of 2700 mg/d of gabapentin resulted in only 10% of patients requiring additional narcotics postoperatively.[18]

The side-effect profile of gabapentin is mild for most patients with dose-limiting side effects related to sedation and dizziness. Various dosing titration regimens have been proposed to avoid these, most conservative titration regiments begin at 300 mg/d and increase according to tolerance.[19]

Pregabalin has also been used for treatment of radiotherapy-related neuropathic pain in patients with HNC[20] and following head and neck–related surgery[21] with good efficacy and similar tolerance to gabapentin. However, evidence for the routine use of pregabalin in the perioperative setting compared with gabapentin is relatively lacking.

Corticosteroids

The efficacy of corticosteroids for pain control has been established for other procedures in otolaryngology,[22] with additional benefits including decreased nausea and swelling (including both airway structures and tissue surrounding microvascular free flap anastomosis). However, steroid use carries considerable risks, including hyperglycemia, psychosis, fluid and electrolyte imbalance, infection, and poor wound healing. A double-blind RCT investigating postoperative dexamethasone versus placebo in 93 patients following HNC resection with free flap reconstruction showed an increase in major complications including wound breakdown/necrosis, infection, venous thrombosis, and postoperative bleeding in the steroid group relative to control.[23]

Local and Regional Analgesia

Support for the routine use of local and regional analgesia for pain following major head and neck procedures remains limited, although protocols for delivering preoperative mandibular nerve blocks with ropivacaine[24] and for parotidectomy have been shown to decrease pain.[25] The utility of these techniques has yet to be used for more extensive head and neck surgeries, however. The continuous infusion of medication to surrounding airway structures and/or free flap pedicles poses obvious risks that warrant careful consideration.

MULTIMODAL ANALGESIA AND ENHANCED RECOVERY AFTER SURGERY

Established in 2010, the ERAS Society aims to optimize all aspects of perioperative care.[26] ERAS protocols improve surgical outcomes. Head and neck oncology recently joined this community.[27,28] According to the ERAS Society, optimal perioperative pain control for major HNC surgery should include the use of an opioid-sparing, multimodal approach consisting of NSAIDs, acetaminophen, gabapentin, local anesthetics, corticosteroids (when appropriate), and opioids for breakthrough pain. With high-level evidence, these are strong recommendations by the ERAS Society.[28] In addition, preemptive analgesia (ie, administered before any noxious stimuli) has become an important aspect of ERAS protocols and is beneficial before major head and neck surgery.[5,6,29]

A recent retrospective cohort study evaluated MMA in the context of the ERAS protocols for head and neck surgery with free tissue transfer.[6] Traditional analgesia in the control group consisted of acetaminophen, hydrocodone-acetaminophen combination, or IV morphine PRN. Study patients received preoperative oral acetaminophen and gabapentin, as well as intraoperative IV acetaminophen. This was followed by postoperative acetaminophen and gabapentin every 8 hours, celecoxib every 12 hours, and ketorolac every 6 hours as needed (for up to 3 days), and IV fentanyl for breakthrough pain. Patients treated with MMA required a median of 10 morphine equivalent doses (MED) compared with 89.6 in the control group over the first 72 hours. Although there were no differences in ambulation, intensive care unit (ICU) or hospital length of stay, or complications (including bleeding), there was a remarkable reduction is discharge opioids. The MMA group was discharged with a median of 0 MEDs compared with 300 in the control group. Discharge medications otherwise included a 5-day course of celecoxib and gabapentin. Although this study population included a select group of patients (excluding those with ongoing opioid use from outside sources, and patients with renal and hepatic failure), it suggests that patients with HNC can achieve great pain control with MMA, significantly reducing the amount of opioids in both the inpatient and outpatient settings without increasing complications.

In concert with MMA, head and neck surgeons should use opioids for breakthrough pain, providing the lowest possible dose that achieves desired pain control. It is recommended that prescribers use institutionally developed prescribing guidelines, procedure-specific recommendations, and promote a culture of opioid stewardship.[5] A sample MMA pathway, provided by Cramer and colleagues[5] based on ERAS principles is depicted in **Fig. 1**.

PROCEDURE-SPECIFIC RECOMMENDATIONS
Transoral Robotic Surgery

Transoral robotic surgery (TORS) has emerged as an important tool for the treatment of oropharyngeal and supraglottic tumors. Strategies to ensure optimal postoperative pain following TORS is critical, as inadequate analgesia can result in unplanned hospital readmissions and increase the risk of bleeding.[30] Unfortunately, evidence-based analgesia regimens following TORS remain lacking. Multiple studies support the use of perioperative steroids in patients undergoing traditional tonsillectomy to reduce pain.[22] Some institutions including ours, have extrapolated from these data and now routinely prescribe perioperative steroids to patients undergoing TORS.[31] One study investigated the effects of an extended perioperative course of corticosteroids for improving pain control following TORS.[32] All patients in the study received a single intraoperative dose of 10-mg dexamethasone and were then randomized to further receive 8-mg every 8 hours, or a placebo, for up to 4 days after surgery. The steroid group reported a sharper decline of visual analog scale (VAS) pain scores over 1 to 3 postoperative days, decreased length of stay by 1 day, and accelerated ability for consumption of solid food at 1- and 3-week follow-up, with no difference in complications.

Pain control regimens for TORS should otherwise include MMA including acetaminophen and gabapentin as with other HNC surgery. The incorporation of NSAIDs in pain management following TORS remains controversial due to the theoretic increased risk of bleeding. However, an increased risk of bleeding has not been demonstrated following traditional tonsillectomy.[33] In addition, Scott and colleagues describe the use of NSAIDS following TORS[31] without an increase in adverse events.

Preoperative
Pre-operative education and develop postoperative pain plan
Risk screen for warning signs of abuse

Immediate Preoperative
Premedication administered in preoperative holding area
1. Acetaminophen once
2. Celecoxib once
3. Gabapentin once

Intraoperative
Pre-incision infiltration of tissues with long acting local anesthetic
Consider post-closure infiltration with additional long acting local anesthetic or placement of pain pump

Postoperative
1. Acetaminophen scheduled
2. Celecoxib scheduled if no significant cardiovascular disease (or NSAIDs)
3. Consider gabapentin if moderate/severe pain
4. If opioids needed consider starting with tramadol (low risk of abuse)

Discharge
If opioids required on discharge then use institutional guidelines for quantity and duration
Monitor for signs of opioid abuse if prescribed using PDMP
Referral to pain specialist if concern for abuse developing

Fig. 1. Sample multimodal analgesia pathway developed using ERAS principles for head and neck surgery. PDMP, prescription drug monitoring program. (*From* Cramer JD, Wisler B, Gouveia CJ. Opioid Stewardship in Otolaryngology: State of the Art Review. Otolaryngol Head Neck Surg. 2018;158(5):817-827; with permission.)

Free Flap Reconstruction

Major head and neck surgery with free flap reconstruction is complex and generates multiple surgical sites. Several MMA regimens have been described (**Table 2**). NSAIDs are an integral part of MMA for major head and neck surgery, although there is a concern that that celecoxib may increase the risk of microvascular complications.[34] However, preclinical studies have shown that celecoxib has no significant negative effects on free tissue transfer survival or healing in a rat model.[35] Furthermore, a retrospective cohort study of 51 patients undergoing free flap surgery who received 200 mg of celecoxib twice daily for a minimum of 5 days starting on postoperative day 1 showed no increased risk of free flap complications compared with retrospective controls who did not receive celecoxib. However, patients receiving celecoxib required less opioids.[15] Another retrospective cohort study examined 65 patients with HNC undergoing free flap reconstruction and found no increase in the rate of adverse effects in the celecoxib and ketorolac receiving groups, but showed a significant decrease in mean MED in the NSAID group.[6]

Gabapentin has also been used in the preemptive analgesic setting for patients with HNC with free flap reconstruction and, similar to postoperative use, has been shown to reduce postoperative pain and nausea, with subsequent decrease in postoperative analgesic and antiemetic usage.[29] Preemptive and postoperative use of gabapentinoids have been used in several MMA regimens for patients with HNC free flap reconstruction with great efficacy.[6,29] Dosing as high as 2700 mg per day (900 mg 3 times a

Table 2
Opioid-sparing analgesic regimens for patients undergoing head and neck free flap surgery

Author, Year	Study Design	Sample Size, n (Treatment Group)	Analgesic Regimen (Comparison Group Regimen)	Pain Outcomes	Other Outcomes
Carpenter et al,[15] 2018	Retrospective cohort	102 (51)	Postop • Celecoxib 200 mg BID ≥ 5 d • Opioids PRN (Historical control group which did not receive celecoxib)	• Decrease of MME by 14/d.	• No difference in complications (flap failure, hematoma, SSI)
Eggerstedt et al,[6] 2019	Retrospective cohort	65 (28)	Preop • Acetaminophen 975 mg • Gabapentin 900 mg Intraop • Acetaminophen 1000 mg IV Postop • Acetaminophen 950 mg Q 8 h • Gabapentin 300 mg Q 8 h • Celecoxib 200 mg Q 12 h • Ketorolac 15 mg IV Q 6 h PRN ≤ 3 d • Fentanyl ORN (Historical control group which received standard opioid-based regimen)	• Decrease in MED over 72 h (10 vs 89.6) • Decrease in mean pain score by DVPRS (2.05 vs 3.66) • Decrease in discharge MED (0 vs 300)	• No difference in LOS, ICU stay, postop bleeding, return to OR, ED visits, or readmissions
Schleiffarth et al,[14] 2014	Retrospective cohort	138 (2)	Postop • Ketorolac 30 mg IV Q 6 h × 5 d[a] (Control group received either 325 mg aspirin or no NSAID per surgeon preference)	• No difference MED/d (48.9 vs 46.6) over 7 d • Higher mean pain score (3.1 vs 2.4 by VAS)	• No difference in postoperative transfusion, flap failure, or return to OR

(continued on next page)

Table 2
(continued)

Author, Year	Study Design	Sample Size, n (Treatment Group)	Analgesic Regimen (Comparison Group Regimen)	Pain Outcomes	Other Outcomes
Chiu et al,[29] 2012	Nonrandomized open labeled trial	50 (25)	Preop • Gabapentin 1200 mg (Control group received no preemptive analgesia)	• Decrease in pain score (1.2 vs 1.7 by VAS) over first 24 h • Decrease in mean morphine use (3.5 vs 11.4)	• Decreased antiemetic use in first 24 h, (0 vs 12.2 mg metoclopramide), no change in LOS or flap failure
Kainulainen et al,[23] 2017; Kainulainen et al,[37] 2018	Prospected, randomized, double-blind trial	93 (51)	Preop • dexamethasone 10 mg IV Postop • Acetaminophen 1 g × 3 doses • Oxycodone PRN • Dexamethasone 10 mg IV Q 8 h on POD1, Q 12 h on POD2, × 1 dose on POD3 (Control group did not receive preop or postop dexamethasone)	• Decrease in total oxycodone administered (81.2 vs 112.1)	• Increased major complications[b], insulin use and lactate levels in steroid group, no change in PONV, LOS, or ICU stay

Abbreviations: BID, twice a day; DVPRS, defense and veterans pain rating score; ED, emergency department; ICU, intensive care unit; Intraop, intraoperative; IV, intravenous; LOS, length of stay; MED, morphine equivalent dose; MME, morphine milligram equivalents; OR, operating room; ORN, osteoradionecrosis; POD, postoperative day; PONV, postoperative nausea and vomiting; Postop, postoperative; Preop, preoperative; PRN, pro re nata; Q, every; SSI, surgical site infection; VAS, visual analog scale.

[a] 15 mg IV Q 6 h for elderly patients and those appearing frail, not recommended use for more than 3 d.

[b] Major complications included flap loss, venous thrombosis, wound necrosis/fistula, infection, postop bleeding, later tracheostomy, and pneumothorax.

Data from Refs.[6,14,15,23,29,37]

day), with no specific up-titration regimen has been described. Despite this, titration should be considered in patients with lower extremity donor sites to limit potential dizziness and prevent increased risk of falls.

There is less robust evidence to support the routine use of corticosteroids for pain control in patients undergoing head and neck free flap surgery. A retrospective cohort study analyzing the routine use of preoperative dexamethasone for large HNC surgeries with free flap reconstruction found a reduction in inflammatory markers and improved hemodynamic stability with no increase in complications.[36] However, these retrospective findings differ from a prospective, double-blind RCT evaluating perioperative dexamethasone use following HNC surgery with free flaps. In this RCT, although dexamethasone was associated with a small reduction in oxycodone administration (81.2 mg vs 112.14 mg over 5 days), it was also associated with an increased risk of major complications (wound breakdown/necrosis, infection, venous thrombosis, and postoperative bleeding.)[23,37] As such, although corticosteroid use following major head and neck surgery with free tissue transfer can improve pain control, the increase in adverse events argue against routine administration.

Head and neck free flap reconstruction surgery introduces an additional donor site, and thus an additional source of acute postoperative pain to be managed. The use of local anesthetic infusions is an increasingly popular method of donor site analgesia following free tissue transfer. A prospective study of patients undergoing fibula free flap surgery for head and neck defects demonstrated that injecting a bolus of Chirocaine (0.125% wt/vol; 20 mL) through a catheter into the fibular donor site at the end of surgery and 8, 16, and 24 hours postoperatively is associated with improved pain control and reduced opioid requirements.[38] At our institution, we routinely uses a continuous infusion of 0.2% ropivacaine at the fibula and anterolateral thigh free tissue donor sites through the ON-Q SELECT-A-FLOW, **Fig. 2**.

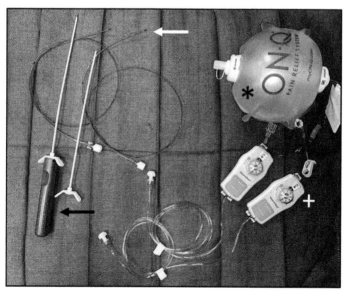

Fig. 2. ON-Q SELECT-A-FLOW system (Halyard Health, Alpharetta, GA) for continuous infusion of 0.2% ropivacaine at donor sites. White arrow = indwelling perforated catheter, black arrow = tunneler and introducer sheath, asterisk = medication containing reservoir, plus = SELECT-A-FLOW adjustment.

SUMMARY AND CLINICAL RECOMMENDATIONS

In conclusion, for the management of acute postoperative pain following major head and neck surgery, we recommend an MMA regimen including preemptive analgesia and postoperative acetaminophen, NSAIDs, gabapentinoids, and locoregional anesthetics as suggested by ERAS. Although the most comprehensive MMA regimens focus on safe and efficacious pain control in patients with HNC undergoing free flaps, we feel that extrapolating these regimens is appropriate for patients who undergo regional, local, or less complex reconstructions as well. **Fig. 1** (from Cramer and colleagues[5]), sets forth an MMA pathway that, based on current evidence, is safe for routine use in patients with HNC, with special considerations as detailed previously. We hope that more procedure-specific MMA regimens arise from ongoing research, particularly for the TORS patient population to address the paucity of reliable and effective opioid-sparing protocols for these patients.

Although opioids will continue to have a role in management of cancer pain, chronic pain, and acute postoperative pain, there is growing literature that provides insight to the prescribing patterns and direction on amount of these rescue analgesics for head and neck procedures.[39] Continued progress in developing optimal combinations, dosages, durations of perioperative analgesia medications, both opioid and nonopioid, is warranted and further exploration of topical, local, and regional anesthesia is still required.

DISCLOSURE

The authors have no financial disclosures.

REFERENCES

1. American Cancer Society. Cancer Facts & Figures 2019. 2019. Available at: https://www.cancer.org/content/dam/cancer-org/research/cancer-facts-and-statistics/annual-cancer-facts-and-figures/2019/cancer-facts-and-figures-2019.pdf. Accessed August 10, 2019.
2. McDermott JD, Eguchi M, Stokes WA, et al. Short- and long-term opioid use in patients with oral and oropharynx cancer. Otolaryngol Head Neck Surg 2019; 160(3):409–19.
3. Macdonald DJ. Anaesthesia for microvascular surgery. A physiological approach. Br J Anaesth 1985;57(9):904–12.
4. Cramer JD, Johnson JT, Nilsen ML. Pain in head and neck cancer survivors: prevalence, predictors, and quality-of-life impact. Otolaryngol Head Neck Surg 2018; 159(5):853–8.
5. Cramer JD, Wisler B, Gouveia CJ. Opioid stewardship in otolaryngology: state of the art review. Otolaryngol Head Neck Surg 2018;158(5):817–27.
6. Eggerstedt M, Stenson KM, Ramirez EA, et al. Association of perioperative opioid-sparing multimodal analgesia with narcotic use and pain control after head and neck free flap reconstruction. JAMA Facial Plast Surg 2019;21(5): 446–51.
7. Du E, Farzal Z, Stephenson E, et al. Multimodal analgesia protocol after head and neck surgery: effect on opioid use and pain control. Otolaryngol Head Neck Surg 2019;161(3):424–30.
8. Saraswathula A, Chen MM, Mudumbai SC, et al. Persistent postoperative opioid use in older head and neck cancer patients. Otolaryngol Head Neck Surg 2019; 160(3):380–7.

9. Memtsoudis SG, Poeran J, Kehlet H. Enhanced recovery after surgery in the United States: from evidence-based practice to uncertain science? JAMA 2019;321(11):1049–50.

10. Smith E, Lange J, Moore C, et al. The role of intravenous acetaminophen in postoperative pain control in head and neck cancer patients. Laryngoscope Investig Otolaryngol 2019;4(2):250–4.

11. Kawakita D, Matsuo K. Alcohol and head and neck cancer. Cancer Metastasis Rev 2017;36(3):425–34.

12. Oltman J, Militsakh O, D'Agostino M, et al. Multimodal analgesia in outpatient head and neck surgery: a feasibility and safety study. JAMA Otolaryngol Head Neck Surg 2017;143(12):1207–12.

13. Leese PT, Hubbard RC, Karim A, et al. Effects of celecoxib, a novel cyclooxygenase-2 inhibitor, on platelet function in healthy adults: a randomized, controlled trial. J Clin Pharmacol 2000;40(2):124–32.

14. Schleiffarth JR, Bayon R, Chang KE, et al. Ketorolac after free tissue transfer: a comparative effectiveness study. Ann Otol Rhinol Laryngol 2014;123(6):446–9.

15. Carpenter PS, Shepherd HM, McCrary H, et al. Association of celecoxib use with decreased opioid requirements after head and neck cancer surgery with free tissue reconstruction. JAMA Otolaryngol Head Neck Surg 2018;144(11):988–94.

16. Gilron I. Review article: the role of anticonvulsant drugs in postoperative pain management: a bench-to-bedside perspective. Can J Anaesth 2006;53(6):562–71.

17. Townsend M, Liou T, Kallogjeri D, et al. Effect of perioperative gabapentin use on postsurgical pain in patients undergoing head and neck mucosal surgery: a randomized clinical trial. JAMA Otolaryngol Head Neck Surg 2018;144(11):959–66.

18. Bar Ad V, Weinstein G, Dutta PR, et al. Gabapentin for the treatment of pain related to radiation-induced mucositis in patients with head and neck tumors treated with intensity-modulated radiation therapy. Head Neck 2010;32(2):173–7.

19. Jordan RI, Mulvey MR, Bennett MI. A critical appraisal of gabapentinoids for pain in cancer patients. Curr Opin Support Palliat Care 2018;12(2):108–17.

20. Jiang J, Li Y, Shen Q, et al. Effect of pregabalin on radiotherapy-related neuropathic pain in patients with head and neck cancer: a randomized controlled trial. J Clin Oncol 2019;37(2):135–43.

21. Liebana-Hermoso S, Manzano-Moreno FJ, Vallecillo-Capilla MF, et al. Oral pregabalin for acute pain relief after cervicofacial surgery: a systematic review. Clin Oral Investig 2018;22(1):119–29.

22. Tolska HK, Hamunen K, Takala A, et al. Systematic review of analgesics and dexamethasone for post-tonsillectomy pain in adults. Br J Anaesth 2019;123(2):e397–411.

23. Kainulainen S, Tornwall J, Koivusalo AM, et al. Dexamethasone in head and neck cancer patients with microvascular reconstruction: No benefit, more complications. Oral Oncol 2017;65:45–50.

24. Plantevin F, Pascal J, Morel J, et al. Effect of mandibular nerve block on postoperative analgesia in patients undergoing oropharyngeal carcinoma surgery under general anaesthesia. Br J Anaesth 2007;99(5):708–12.

25. Charous S. Use of the ON-Q pain pump management system in the head and neck: preliminary report. Otolaryngol Head Neck Surg 2008;138(1):110–2.

26. Ljungqvist O, Young-Fadok T, Demartines N. The history of enhanced recovery after surgery and the ERAS society. J Laparoendosc Adv Surg Tech A 2017;27(9):860–2.

27. Huber GF, Dort JC. Reducing morbidity and complications after major head and neck cancer surgery: the (future) role of enhanced recovery after surgery protocols. Curr Opin Otolaryngol Head Neck Surg 2018;26(2):71–7.

28. Dort JC, Farwell DG, Findlay M, et al. Optimal perioperative care in major head and neck cancer surgery with free flap reconstruction: a consensus review and recommendations from the enhanced recovery after surgery society. JAMA Otolaryngol Head Neck Surg 2017;143(3):292–303.

29. Chiu TW, Leung CC, Lau EY, et al. Analgesic effects of preoperative gabapentin after tongue reconstruction with the anterolateral thigh flap. Hong Kong Med J 2012;18(1):30–4.

30. Hay A, Migliacci J, Karassawa Zanoni D, et al. Haemorrhage following transoral robotic surgery. Clin Otolaryngol 2018;43(2):638–44.

31. Scott SI, Madsen AKO, Rubek N, et al. Time course of subacute pain after transoral robotic surgery (TORS) for oropharyngeal squamous cell carcinoma versus traditional bilateral tonsillectomy in adults - a case-control study. Acta Otolaryngol 2018;138(9):837–42.

32. Clayburgh D, Stott W, Bolognone R, et al. A randomized controlled trial of corticosteroids for pain after transoral robotic surgery. Laryngoscope 2017;127(11):2558–64.

33. Nikanne E, Kokki H, Salo J, et al. Celecoxib and ketoprofen for pain management during tonsillectomy: a placebo-controlled clinical trial. Otolaryngol Head Neck Surg 2005;132(2):287–94.

34. Al-Sukhun J, Koivusalo A, Tornwall J, et al. COX-2 inhibitors and early failure of free vascular flaps. N Engl J Med 2006;355(5):528–9.

35. Wax MK, Reh DD, Levack MM. Effect of celecoxib on fasciocutaneous flap survival and revascularization. Arch Facial Plast Surg 2007;9(2):120–4.

36. Imai T, Kurosawa K, Yamaguchi K, et al. Enhanced recovery after surgery program with dexamethasone administration for major head and neck surgery with free tissue transfer reconstruction: initial institutional experience. Acta Otolaryngol 2018;138(7):664–9.

37. Kainulainen S, Lassus P, Suominen AL, et al. More harm than benefit of perioperative dexamethasone on recovery following reconstructive head and neck cancer surgery: a prospective double-blind randomized trial. J Oral Maxillofac Surg 2018;76(11):2425–32.

38. Ferri A, Varazzani A, Valente A, et al. Perioperative pain management after fibular free flap harvesting for head-and-neck reconstruction using mini-catheters to inject local anesthetic: A pilot study. Microsurgery 2018;38(3):295–9.

39. Pang J, Tringale KR, Tapia VJ, et al. Opioid prescribing practices in patients undergoing surgery for oral cavity cancer. Laryngoscope 2018;128(10):2361–6.

Assessment and Management of Postoperative Pain Associated with Sleep Apnea Surgery

Jonathan A. Waxman, MD, PhD*, Kerolos G. Shenouda, MD, Ho-Sheng Lin, MD

KEYWORDS

- OSA • Surgery • Postoperative • Pain • Opioids

KEY POINTS

- Given the risks of opioid use by patients with obstructive sleep apnea (OSA), special attention to opioid risk reduction and avoidance is warranted.
- There is a growing body of evidence that supports the safe and effective use of nonopioids and nonpharmacologic management of postoperative pain following OSA surgery.
- Strategies for managing postoperative pain should include the use of local anesthetic infiltration, nonsteroidal antiinflammatory drugs, acetaminophen, topical analgesics, surgical wound cooling, and when necessary, safer opioid medications, such as tramadol and intranasal butorphanol.

INTRODUCTION

Obstructive sleep apnea (OSA) is a highly prevalent disorder in which individuals experience periodic repetitive episodes of complete or partial obstruction of the upper airway during sleep. In the United States, OSA affects at least 10% of men and 3% of women older than 30 years.[1] OSA is associated with cardiovascular disease, stroke, diabetes, and cognitive dysfunction, contributing to decreased work productivity and quality of life, as well as increased risk of workplace disability and car accidents.[2–4] Consequently, OSA results in a socioeconomic cost comparable to that of smoking.[5]

The gold-standard treatment of OSA is continuous positive airway pressure (CPAP), which attempts to maintain airway patency by blowing a stream of air through the nose or mouth. Although effective, CPAP is difficult to tolerate for many, resulting in poor

Department of Otolaryngology, Head and Neck Surgery, Wayne State University, 4201 St. Antoine, 5E-UHC, Detroit, MI 48201, USA
* Corresponding author.
E-mail address: jwaxman@med.wayne.edu

Otolaryngol Clin N Am 53 (2020) 765–777
https://doi.org/10.1016/j.otc.2020.05.006
0030-6665/20/© 2020 Elsevier Inc. All rights reserved.

long-term adherence.[6] For patients who fail CPAP, surgery may be offered. OSA surgery aims to restore airway patency by removing or displacing obstructing tissue at one or more levels along the upper airway or by increasing the size of the airway via reconstructive techniques. The recognition that obstruction may occur at more than one anatomic level led to multilevel surgical approaches in which multiple surgical procedures are performed at the nasal, soft-palate, oropharyngeal, and/or hypopharyngeal levels.[7]

Surgery for OSA can be extremely painful postoperatively. In a study of adult patients with OSA who underwent nasal, pharyngeal, or combination surgery, the most common adverse outcome was emergency room visit for pain-related diagnoses.[8] Postoperative pain may also be a significant reason why patients avoid surgery.[9] When OSA surgery is performed, postoperative pain is commonly treated with opioids analgesics. In a recent survey of prescribing patterns among otolaryngologists, tonsillectomy and uvulopalatopharyngoplasty (UPPP) had the highest average number of tablets of pain medication prescribed of all surgical procedures assessed.[10] Given the present epidemic of opioid addiction in the US, opioid stewardship is a particularly important issue for otolaryngologists who perform sleep surgery.[11] In addition, the use of opioids by OSA patients deserves special attention, as OSA may be a risk factor for opioid-induced respiratory depression.[12] Moreover, OSA patients may experience increased postoperative pain intensity and decreased pain tolerance.[13] The mechanisms that underlie these associations are poorly understood, and the effect of OSA surgery on pain sensing has not been well studied.

The aim of this work is to review and synthesize the literature encompassing the assessment and management of postoperative pain in adults following OSA surgery, with an emphasis on opioid risk-reduction and avoidance.

ASSESSMENT OF POSTOPERATIVE PAIN
Uvulopalatopharyngoplasty, Modifications, and Variations

UPPP, the most common surgical procedure for OSA, was first reported as a surgical correction of anatomic abnormalities in OSA by Fujita and colleagues[14] in 1981. Although high success rates were initially reported, subsequent studies demonstrated poor outcomes for UPPP in isolation when used to treat OSA in all but a select group of patients.[15] Consequently, variations of UPPP, as well as palatopharyngeal reconstructive procedures, have been introduced.

Early variations to conventional UPPP include coblation- and laser-assisted uvulopalatoplasty (LAUP), which may be staged procedures, and may take place in an outpatient setting. In studies evaluating LAUP, postoperative pain visual analogue scale (VAS) scores were in the moderate to severe range.[16–23] Pain associated with LAUP may be significantly less than traditional UPPP[17,19,22,23] but worse compared with coblation and radiofrequency (RF) palate surgery.[16,18,22,23] LAUP may also require a shorter duration of pain medication use than UPPP but a longer duration compared with RF palate surgery. In these studies, patients received a nonsteroidal antiinflammatory drug (NSAID) and/or acetaminophen, and/or narcotic pain medications, and/or corticosteroids for pain control.

In a study that described a modified UPPP using a microdebrider, postoperative VAS pain scores were in the low to moderate range, much less than those associated with traditional UPPP.[24] Patients received acetaminophen with codeine.

Several palatal reconstructive procedures have been proposed for lateral pharyngeal wall collapse. Lateral pharyngoplasty was the first such procedure. Postoperative pain after LP is reported as moderate and not significantly different than UPPP.[25–27] In studies, pain medications used for LP include NSAIDs, tramadol patient-controlled analgesia (PCA), and pethidine.

Expansion sphincter pharyngoplasty (ESP) was introduced to address lateral pharyngeal wall collapse while minimizing the relatively high rates of dysphagia reported after lateral pharyngoplasty. A randomized controlled trial (RCT) that compared ESP with UPPP using NSAIDs for pain relief showed no significant difference in the use of analgesics postoperatively.[28] A recent prospective study evaluating a modified ESP technique in patients who received acetaminophen, NSAIDs, tramadol, and steroids reported significant postoperative pain in more than half of patients.[29]

In a prospective study evaluating soft palatal webbing flap palatopharyngoplasty, a procedure designed to simultaneously address both lateral pharyngeal wall and soft palatal collapse, patients who received acetaminophen for pain control reported moderate VAS pain scores in the first week that subsided by the end of the second week after surgery.[30]

Anterior palatoplasty (AP) was introduced as a modification to a palatal stiffening procedure using electrocautery designed to create a palatal scar and fibrosis, resulting in an increase in the anteroposterior distance of the velopharynx.[31] Postoperative VAS pain scores for AP are in the moderate to high range with or without tonsillectomy.[27,31–36] With NSAIDs and possibly narcotic pain medication, pain reportedly resolves by 2 weeks following surgery. One study comparing AP with LP found no significant difference in postoperative pain when patients received tramadol PCA and pethidine.[27] A retrospective study that looked at combined AP and ESP reported pain medication use that lasted about 5 days on average.[37]

The uvulopalatal flap (UPF) technique is a reversible technique that was designed to achieve the same anatomic results of the UPPP while reducing the risks of velopharyngeal insufficiency.[38] UPF results in moderate postoperative pain.[17,34–36,39] Compared with UPPP, UPF results in less intense pain of shorter duration among patients who received an NSAID.[17] Three RCTs that compared UPF with AP found that UPF resulted in significantly more postoperative pain.[34–36] Patients received acetaminophen in 2 of the studies and IV tramadol and acetaminophen in the third.

Z-palatoplasty (ZPP) is a modified UPPP designed to create a scar contracture that ensures widening of the anteroposterior and lateral oropharynx at the level of the palate, particularly in individuals without tonsils. Compared with UPPP, ZPP results in a significantly shorter duration of pain medication use among patients taking acetaminophen with codeine.[40]

Other palatal reconstructive techniques have been devised to reposition or displace the palatopharyngeus muscle in a more lateral and anterior position to enlarge the retropalatal space, including relocation pharyngoplasty (RP),[41] barbed reposition pharyngoplasty (BRP),[42] barbed palatoplasty (BP),[37] the velo-uvulo-pharyngeal lift,[43] barbed Roman blinds technique,[44] and the Alianza technique.[45] Studies describing these techniques report postoperative pain in the moderate range that decreased to mild by postoperative day 7. In a retrospective study comparing BP with combined AP and ESP, patients who underwent BP used pain medications for a significantly shorter duration than for combined AP and ESP.

Radiofrequency/Coblation Tongue Base Reduction

The tongue base is a common site of obstruction in patients with OSA. Traditional midline glossectomy and open procedures are rarely, if ever, performed due to significant morbidity. Alternatively, minimally invasive techniques were developed to address tongue base obstruction, including submucosal minimally invasive lingual excision (SMILE), RF tongue base reduction (RFTBR), and robot-assisted tongue base resection procedures.

Postoperative pain VAS scores for RFTBR range from mild to moderate, and durations of pain medication use range from 2 to 4 days.[46–51] Reported pain regimens include NSAIDs only, NSAIDs and steroids, and narcotics and NSAIDs. One study that compared RFTBR with SMILE reported no significant difference in postoperative pain.[51] Another study found that RFTBR resulted in significantly less postoperative pain than SMILE.[50]

In a study examining postoperative outcomes of multilevel surgery involving RFTBR, patients also underwent nasal surgery when appropriate, palatal stiffening implants, and partial uvulectomy.[52] The number of postoperative days that narcotic pain medication was used ranged from 0 to 4. Another study that involved RFTBR as well as RF ablation of the inferior turbinates, soft palate, genioglossus, and tonsils demonstrated very low overall postoperative VAS scores.[53]

Hyoid Suspension

Hyoid suspension and its variants involve repositioning the hyoid bone using fascia, sutures, or wires to expand the retrolingual airway. With the use of an NSAID, postoperative pain following hyoid surgery is low to moderate and decreases to mild by postoperative day 5 to 7.[54–56]

Transoral Robotic Surgery

Transoral robotic surgery (TORS) for OSA was introduced to provide a minimally invasive technique with better access, exposure, and visualization of oropharyngeal and supraglottic structures. Studies that evaluated TORS in combination with ESP report low postoperative pain that is not significantly different than TORS plus UPPP or TORS plus BRP.[57,58] Another study retrospectively compared TORS with ZPP with RFTBR with ZPP and SMILE with ZPP.[59] Postoperative day 1 pain was in the severe range for all 3 procedures.

Hypoglossal Nerve Stimulation

Direct stimulation of the hypoglossal nerve to protrude the tongue and expand the pharyngeal airway during sleep is a relatively new and promising surgical approach to the treatment of OSA. Because the procedure involves only small incisions over the neck and chest with minimal dissection, low postoperative pain is expected. In several studies, mild pain was reported in 14% to 26% of patients, whereas moderate to severe pain was reported in 2% to 4% of patients.[60–62] A recent systematic review of hypoglossal nerve stimulation (HNS) for OSA found that only 6.2% of patients reported postoperative pain.[63]

NONOPIOID TREATMENT OF POSTOPERATIVE PAIN
Vitamin C

One RCT demonstrated improved pain scores and reduced opioid analgesic utilization after preoperative vitamin C. It is unclear if this effect lasted more than 24 hours postoperatively.[64]

Local Anesthetics

Local infiltration with anesthetic agents has significant potential for decreasing immediate postoperative pain and can potentially decrease overall narcotic use. One prospective analysis found that bupivacaine infiltration resulted in significant improvement in postoperative pain during swallow and at rest. Similarly, lidocaine infiltration was found to be superior to placebo.[65] Another RCT demonstrated the advantageous effects of ropivacaine infiltration at rest and during swallowing, including decreased morphine PCA consumption.[66]

Local glossopharyngeal nerve blocks, however, do not seem to confer similar benefits.[63] A novel technique for continuous lesser palatine nerve local anesthesia infiltration using a tunneled catheter after UPPP provided some benefit but is challenging to perform and complications are unclear.[67]

Corticosteroids

Corticosteroids are known for their antiinflammatory and antiemetic effects. One prospective study tested the analgesic effects of unilateral local wound infiltration with triamcinolone in UPPP patients and found lower VAS scores on the test side.[68] One the other hand, systemic corticosteroids have not proved as efficacious in UPPP patients.[69]

Sucralfate

Sucralfate has been used for decades in the treatment of peptic ulcer disease. It is thought to provide a protective coating by binding exposed protein of damaged cells. It also promotes local production of prostaglandin E2, which increases blood flow, mucous production, and surface migration of cells and accelerates healing. Two RCTs found that sucralfate improved postoperative pain outcomes, decreased analgesic requirement, accelerated mucosal healing, and resulted in early return to regular daily activities.[70,71]

Dexmedetomidine

Dexmedetomidine is an alpha-2-adrenergic agonist with sedative and analgesic properties. Its use for intraoperative anesthesia during upper airway surgery for OSA has been shown to be safe, with a stable hemodynamic profile; however, its opioid-sparing properties have not been shown to decrease narcotic use intraoperatively.[72] Conversely, postoperative infusion of dexmedetomidine is associated with improved VAS scores, decreased morphine utilization, longer time to first analgesic request, and less side effects in UPPP patients.[73] Moreover, use of dexmedetomidine may result in significantly lower incidence of oxyhemoglobin desaturation and bradypnea.

Nonsteroidal Antiinflammatory Drugs

NSAIDs are effective analgesics because of their ability to inhibit inflammatory prostaglandins via inhibition of the cyclooxygenase-2 (COX2) enzyme. However, their use in upper airway surgery has traditionally been guarded due to a presumed increased risk of postoperative hemorrhage.

Ketoprofen is a phenylpropionic acid-derivative NSAID that has been in clinical use since 1973. It seems to take effect rapidly and is believed to decrease the respiratory depressive effects of opioids. It is also less likely to disturb hemostatic function compared with several other NSAIDs. Its use with UPPP has been examined in several studies. One study found ketoprofen to provide sufficient analgesia in 90% of patients after UPPP for up to 2 weeks postoperatively.[74] However, this effect was not long-lasting, as its half-life is only 2 hours. An increased risk of postoperative bleeding has not been found.[75] An RCT that examined the effects of ketorolac versus ketoprofen after UPPP found that ketorolac resulted in lower VAS pain scores and less opioid use than ketoprofen without a difference in the rate of complications.[76] No increased risk of postoperative hemorrhage was found with ketorolac. Similar findings were confirmed when ketorolac was compared with mefenamic acid.[77]

Parecoxib and celecoxib belong to a subclass of NSAIDs that selectively bind and inhibit COX2. Celecoxib in combination with pregabalin was shown to decrease VAS pain scores and postoperative opioid consumption when given preemptively 1 hour preoperatively before maxillomandibular advancement with or without concomitant genioglossus advancement.[78] Another study examined the role of parecoxib after UPPP in patients with OSA and found significantly improved VAS pain scores at rest and during swallowing, without an increase in adverse reactions.[79]

Lastly, the use of diclofenac after UPPP was associated with less rescue analgesic consumption and significantly lower VAS pain scores compared with placebo.[80] There was no increase in side effect profile or bleeding time associated with diclofenac.

OPIOID TREATMENT OF POSTOPERATIVE PAIN
Intranasal Butorphanol

Butorphanol, a synthetic opioid agonist-antagonist, is a potent narcotic. Its analgesic potency is 15 to 23 times greater than that of meperidine. It does not appear to cause dose-related respiratory depression and seldom causes physical dependence. Intranasal (IN) butorphanol is easy to administer, especially in patients experiencing severe oral pain, and is rapidly absorbed.

Several studies have examined the impact of IN butorphanol on postoperative pain in UPPP. In a study that compared IN butorphanol, IV butorphanol, and IN fentanyl, those treated with IN butorphanol experienced less nausea and vomiting, less postoperative pain, and less postoperative cognitive dysfunction.[81] Another RCT found that IN butorphanol was equivalent to mefenamic acid and intramuscular meperidine in terms of postoperative pain control and pain-associated morbidities.[82] Finally, a prospective cohort study examined the use of IN butorphanol, ibuprofen, and magic mouthwash in patients who underwent LAUP and nasal turbinate coblation.[83] The intervention was found to cause a 50% reduction in pain within an average of 48 minutes, with 30% of patients requiring no additional interventions.

Fentanyl

In one study that examined the use of fentanyl to treat OSA surgery postoperative pain, patients who underwent either UPPP or tonsillectomy received loading and continuous doses of ketoprofen in addition to fentanyl PCA.[84] There were no reported adverse side effects that warranted drug discontinuation. In addition, there were no reported episodes of increased respiratory depression or significant sedation.

Hydrocodone and Oxycodone

There is a paucity of research examining the use of oxycodone and hydrocodone in OSA surgery patients. One retrospective analysis comparing narcotic use alone versus use in addition to ketorolac or gabapentin reported no differences in pain-related phone or clinic encounters or in complication rates.

NONPHARMACOLOGIC TREATMENT OF POSTOPERATIVE PAIN
Autologous Platelet-Rich Fibrin

Platelet-rich fibrin (PRF) is an immune and platelet concentrate in a single-fibrin membrane, which is believed to contain up to 60 different biologically active substances. Topical application of PRF theoretically mimics and supports physiologic wound healing. Its use has been studied in numerous clinical settings.[85] In a study of patients undergoing RP who received PRF, there was a significant reduction in VAS pain scores, time required to return to a normal diet, and rate of wound dehiscence.[86]

Cooling Techniques

Cooling is one of the oldest methods of pain control. Immediate cooling of thermal injuries reduces pain, decreases injury to tissues, and promotes quicker healing. In an RCT evaluating surgical wound cooling after UPPP and tonsillectomy, 5 minutes of cooling was associated with a significant reduction in the average daily and overall pain VAS scores.

DISCUSSION

OSA is a highly prevalent disorder with significant comorbidities that often requires painful surgical treatment in individuals who are unable to tolerate treatment with CPAP. Postoperative pain has traditionally been managed with opioid pain medications. However, there is a growing body of evidence that supports a detrimental impact of opioids on patients with OSA. In particular, people with OSA are at increased risk of opioid-induced respiratory depression or central apnea and may have increased pain sensitivity and decreased pain tolerance. Therefore, the issue of postoperative pain management is a particularly important aspect of safe and quality care for patients with OSA. In 2014, the American Society of Anesthesiologists published a set of evidence-based practice guidelines for perioperative management of patients with OSA that offers some guidance on general postoperative pain management for patients with OSA.[87] Among their recommendations, the investigators advocate for the reduction or elimination of opioid medications via the use of regional analgesic techniques, NSAIDs, and other modalities, such as ice or transcutaneous electrical nerve stimulation. However, there is presently no widespread consensus specifically regarding the management of pain after OSA surgery.

A review of the literature revealed widely varying postoperative pain levels depending on the type of surgery. In general, procedures that are limited to mucosa and do not include tonsillectomy produce less postoperative pain. A diversity of pain medications and pain management approaches used to treat postoperative pain after OSA surgery was also observed. Because of significant heterogeneity and incomplete reporting, it is difficult to systematically compare postoperative pain and pain relief across studies. Moreover, it is unclear whether reports of pain reflect analgesic suppressed pain levels or pain that subsequently required analgesia. Nonetheless, numerous studies of a variety of types of OSA surgery report that postoperative pain scores for patients who received narcotic pain medications are similar to postoperative pain scores of patients who used nonnarcotic medications. This suggests that postoperative pain for many patients might be effectively managed with nonopioids, even for the most painful surgeries, such as UPPP and tongue base resection.

Numerous studies have assessed postoperative pain outcomes using nonopioid medications, including NSAIDs (ibuprofen, diclofenac, naproxen, and celecoxib), acetaminophen, and corticosteroids and collectively suggest a minimal detrimental impact on postoperative complications.[17–19,25,30,31,34,35,49,51,54,56,88] In several studies, patients were given tramadol in addition to other nonopioid medications.[27,29,36]

Evidence for nonopioid postoperative pain control is provided by numerous studies that demonstrate improved postoperative pain and decreased opioid use with NSAIDs, including ketorolac,[76,77] diclofenac,[80] and COX2 inhibitors.[78,79] The use of NSAIDs does not seem to significantly increase the risk of postoperative bleeding.

Several other analgesic adjuncts with opioid-sparing properties, including sucralfate, pregabalin, and dexmedetomidine, may also provide significant pain relief. High-level evidence supports the use of topical sucralfate to reduce analgesic requirements following UPPP and LAUP.[70,71] One RCT showed that a one-time preoperative oral dose of pregabalin and celecoxib before maxillomandibular advancement surgery decreased postoperative pain and reduced postoperative narcotic used.[78] Another study reported that dexmedetomidine resulted in lower postoperative pain and decreased opioid consumption.[73] It also significantly lowered the incidence of oxyhemoglobin desaturation and bradypnea, a particularly important finding given the increased risk of opioid-induced respiratory depression in patients with OSA. In addition, novel nonpharmacologic approaches have shown promising results, such as topical PRF[86] and IV vitamin C[64]; however, further study is required.

Several studies support the use of intraoperative local infiltration of bupivacaine or ropivacaine to help alleviate postoperative pain and reduce opioid use after OSA surgery.[65,66] Local wound infiltration with triamcinolone acetonide may also help to reduce surgical pain.[68] In addition, one RCT showed that simple intraoperative ice pack administration results in significantly reduced pain following UPPP.[89]

Because patients with a history of OSA may experience pain more intensely and have a lower pain tolerance than the general population, the use of opioid pain medications may be necessary for some individuals. Butorphanol, a potent narcotic that does not seem to cause dose-related respiratory depression and seldom causes physical dependence has gained interest in the management of postoperative pain for patients with OSA. Several studies have demonstrated equivalent or better pain control after OSA surgery compared with other narcotic pain medications.[81–83]

This review demonstrates the existence of a body of evidence that supports the use of nonopioid analgesics and nonpharmacologic approaches to the management of postoperative pain following surgery for OSA. The risks of opioids for people with OSA are significant, and in light of the growing epidemic of opioid misuse and abuse, special attention to opioid risk-reduction and avoidance is warranted in this population.

SUMMARY

Strategies for managing postoperative pain should emphasize the use of multimodal analgesic therapy, including long-acting local anesthetic infiltration, NSAIDs, acetaminophen, topical analgesics, and surgical wound cooling. In cases where necessary, opioid medications may be used; however, safer medications such as tramadol and IN butorphanol should be considered.

DISCLOSURE

The authors report no financial or other relationships that may lead to a conflict of interest.

REFERENCES

1. Peppard PE, Young T, Barnet JH, et al. Increased prevalence of sleep-disordered breathing in adults. Am J Epidemiol 2013. https://doi.org/10.1093/aje/kws342.
2. Levy P, Tamisier R, Arnaud C, et al. Sleep deprivation, sleep apnea and cardiovascular diseases. Front Biosci (Elite Ed) 2012;4:2007–21.
3. Moyer CA, Sonnad SS, Garetz SL, et al. Quality of life in obstructive sleep apnea: a systematic review of the literature. Sleep Med 2001;2(6):477–91.
4. Garbarino S, Guglielmi O, Sanna A, et al. Risk of occupational accidents in workers with obstructive sleep apnea: systematic review and meta-analysis. Sleep 2016;39(6):1211–8.

5. Phillipson EA. Sleep apnea–a major public health problem. N Engl J Med 1993; 328(17):1271–3.
6. Rotenberg BW, Murariu D, Pang KP. Trends in CPAP adherence over twenty years of data collection: a flattened curve. J Otolaryngol Head Neck Surg 2016; 45(1):43.
7. Lin H-C, Friedman M, Chang H-W, et al. The efficacy of multilevel surgery of the upper airway in adults with obstructive sleep apnea/hypopnea syndrome. Laryngoscope 2008;118(5):902–8.
8. Baugh R, Burke B, Fink B, et al. Safety of outpatient surgery for obstructive sleep apnea. Otolaryngol Head Neck Surg 2013;148(5):867–72.
9. Gasparini G, Torroni A, Di Nardo F, et al. OSAS surgery and postoperative discomfort: phase I surgery versus phase II surgery. Biomed Res Int 2015; 2015:439847.
10. Murphey AW, Munawar S, Nguyen SA, et al. Opioid prescribing patterns within otolaryngology. World J Otorhinolaryngol Head Neck Surg 2019;5(2):112–6.
11. Cramer JD, Wisler B, Gouveia CJ. Opioid Stewardship in Otolaryngology: State of the Art Review. Otolaryngol Head Neck Surg 2018;158(5):817–27.
12. Cozowicz C, Chung F, Doufas AG, et al. Opioids for acute pain management in patients with obstructive sleep apnea: a systematic review. Anesth Analg 2018; 127(4):988–1001.
13. Charokopos A, Card ME, Gunderson C, et al. The association of obstructive sleep apnea and pain outcomes in adults: a systematic review. Pain Med 2018; 19(suppl_1):S69–75.
14. Fujita S, Conway W, Zorick F, et al. Surgical correction of anatomic abnormalities in obstructive sleep apnea syndrome: uvulopalatopharyngoplasty. Otolaryngol Head Neck Surg 1981;89(6):923–34.
15. Friedman M, Ibrahim H, Bass L. Clinical staging for sleep-disordered breathing. Otolaryngol Head Neck Surg 2002;127(1):13–21.
16. Belloso A, Morar P, Tahery J, et al. Randomized-controlled study comparing postoperative pain between coblation palatoplasty and laser palatoplasty. Clin Otolaryngol 2006;31(2):138–43.
17. Cekin E, Cincik H, Ulubil SA, et al. Comparison of uvulopalatopharyngoplasty and uvulopalatal flap in Turkish military personnel with primary snoring. Mil Med 2009; 174(4):432–6.
18. Lim DJ, Kang SH, Kim BH, et al. Treatment of primary snoring using radiofrequency-assisted uvulopalatoplasty. Eur Arch Otorhinolaryngol 2007; 264(7):761–7.
19. Osman EZ, Osborne JE, Hill PD, et al. Uvulopalatopharyngoplasty versus laser assisted uvulopalatoplasty for the treatment of snoring: an objective randomised clinical trial. Clin Otolaryngol Allied Sci 2000;25(4):305–10.
20. Pavelec V, Polenik P. Use of Er,Cr:YSGG versus standard lasers in laser assisted uvulopalatoplasty for treatment of snoring. Laryngoscope 2006;116(8):1512–6.
21. Terris DJ, Coker JF, Thomas AJ, et al. Preliminary findings from a prospective, randomized trial of two palatal operations for sleep-disordered breathing. Otolaryngol Head Neck Surg 2002;127(4):315–23.
22. Rombaux P, Hamoir M, Bertrand B, et al. Postoperative pain and side effects after uvulopalatopharyngoplasty, laser-assisted uvulopalatoplasty, and radiofrequency tissue volume reduction in primary snoring. Laryngoscope 2003;113(12): 2169–73.
23. Troell RJ, Powell NB, Riley RW, et al. Comparison of postoperative pain between laser-assisted uvulopalatoplasty, uvulopalatopharyngoplasty, and radiofrequency

volumetric tissue reduction of the palate. Otolaryngol Head Neck Surg 2000; 122(3):402–9.

24. Huang T-W, Cheng P-W. Microdebrider-assisted extended uvulopalatoplasty: an effective and safe technique for selected patients with obstructive sleep apnea syndrome. Arch Otolaryngol Head Neck Surg 2008;134(2):141–5.

25. Cahali MB. Lateral pharyngoplasty: a new treatment for obstructive sleep apnea hypopnea syndrome. Laryngoscope 2003;113(11):1961–8.

26. Cahali MB, Formigoni GGS, Gebrim EMMS, et al. Lateral pharyngoplasty versus uvulopalatopharyngoplasty: a clinical, polysomnographic and computed tomography measurement comparison. Sleep 2004;27(5):942–50.

27. Akcam T, Arslan HH, Deniz S, et al. Comparison of early postoperative pain among surgical techniques for obstructive sleep apnea. Eur Arch Otorhinolaryngol 2012;269(11):2433–40.

28. Pang KP, Woodson BT. Expansion sphincter pharyngoplasty: a new technique for the treatment of obstructive sleep apnea. Otolaryngol Head Neck Surg 2007; 137(1):110–4.

29. Despeghel A-S, Mus L, Dick C, et al. Long-term results of a modified expansion sphincter pharyngoplasty for sleep-disordered breathing. Eur Arch Otorhinolaryngol 2017;274(3):1665–70.

30. Elbassiouny AMME. Modified barbed soft palatal posterior pillar webbing flap palatopharyngoplasty. Sleep Breath 2016;20(2):829–36.

31. Pang KP, Terris DJ. Modified cautery-assisted palatal stiffening operation: new method for treating snoring and mild obstructive sleep apnea. Otolaryngol Head Neck Surg 2007;136(5):823–6.

32. Ugur KS, Ark N, Kurtaran H, et al. Anterior palatoplasty for selected mild and moderate obstructive sleep apnea: preliminary results. Eur Arch Otorhinolaryngol 2014;271(6):1777–83.

33. Adzreil B, Wong EHC, Saraiza AB, et al. The effectiveness of combined tonsillectomy and anterior palatoplasty in the treatment of snoring and obstructive sleep apnoea (OSA). Eur Arch Otorhinolaryngol 2017;274(4):2005–11.

34. Marzetti A, Tedaldi M, Passali FM. Preliminary findings from our experience in anterior palatoplasty for the treatment of obstructive sleep apnea. Clin Exp Otorhinolaryngol 2013;6(1):18–22.

35. Haytoğlu S, Arikan OK, Muluk NB, et al. Comparison of anterior palatoplasty and uvulopalatal flap placement for treating mild and moderate obstructive sleep apnea. Ear Nose Throat J 2018;97(3):69–78.

36. Yüksel E, Mutlu M, Bayır Ö, et al. Comparison of postoperative pain scores and dysphagia between anterior palatoplasty and uvulopalatal flap surgeries. Acta Otolaryngol 2018;138(12):1092–8.

37. Babademez MA, Gul F, Teleke YC. Barbed palatoplasty vs. expansion sphincter pharyngoplasty with anterior palatoplasty. Laryngoscope 2019. https://doi.org/10.1002/lary.28136.

38. Powell N, Riley R, Guilleminault C, et al. A reversible uvulopalatal flap for snoring and sleep apnea syndrome. Sleep 1996;19(7):593–9.

39. Neruntarat C. Uvulopalatal flap for obstructive sleep apnea: short-term and long-term results. Laryngoscope 2011;121(3):683–7.

40. Friedman M, Ibrahim HZ, Vidyasagar R, et al. Z-palatoplasty (ZPP): a technique for patients without tonsils. Otolaryngol Head Neck Surg 2004;131(1):89–100.

41. Li H-Y, Lee L-A. Relocation pharyngoplasty for obstructive sleep apnea. Laryngoscope 2009;119(12):2472–7.

42. Vicini C, Hendawy E, Campanini A, et al. Barbed reposition pharyngoplasty (BRP) for OSAHS: a feasibility, safety, efficacy and teachability pilot study. "We are on the giant's shoulders. Eur Arch Otorhinolaryngol 2015;272(10):3065–70.

43. Mantovani M, Minetti A, Torretta S, et al. The velo-uvulo-pharyngeal lift or "roman blinds" technique for treatment of snoring: a preliminary report. Acta Otorhinolaryngol Ital 2012;32(1):48–53.

44. Mantovani M, Rinaldi V, Torretta S, et al. Barbed Roman blinds technique for the treatment of obstructive sleep apnea: how we do it? Eur Arch Otorhinolaryngol 2016;273(2):517–23.

45. Mantovani M, Carioli D, Torretta S, et al. Barbed snore surgery for concentric collapse at the velum: The Alianza technique. J Craniomaxillofac Surg 2017; 45(11):1794–800.

46. Powell NB, Riley RW, Guilleminault C. Radiofrequency tongue base reduction in sleep-disordered breathing: A pilot study. Otolaryngol Head Neck Surg 1999; 120(5):656–64.

47. Woodson BT, Nelson L, Mickelson S, et al. A multi-institutional study of radiofrequency volumetric tissue reduction for OSAS. Otolaryngol Head Neck Surg 2001; 125(4):303–11.

48. Stuck BA, Maurer JT, Verse T, et al. Tongue base reduction with temperature-controlled radiofrequency volumetric tissue reduction for treatment of obstructive sleep apnea syndrome. Acta Otolaryngol 2002;122(5):531–6.

49. Stuck BA, Starzak K, Hein G, et al. Combined radiofrequency surgery of the tongue base and soft palate in obstructive sleep apnoea. Acta Otolaryngol 2004;124(7):827–32.

50. Friedman M, Soans R, Gurpinar B, et al. Evaluation of submucosal minimally invasive lingual excision technique for treatment of obstructive sleep apnea/hypopnea syndrome. Otolaryngol Head Neck Surg 2008;139(3):378–84 [discussion: 385].

51. Babademez MA, Yorubulut M, Yurekli MF, et al. Comparison of minimally invasive techniques in tongue base surgery in patients with obstructive sleep apnea. Otolaryngol Head Neck Surg 2011;145(5):858–64.

52. Friedman M, Lin H-C, Gurpinar B, et al. Minimally invasive single-stage multilevel treatment for obstructive sleep apnea/hypopnea syndrome. Laryngoscope 2007; 117(10):1859–63.

53. De Vito A, Frassineti S, Panatta ML, et al. Multilevel radiofrequency ablation for snoring and OSAHS patients therapy: long-term outcomes. Eur Arch Otorhinolaryngol 2012;269(1):321–30.

54. Stuck BA, Neff W, Hörmann K, et al. Anatomic changes after hyoid suspension for obstructive sleep apnea: an MRI study. Otolaryngol Head Neck Surg 2005; 133(3):397–402.

55. Richard W, Timmer F, van Tinteren H, et al. Complications of hyoid suspension in the treatment of obstructive sleep apnea syndrome. Eur Arch Otorhinolaryngol 2011;268(4):631–5.

56. Hamans E, Stuck BA, de Vries N, et al. Hyoid expansion as a treatment for obstructive sleep apnea: a pilot study. Sleep Breath 2013;17(1):195–201.

57. Vicini C, Montevecchi F, Campanini A, et al. Clinical outcomes and complications associated with TORS for OSAHS: a benchmark for evaluating an emerging surgical technology in a targeted application for benign disease. ORL J Otorhinolaryngol Relat Spec 2014;76(2):63–9.

58. Cammaroto G, Montevecchi F, D'Agostino G, et al. Palatal surgery in a transoral robotic setting (TORS): preliminary results of a retrospective comparison between

uvulopalatopharyngoplasty (UPPP), expansion sphincter pharyngoplasty (ESP) and barbed repositioning pharyngoplasty (BRP). Acta Otorhinolaryngol Ital 2017;37(5):406–9.

59. Friedman M, Hamilton C, Samuelson CG, et al. Transoral robotic glossectomy for the treatment of obstructive sleep apnea-hypopnea syndrome. Otolaryngol Head Neck Surg 2012;146(5):854–62.

60. Eastwood PR, Barnes M, Walsh JH, et al. Treating obstructive sleep apnea with hypoglossal nerve stimulation. Sleep 2011;34(11):1479–86.

61. Strollo PJ, Soose RJ, Maurer JT, et al. Upper-airway stimulation for obstructive sleep apnea. N Engl J Med 2014;370(2):139–49.

62. Friedman M, Jacobowitz O, Hwang MS, et al. Targeted hypoglossal nerve stimulation for the treatment of obstructive sleep apnea: Six-month results. Laryngoscope 2016;126(11):2618–23.

63. Kompelli AR, Ni JS, Nguyen SA, et al. The outcomes of hypoglossal nerve stimulation in the management of OSA: A systematic review and meta-analysis. World J Otorhinolaryngol Head Neck Surg 2019;5(1):41–8.

64. Ayatollahi V, Dehghanpour Farashah S, Behdad S, et al. Effect of intravenous vitamin C on postoperative pain in uvulopalatopharyngoplasty with tonsillectomy. Clin Otolaryngol 2017;42(1):139–43.

65. Haytoğlu S, Arikan OK, Muluk NB, et al. Relief of pain at rest and during swallowing after modified cautery-assisted uvulopalatopharyngoplasty: bupivacaine versus lidocaine. J Craniofac Surg 2015;26(3):e216–23.

66. Li L, Feng J, Xie S, et al. Preemptive submucosal infiltration with ropivacaine for uvulopalatopharyngoplasty. Otolaryngol Head Neck Surg 2014;151(5):874–9.

67. Ponstein NA, Kim T-WE, Hsia J, et al. Continuous lesser palatine nerve block for postoperative analgesia after uvulopalatopharyngoplasty. Clin J Pain 2013; 29(12):e35–8.

68. Hirunwiwatkul P. Pain-relieving effect of local steroid injection in uvulopalatopharyngoplasty. J Med Assoc Thai 2001;84(Suppl 1):S384–90.

69. Williams PM, Strome M, Eliachar I, et al. Impact of steroids on recovery after uvulopalatopharyngoplasty. Laryngoscope 1999;109(12):1941–6.

70. Zodpe P, Cho JG, Kang HJ, et al. Efficacy of sucralfate in the postoperative management of uvulopalatopharyngoplasty: a double-blind, randomized, controlled study. Arch Otolaryngol Head Neck Surg 2006;132(10):1082–5.

71. Kyrmizakis DE, Papadakis CE, Bizakis JG, et al. Sucralfate alleviating post-laser-assisted uvulopalatoplasty pain. Am J Otolaryngol 2001;22(1):55–8.

72. Chawla S, Robinson S, Norton A, et al. Peri-operative use of dexmedetomidine in airway reconstruction surgery for obstructive sleep apnoea. J Laryngol Otol 2010; 124(1):67–72.

73. Abdelmageed WM, Elquesny KM, Shabana RI, et al. Analgesic properties of a dexmedetomidine infusion after uvulopalatopharyngoplasty in patients with obstructive sleep apnea. Saudi J Anaesth 2011;5(2):150–6.

74. Nikanne E, Virtaniemi J, Aho M, et al. Ketoprofen for postoperative pain after uvulopalatopharyngoplasty and tonsillectomy: two-week follow-up study. Otolaryngol Head Neck Surg 2003;129(5):577–81.

75. McClain K, Williams AM, Yaremchuk K. Ketorolac usage in tonsillectomy and uvulopalatopharyngoplasty patients. Laryngoscope 2019. https://doi.org/10.1002/lary.28077.

76. Patrocínio LG, Rangel M de O, Marques Miziara GS, et al. A comparative study between ketorolac and ketoprofen in postoperative pain after uvulopalatopharyngoplasty. Braz J Otorhinolaryngol 2007;73(3):339–42.

77. Lee L-A, Wang P-C, Chen N-H, et al. Alleviation of wound pain after surgeries for obstructive sleep apnea. Laryngoscope 2007;117(9):1689–94.
78. Cillo JE, Dattilo DJ. Pre-emptive analgesia with pregabalin and celecoxib decreases postsurgical pain following maxillomandibular advancement surgery: a randomized controlled clinical trial. J Oral Maxillofac Surg 2014;72(10):1909–14.
79. Xie G-L, Chu Q-J, Liu C-L. Application of parecoxib in post-uvulopalatopharyngoplasty analgesia. J Int Med Res 2013;41(5):1699–704.
80. Ejnell H, Björkman R, Wåhlander L, et al. Treatment of postoperative pain with diclofenac in uvulopalatopharyngoplasty. Br J Anaesth 1992;68(1):76–80.
81. Yang L, Sun D, Wu Y, et al. Intranasal administration of butorphanol benefits old patients undergoing H-uvulopalatopharyngoplasty: a randomized trial. BMC Anesthesiol 2015;15:20.
82. Huang H-C, Lee L-A, Fang T-J, et al. Transnasal butorphanol for pain relief after uvulopalatopharyngoplasty - a hospital-based,randomized study. Chang Gung Med J 2009;32(4):390–9.
83. Madani M. Effectiveness of Stadol NS (butorphanol tartrate) with ibuprofen in the treatment of pain after laser-assisted uvulopalatopharyngoplasty. J Oral Maxillofac Surg 2000;58(10 Suppl 2):27–31.
84. Virtaniemi J, Kokki H, Nikanne E, et al. Ketoprofen and fentanyl for pain after uvulopalatopharyngoplasty and tonsillectomy. Laryngoscope 1999;109(12):1950–4.
85. Miron RJ, Zucchelli G, Pikos MA, et al. Use of platelet-rich fibrin in regenerative dentistry: a systematic review. Clin Oral Investig 2017;21(6):1913–27.
86. Elkahwagi M, Elokda M, Elghannam D, et al. Role of autologous platelet-rich fibrin in relocation pharyngoplasty for obstructive sleep apnoea. Int J Oral Maxillofac Surg 2019. https://doi.org/10.1016/j.ijom.2019.05.008.
87. American Society of Anesthesiologists Task Force on Perioperative Management of patients with obstructive sleep apnea. Practice guidelines for the perioperative management of patients with obstructive sleep apnea: an updated report by the American Society of Anesthesiologists Task Force on Perioperative Management of patients with obstructive sleep apnea. Anesthesiology 2014;120(2):268–86.
88. Verse T, Pirsig W, Stuck BA, et al. Recent developments in the treatment of obstructive sleep apnea. Am J Respir Med 2003;2(2):157–68.
89. Rotenberg BW, Wickens B, Parnes J. Intraoperative ice pack application for uvulopalatoplasty pain reduction: a randomized controlled trial. Laryngoscope 2013; 123(2):533–6.

Perioperative Analgesia for Thyroid and Parathyroid Surgery: A Review of Current Practices

Vaninder K. Dhillon, MD[a],*, Babak Jahan-Parwar, MD[b],
David S. Cohen, MD[c]

KEYWORDS

- General anesthesia • Local anesthesia • Nerve block • Thyroid surgery
- Parathyroid surgery • Pain control • NSAIDS • ERAS

KEY POINTS

- Perioperative analgesia for endocrine surgery of the head and neck includes general anesthesia, local anesthesia, oral, and multimodality techniques for pain control.
- General anesthesia should avoid long-acting paralytics because of intraoperative recurrent laryngeal nerve monitoring.
- Consider the use of perioperative steroids to reduce postoperative pain in the immediate postoperative period.
- Recognize that local anesthesia includes cervical nerve blocks for patients undergoing surgery.
- Multimodal analgesia, including expedited recovery after surgery algorithms, is key for optimal pain control.

INTRODUCTION

Endocrine surgery of the head and neck includes removal of the thyroid and parathyroid glands with or without central or lateral neck dissection. Paradigm shifts, including increased same-day surgical discharges and heightened scrutiny of hospital bed utilization and associated cost, have influenced perioperative management of patients. Furthermore, the current epidemic surrounding opioid overuse and abuse has focused research and institutional efforts on minimizing opioid use. These factors have led to

[a] Department of Otolaryngology, Johns Hopkins University, 6420 Rockledge Drive, Suite 4920, Bethesda, MD 20817, USA; [b] Department of Head and Neck Surgery, Southern California Permanente Medical Group, 1101 Baldwin Park Boulevard, Baldwin Park, CA 91706, USA; [c] Department of Head and Neck Surgery, Southern California Permanente Medical Group, 25825 South Vermont Avenue, 3rd Floor Parkview Building, Harbor City, CA 90710, USA
* Corresponding author.
E-mail address: vdhillo2@jhmi.edu

Otolaryngol Clin N Am 53 (2020) 779–787
https://doi.org/10.1016/j.otc.2020.05.007
0030-6665/20/© 2020 Elsevier Inc. All rights reserved.

the development of multimodality algorithms aimed at optimizing pain control for outpatient surgery.

This article discusses perioperative analgesia for thyroid and parathyroid surgery during preoperative, intraoperative, and postoperative periods. Multimodality approaches, including expedited recovery after surgery (ERAS), will be addressed. The authors review current evidence regarding pain management and consider best practices regarding analgesia for head and neck endocrine surgical patients.

PERIOPERATIVE AND MULTIMODAL ANALGESIA

Multimodal analgesia (MMA) combines local anesthesia with preoperative, perioperative, and/or postoperative administration of N-acetyl-p-amino-phenol (APAP) derivatives (such as acetaminophen), nonsteroidal antiinflammatory drugs (NSAIDs), ketamine, and/or gamma-amino-butyric-acid (GABA) analogues. A synergistic or cumulative effect may exist with MMA, providing superior analgesia compared with single modality therapy.

The concept of preemptive analgesia to prevent central sensitization, thereby improving postoperative pain management, is demonstrated in multiple studies. This has led to adoption of MMA for pain management, including nonopiate alternatives.[1] Militsakh and colleagues[2] studied an MMA regimen in thyroid and parathyroid surgery patients of preoperative acetaminophen, NSAIDS, and gabapentin, coupled with postoperative acetaminophen and ibuprofen, which demonstrated decreased opioid use without change in bleeding complications. In addition, celecoxib has been heralded as an NSAID that does not increase bleeding risk, due to selective COX-2 inhibition. Although it has been shown to decrease total opioid use when given preoperatively as a single dose in other head and neck surgeries,[3] its specific effect regarding endocrine surgery has not been identified.

The role of perioperative administration of corticosteroids in reducing postoperative pain or temporary recurrent laryngeal nerve palsy is controversial. Early studies demonstrated improvement in voice outcomes with perioperative steroid use.[4] Additional studies have conflicting findings, with some studies demonstrating no change in pain or voice[5] and other studies suggesting improvement in pain control with perioperative steroid use.[6]

INTRAOPERATIVE TECHNIQUES AND AGENTS
General Anesthesia

Thyroid and parathyroid surgery is traditionally completed under general anesthesia for airway security, as well as concern for potential hematoma postoperatively that may complicate emergent intubation.[7,8] Despite this, cases under local anesthesia alone have been reported in resource-limited locations and are feasible.[9] Induction of general anesthesia is completed with multiple anesthetic agents, but typical techniques use an opioid (eg, fentanyl) administered before a sedative-hypnotic agent (eg, propofol) to achieve optimal synergistic effect.[10] Intravenous induction causes less nausea/vomiting than inhalational agents and is thus preferred.[10] Furthermore, dexmedetomidine (Precedex) has been shown to reduce postoperative nausea in patients undergoing general anesthesia and can decrease intraoperative and postoperative pain in patients undergoing nasal surgery.[11] The effects of dexmedetomidine in thyroid and parathyroid surgical patients need further investigation.

Laryngeal Anesthesia

Laryngeal anesthesia is an important concern due to trauma associated with intubation and endotracheal tube presence. The use of intraoperative nerve monitoring has become more prevalent during thyroid or parathyroid surgery,[12] and because monitoring technology requires electromyography, long-term neuromuscular blockade must be avoided. A short-acting neuromuscular blocking agent may be used for induction, but the effect must not persist past this period to allow for accurate nerve monitoring. The placement of endotracheal tube must also be precise to ensure electrodes are contacting each vocal fold. Topical anesthesia to the larynx may prevent laryngospasm associated with endotracheal tube presence.

Postoperative sore throat (POST) secondary to intubation is a known risk to endocrine surgery. Recently, studies have examined the effect of tracheal topical anesthesia on immediate postoperative pain. Use of a smaller-diameter endotracheal tube has been associated with decreased POST between size 7.0 versus 6.0 tubes (51.1% vs 27.1%).[13] Kim and colleagues randomized benzydamine hydrochloride (BH), 10% lidocaine, and normal saline spray on endotracheal tube cuffs in total thyroidectomy patients to evaluate POST. In 87 patients, BH spray reduced the incidence and severity of POST at 12 hours compared with other groups.[14] In addition, the use of nasogastric tubes intraoperatively has strong association with POST (adjusted odds ratio = 0.41, 95% confidence interval: 0.174, 0.965; P = .041).[15]

Local Anesthesia

Cervical nerve blocks and local anesthesia to the incision are effective in managing perioperative pain for thyroid and parathyroid surgery. The injection of lidocaine, bupivacaine, or ropivicaine into the skin before incision is effective in postoperative pain control, decreasing pain scores, and improving overall patient satisfaction.[16] Biery and Pellitteri[17] found that MMA including preincision local wound infiltration with bupivacaine and outpatient ibuprofen/acetaminophen provided sufficient pain control after thyroidectomy and parathyroidectomy in more than 98% of patients.

In addition to subdermal injection at the operative site, bilateral superficial cervical plexus block (BSCPB) seems to improve postoperative pain control.[18] BSCPBs are local anesthetic blocks to the emerging branches of the superficial cervical plexus (lesser occipital, greater auricular, transverse cervical, and supraclavicular nerves). Complication rates with this technique are low with little risk to deeper structures. A recent meta-analysis demonstrated BSCPB offers greater analgesic efficacy after thyroid surgery, with reduction in subjective pain score and longer time to first postoperative dose of narcotic medication compared with narcotics alone.[19] Also, it seems that preoperative block is more efficacious than postoperative.[19]

Pharmacologic treatments

Opioids (oxycodone, hydrocodone, morphine, tramadol) Opioids have long been the mainstay of postoperative analgesia regimens for head and neck endocrine procedures; however, recognition of their addictive potential in combination with monetary and societal cost of addiction has driven a trend toward minimization or elimination of opioid use. The most common opioid prescribed depends on center-specific preferences and includes oxycodone, oxycodone/acetaminophen, hydrocodone/acetaminophen, and tramadol.

Lou and colleagues[20] found 93% of patients undergoing thyroidectomy or parathyroidectomy required 20 or fewer oral morphine equivalents at first postoperative visit. Furthermore, Tharakan and colleagues[21] found 80% of thyroidectomy and parathyroidectomy patients required 15 or less oral morphine equivalents with half of patients not requiring opioid use at all. Similarly, Sada and colleagues[22] found more than half of parathyroidectomy patients did not require opioids postoperatively whatsoever.

Tramadol is a different opioid with dual mechanisms of action. The reduced u-opioid receptor activation as well as the serotonin and norepinephrine reuptake inhibition may create a favorable profile for pain control.[23] Tramadol has been reported to have lower abuse potential than traditional opioids.[24] Multiple studies have found age less than 45 years, maximum pain score postoperatively, and preoperative opioid use were independent predictors of postoperative opioid use.[20–25]

Nonsteroidal antiinflammatory drugs NSAIDS are also considered mainstay in pain management; however, due to concern for bleeding complications, widespread adoption for perioperative use has been slow in surgeries of the head and neck. In a prospective randomized control trial, Nguyen and colleagues[26] concluded that ibuprofen provided equally effective pain control compared with hydrocodone/acetaminophen in outpatient otolaryngology procedures, including thyroidectomy and parathyroidectomy, with decreased opioid requirement. In a comparison of lornoxicam and low-dose tramadol for postthyroidectomy analgesia, Yücel and colleagues[27] found pain scores were lower in the first hour and time to postoperative analgesic use was longer with lornoxicam compared with low-dose tramadol, with higher rates of nausea and vomiting in the tramadol group. Recent studies have also demonstrated reduced opioid consumption associated with single preoperative dose of intravenous (IV) ibuprofen.[28] Despite this, consensus has not been reached.

The intraoperative use of ketorolac (Torodol) for surgery has been widely implemented, but the adoption in head and neck surgeries has been delayed due to concern for increased bleeding risk. Some studies have demonstrated similar analgesic effect when combined with fentanyl and ondansetron compared with opioid alone, as well as lower rates of postoperative nausea, vomiting, and dizziness.[29] Postoperative bleeding after thyroidectomy has been associated with NSAID use postoperatively,[30] although its clinical significance has been debated.[31] Despite their utility, NSAIDS have side effects and must be used with caution in patients with renal insufficiency, gastric ulcers, or history of gastric bypass surgery.

N-acetyl-p-amino-phenol (paracetamol, acetaminophen) IV and oral administration of APAP derivatives have been used for postoperative analgesia after thyroid and parathyroid surgery for years. IV paracetamol was shown to reduce postoperative pain scores, opioid requirement, and incidence of nausea and vomiting, while prolonging time to first analgesic after thyroidectomy.[32] Hong and colleagues[33] found IV paracetamol reduced postoperative pain and rescue analgesic demand after robotic transaxillary thyroidectomy. A Kaiser Permanente study found in 469 thyroid and parathyroid surgeries that postoperative analgesic regimen of oral acetaminophen alone was sufficient to prevent opioid use after discharge in more than 90% of cases (David S. Cohen, 2019, unpublished data).

Gamma-amino-butyric-acid analogs (gabapentin, pregabalin) Gabapentinoids have been postulated to desensitize patients to painful stimuli, thereby reducing the need for other analgesic medication. Hema and colleagues[34] found oral gabapentin was effective as a preventative analgesic in reducing postoperative pain scores, total tramadol consumption, and prolonged time to rescue analgesic after thyroidectomy. Sanders and Dawes[35] demonstrated gabapentin seems to have a beneficial effect on perioperative pain relief and analgesic consumption in head and neck surgeries, including thyroidectomy. Lee and colleagues[36] showed that preoperative oral gabapentin reduced the intensity and incidence of sore throat after thyroid surgery. Despite this, other studies have suggested that groups receiving a preoperative dose of gabapentin may actually have an increased opioid or APAP consumption.[37] For this reason, additional studies specific to thyroid and parathyroid surgery are needed.

Ketamine

Ketamine has been studied as local wound irrigation and IV infusion for analgesia in many surgeries, including parathyroid and thyroid surgery.[38] According to Abd El-Rahman and colleagues,[39] local wound instillation of ketamine reduced pain scores, total morphine consumption, and time to first analgesic. Kim and colleagues[40] found IV infusion of ketamine intraoperatively reduced postoperative pain associated with axillary approach for thyroidectomy. Similarly, Lee and colleagues[41] noted reduced pain scores compared with placebo after IV ketamine infusion following robotic thyroidectomy.

DISCUSSION

The authors theorize that postoperative pain after thyroid and parathyroid surgery is derived primarily from 3 sources: (1) sore throat from laryngeal or tracheal trauma during intubation or intraoperatively from endotracheal or nasogastric tube presence, (2) posterior neck discomfort from cervical positioning in extended position typical for head and neck endocrine surgeries, and (3) anterior neck pain from the skin incision itself or trauma from dissection, retraction, or muscle division. Studies examining efficacy of postoperative pain regimens do not distinguish between these sources of postoperative pain. Distinguishing the source of discomfort may help improve

Table 1
Summary of analgesia types used for thyroid or parathyroid surgery

Intraoperative anesthesia	
General	IV induction with propofol and IV opioids
NMDA selective antagonists	IV ketamine
NSAIDS	IV ketorolac
Topical laryngeal	Lidocaine, benzydamine hydrochloride
Local injectable	Lidocaine with epinephrine, bupivacaine, or ropivacaine injection, superior cervical nerve block (SCPB)
Pharmacologic treatment	
APAP derivatives	Acetaminophen, paracetamol
Opiates	Oxycodone/acetaminophen, hydrocodone/acetaminophen, morphine, and tramadol
NSAIDs	Celecoxib (COX 2), lornoxicam/meloxicam (COX2 >COX1) ibuprofen, naproxen (COX2 + COX1)
N-acetyl-p-amino-phenol	Paracetamol, acetaminophen
Gamma-amino-butyric-acid analogues	Gabapentin, pregabalin
Multimodal analgesia (MMA)	APAP, NSAIDs, GABA analogues, topical laryngeal anesthesia, and local anesthesia including SCPB

postoperative pain management. For this reason, additional research with specific attention to the cause of pain may help elucidate a more optimal algorithm.

Methods used to decrease laryngeal or oropharyngeal trauma associated with intubation are key to minimizing POST. These practices should include small-sized endotracheal tubes and eliminating routine use of nasogastric tubes or esophageal temperature probes if possible. Avoiding such equipment or practice may reduce postoperative sore throat and warrants additional research.

Neck extension is helpful for exposure to the mediastinum or substernal area for dissection. Care must be taken to support the neck in patients with limited cervical mobility or cervical degenerative joint disease to avoid postoperative pain from traction. Alternative therapies such as cervical kinesio taping[42] and electroacupuncture[43] have shown promising results in reducing postoperative pain and analgesic use after thyroidectomy. Randomized controlled trials are necessary to confirm such findings.

Table 1 is a summary of perioperative analgesia for thyroid and parathyroid surgical patients discussed in this article. In determining the best way to treat postoperative pain, it may be important to identify the source of pain in order to better adopt analgesic or pain management to target that type of pain.

SUMMARY

Undoubtedly, there has been a transition to nonopiate pain control in thyroid and parathyroid surgery. Patients who undergo surgery have been safely discharged the same day, alleviating hospital costs and bed utilization.[44–46] With this trend, there has been increased attention to MMA, including ERAS incorporating NSAIDs, GABA analogues, and local anesthesia techniques such as BSCPB. One major hurdle to broad implementation has been concern for side effects, specifically postoperative bleeding complications such as neck hematoma. Although evidence for clinically significant risk is lacking, additional research is required to determine if an optimal multimodality regime can be discovered without an increase in surgical complications. Postoperative pain after thyroid and parathyroid surgery is derived primarily from 3 sources: (1) sore throat from laryngeal or tracheal trauma during intubation or intraoperatively from endotracheal or nasogastric tube presence, (2) posterior neck discomfort from cervical positioning in extended position typical for head and neck endocrine surgeries, and (3) anterior neck pain from the skin incision itself or trauma from dissection, retraction, or muscle division. Further studies examining efficacy of postoperative pain regimens should distinguish between these sources of postoperative pain.

DISCLOSURE

The authors have nothing to disclose.

REFERENCES

1. Grape S, Trimer MR. Do we need preemptive analgesia for the treatment of postoperative pain? Best Pract Res Clin Anaesthesiol 2007;21(1):51–63.

2. Militsakh O, Lydiatt W, Lydiatt D, et al. Development of multimodal analgesia pathways in outpatient thyroid and parathyroid surgery and association with postoperative opioid prescription patterns. JAMA Otolaryngol Head Neck Surg 2018; 144(11):1023–9.

3. Carpenter PS, Shepherd HM, McCrary H, et al. Association of celecoxib use with decreased opioid requirements after head and neck cancer surgery with free tissue reconstruction. JAMA Otolaryngol Head Neck Surg 2018;144(11):988–94.
4. Schietroma M, Cecilia E, Carlei F, et al. Dexamethasone for the prevention of recurrent laryngeal nerve palsy and other complications after thyroid surgery. JAMA Otolaryngol Head Neck Surg 2013;139(5):471–8.
5. Noel JE, Kligerman MP, Megwalu UC, et al. Intraoperative corticosteroids for voice outcomes among patients undergoing thyroidectomy: a systematic review and meta-analysis. Otolaryngol Head Neck Surg 2018;159(5):811–6.
6. Ahmad R, Changeez M, Tameez Ud Din A, et al. Role of Prophylactic Dexamethasone Before Thyroidectomy in Reducing Postoperative Pain, Nausea and Vomiting. Cureus 2019;11(5):e4735.
7. Bacuzzi A, Dionigi G, Del Bosco A, et al. Anaesthesia for thyroid surgery: perioperative management. Int J Surg 2008;6(Suppl 1):S82–5.
8. Bajwa SJ, Sehgal V. Anesthesia and thyroid surgery: the never ending challenges. Indian J Endocrinol Metab 2013;17:228–34.
9. Latifi R, Harper J, Rivera R. Total thyroidectomy for giant goiter under local anesthesia and Ketamine in a surgical mission. Int J Surg Case Rep 2015;8C:52–4.
10. Whitwam JG. Co-inducation of anaesthsia: day-case surgery. Eur J Anaesthesiol Suppl 1995;12:25–34.
11. Hwang SH, Lee HS, Joo YH, et al. Efficacy of dexmedetomidine on perioperative morbidity during nasal surgery: a meta-analysis. Laryngoscope 2018;128(3): 573–80.
12. Randolph G, Dralle H, Abdullah H, et al. Electrophysiologic recurrent laryngeal nerve monitoring during thyroid and parathyroid surgery: international standards guideline statement. Laryngoscope 2010;121(Suppl 1):S1–16.
13. Jaensson M, Olowsson LL, Nilsson U. Endotracheal tube size and sore throat following surgery: a randomized-controlled study. Acta Anaesthesiol Scand 2010;54(2):147–53.
14. Kim D, Jeong H, Kwon J, et al. The effect of benzydamine hydrochloride on preventing postoperative sore throat after total thyroidectomy: a randomized-controlled trial. Can J Anaesth 2019;66(8):934–42.
15. Biruk MG, Endale GG, Tadesse BM. Risk factors for postoperative throat pain after general anaesthesia with endotracheal intubation at the University of Gondar Teaching Hospital, Northwest Ethiopia, 2014. Pan Afr Med J 2017;27:127.
16. Hadri B, Emini L, Krasniqi I. Post thyroidectomy wound infiltration for postoperative pain relief. Eur J Anaesthesiol 2014;(31):229.
17. Biery J, Pellitteri PK. Effectiveness of nonopioid/non-narcotic postoperative pain management regimen for patients undergoing thyroidectomy and/or parathyroidectomy. J Am Coll Surg 2018;227(4, Supplement 2):e17.
18. Woolf CJ, Chong MS. Preemptive analgesia treating postoperative pain by preventing the establishment of central sensitization. Anesth Analg 1993;77:362e79.
19. Mayhew D, Sahgal N, Khirwadkar R, et al. Analgesic efficacy of bilateral superficial cervical plexus block for thyroid surgery: meta-analysis and systematic review. Br J Anaesth 2018;120(2):241e251.
20. Lou I, Chennell TB, Schaefer SC, et al. Optimizing outpatient pain management after thyroid and parathyroid surgery: a two-institution experience. Ann Surg Oncol 2017;24(7):1951–7.
21. Tharakan T, Jiang S, Fastenberg J, et al. Postoperative pain control and opioid usage patterns among patients undergoing thyroidectomy and parathyroidectomy volume. Otolaryngol Head Neck Surg 2019;160(3):394–401.

22. Sada A, Ubl DS, Thiels CA, et al. Optimizing Opioid-Prescribing Practices After Parathyroidectomy. J Surg Res 2020;(245):107 e11.

23. Uhlmann RA, Henry A, Reinhart MD, et al. A review of postoperative pain management for thyroid and parathyroid surgery. J Surg Res 2019;241:107–11.

24. Babalonis S, Lofwall MR, Nuzzo PA, et al. Liability and reinforcing efficacy of oral tramadol in humans. Drug Alcohol Depend 2013;129(1–2):116–24.

25. Long SM, Lumley CJ, Zeymo A, et al. Prescription and usage pattern of opioids after thyroid and parathyroid surgery. Otolaryngol Head Neck Surg 2019;160(3):388–93.

26. Nguyen KK, Liu YF, Chang C, et al. A randomized single-blinded trial of ibuprofen- versus opioid-based primary analgesic therapy in outpatient otolaryngology surgery. Otolaryngol head neck Surg 2019;160(5):839–46.

27. Yücel A, Yazıcı A, Müderris T, et al. Comparison of lornoxicam and low-dose tramadol for management of post-thyroidectomy pain. Agri 2016;28(4):183–9.

28. Mutlu V, Ince I. Preemptive intravenous ibuprofen application reduces pain and opioid consumption following thyroid surgery. Am J Otolaryngol 2019;40(1):70–3.

29. Kim SY, Kim EM, Nam KH, et al. Postoperative intravenous patient-controlled analgesia in thyroid surgery: comparison of fentanyl and ondansetron regimens with and without the nonsteriodal anti-inflammatory drug ketorolac. Thyroid 2008;18(12):1285–90.

30. Lee M, Rhee J, Kim Y 2, et al. Perioperative risk factors for post-thyroidectomy hematoma: Significance of pain and ketorolac usage. Head Neck 2019;41(10):3656–60.

31. Chin CJ, Franklin JH, Turner B, et al. Ketorolac in thyroid surgery: quantifying the risk of hematoma. J Otolaryngol Head Neck Surg 2011;40(3):196–9.

32. Arslan M, Çiçek R, Celep B, et al. Comparison of the analgesic effects of intravenous paracetamol and lornoxicam in postoperative pain following thyroidectomies. Agri 2011;23(4):160–6.

33. Hong JY, Kim WO, Chung WY, et al. Paracetamol reduces postoperative pain and rescue analgesic demand after robot-assisted endoscopic thyroidectomy by the transaxillary approach. World J Surg 2010;34(3):521–6.

34. Hema VR, Ramadas KT, Biji KP, et al. A prospective, observational study to evaluate the role of gabapentin as preventive analgesic in thyroidectomy under general anesthesia. Anesth Essays Res 2017;11(3):718–23.

35. Sanders JG, Dawes PJ. Gabapentin for perioperative analgesia in otorhinolaryngology-head and neck surgery: systematic review. Otolaryngol Head Neck Surg 2016;155(6):893–903.

36. Lee JH, Lee HK, Chun NH, et al. The prophylactic effects of gabapentin on postoperative sore throat after thyroid surgery. Korean J Anesthesiol 2013;64(2):138–42.

37. Sanders JG, Cameron C, Dawes PJD. Gabapentin in the management of pain following tonsillectomy: a randomized double-blind placebo-controlled trial. Otolaryngol Head Neck Surg 2017;157(5):781–90.

38. Brinck EC, Tiippana E, Heesen M, et al. Perioperative intravenous ketamine for acute postoperative pain in adults. Cochrane Database Syst Rev 2018;(12):CD012033.

39. Abd El-Rahman AM, El Sherif FA. Efficacy of postoperative analgesia of local ketamine wound instillation following total thyroidectomy: a randomized, double-blind, controlled clinical trial. Clin J Pain 2018;34(1):53–8.

40. Kim DH, Choi J, Kim B-G, et al. Prospective, randomized, and controlled trial on ketamine infusion during bilateral axillo-breast approach (BABA) robotic or

endoscopic thyroidectomy: Effects on postoperative pain and recovery profiles. Medicine 2016;95:e5485.

41. Lee J, Park H-P, Jeong M-H, et al. Efficacy of ketamine for postoperative pain following robotic thyroidectomy: a prospective randomised study. J Int Med Res 2018;46(3):1109–20.

42. Genç A, Çelik SU, Genç V, et al. The effects of cervical kinesiotaping on neck pain, range of motion, and disability in patients following thyroidectomy: a randomized, double-blind, sham-controlled clinical trialTurk. J Med Sci 2019;49(4): 1185–91.

43. Zhang C, Zhou M, Li M. Clinical study of electroacupuncture on perioperative analgesia in patients with thyroid surgery under cervical plexus block. Zhongguo Zhen Jiu 2018;38(12):1261–5 [in Chinese].

44. Mowschenson PM, Hodin RA. Outpatient thyroid and parathyroid surgery: a prospective study of feasibility, safety, and costs. Surgery 1995;118(6):1051–3 [discussion: 1053–4].

45. Terris DJ, Snyder S, Carneiro-Pla D, et al. American Thyroid Association statement on outpatient thyroidectomy. Thyroid 2013;23(10):1193–202.

46. Orosco RK. Ambulatory thyroidectomy: a multistate study of revisits and complications. Otolaryngol Head Neck Surg 2015;31:1017–23.

Perioperative Analgesia for Sinus and Skull-Base Surgery

Brandon K. Nguyen, MD[a], Peter F. Svider, MD[b], Wayne D. Hsueh, MD[a],
Adam J. Folbe, MD[c,d],*

KEYWORDS

- Perioperative analgesia • Pain • Sinus surgery • Skull base
- Endoscopic sinus surgery • Endoscopy

KEY POINTS

- Perioperative evaluation and history are critical components for analgesic control. Physicians should use a team-based approach with their patients and provide clear postoperative pain expectations.
- Nonopioid alternatives are efficacious for sinus and skull-base surgery and should be prescribed in a multimodal approach. Opioids should be reserved for breakthrough management.
- Acetaminophen, gabapentin, and alpha-2 agonists are reliable preoperative medications that may provide reduction of required postoperative analgesics.
- Geriatric, pediatric, and chronic pain patients require careful consideration when creating a pain management plan. A multidisciplinary approach may prevent overtreatment or undertreatment of postoperative pain.

INTRODUCTION

Over the last 30 years, sinus surgery has been at the forefront of technological innovation. Procedures once limited to open approaches now use advanced surgical instrumentation, high-definition scopes, and intraoperative surgical navigation. With these advances in tools and technique, sinus surgery is now generally associated with low levels of postoperative pain.[1–3] Despite this, postoperative pain is of considerable interest and concern for patients undergoing surgery with many patients citing the possibility of pain as a potential barrier to undergo surgery.[4–6]

Otolaryngologists have recognized the need for postoperative pain control and the consequences of inadequate analgesia, and as a result, many now provide aggressive

[a] Department of Otolaryngology–Head and Neck Surgery, Rutgers New Jersey Medical School, Newark, NJ, USA; [b] Hackensack Meridian Health, Hackensack University Medical Center, Hackensack, NJ, USA; [c] Department of Otolaryngology, William Beaumont Hospital, Royal Oak, MI, USA; [d] Barbara Ann Karmanos Cancer Institute, Detroit, MI, USA
* Corresponding author. 4201 St. Antoine 5E UHC, Detroit, MI 48201.
E-mail address: afolbe@gmail.com

Otolaryngol Clin N Am 53 (2020) 789–802
https://doi.org/10.1016/j.otc.2020.05.008
0030-6665/20/© 2020 Elsevier Inc. All rights reserved.

postoperative analgesia. A recent study of otolaryngologists prescribing patterns reported more than 90% of otolaryngologists writing for at least 1 form of opioids following functional endoscopic sinus surgery.[7] In 2015, with regards to Medicare beneficiaries alone, otolaryngologists wrote nearly 1,000,000 days' worth of opioid prescriptions; furthermore, sinus surgeons who wrote a greater amount of opioid prescriptions also tended to write lengthier courses.[8,9] In light of these considerations, there have not been any explicit guidelines regarding postoperative pain control following sinus surgery, and thus regimens vary widely. In a recent study, 22% of polled sinus surgeons reported that they did not know if they practiced evidence-based medicine in regards to postoperative analgesia.[7] The authors hope that this review provides pragmatic evidence-based algorithms with which they can update their own practice patterns.

OPIOID CRISIS

In the 1990s, an initiative to make pain the "fifth vital sign" was undertaken, leading to increased focus on alleviating patient pain and the subsequent escalation of opioid prescriptions.[10] In the last 2 decades, more than 700,000 people have died of a drug overdose.[11,12] In 2017 alone, more than 70,000 people died of drug overdoses, making accidental overdose a leading cause of injury-related death in the United States.[11–13] The National Survey on Drug Use and Health estimates that more than 10 million people in the United States used prescription opioids for nonmedical use in 2016.[14] Surgeons have played a large role in this epidemic with more than 36% of prescription opioids originating from surgical specialties.[15] Among sinus surgeons alone, more than 20,000 opioid prescriptions were written in 2015.[9] In this current health care climate, it is increasingly necessary for otolaryngologists to reevaluate their analgesic practices and use nonopioid alternatives when appropriate.

PREOPERATIVE PAIN MANAGEMENT

A preoperative discussion of patient expectations of pain, likely course, and modalities used for alleviating pain is of utmost importance. The American Pain Society (APS) and American Society of Anesthesiologists (ASA) recommend an individualized, patient-centered dialogue on pain management because this education has been shown to reduce postoperative opioid consumption, pain anxiety, and length of stay.[16–18] As patients are further educated on negative effects of narcotics, a vast majority will decline opioids in favor of nonopioid alternatives.[19] In addition, when possible, verbal and written communication should be used in conjunction in order to encourage patient participation in their care.[20] In these discussions, providers should take careful note of medical and psychiatric comorbidities, medications, histories of chronic pain or substance abuse, and past postoperative pain regimens if available.

SCREENING FOR ABUSE

Prescription Drug Monitoring Programs (PDMPs) were established as an attempt to create a centralized and structured platform with the aim of mitigating diversion and misuse of opioids and other medications of interest (**Fig. 1**). These programs track

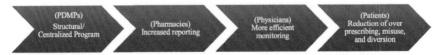

Fig. 1. Current framework theory for PDMP.

information, such as which medication was prescribed, dose, date of prescription, prescribing physician, pharmacy, and other relevant information, to provide prescribers and pharmacists more information before distributing medications. PDMPs were first established in 1939; however, they have only recently started gaining traction across the United States. As of 2019, PDMPs were active in 49 states with Missouri actively creating legislation for its own program.[21,22]

There are clear benefits to having such programs available to prescribers. The information provided can help physicians develop a better understanding of a patient's medication history, which may further help tailor a patient's pain control plan. In addition, this information can help avoid polypharmacy and "doctor shopping," the process in which patients visit different physicians to obtain multiple prescriptions. Despite these benefits, the literature evaluating the effectiveness of these programs remains indeterminate. PDMPs vary greatly across states, and laws mandating their use fluctuate as well. In a recent study assessing PDMP use, only 22 of the 49 states legally mandated prescribers query their systems before writing for medications of interest.[23] Because of the lack consistency among these programs, it is hard to say what impact these systems have had on the opioid epidemic. Increased and consistent use of PDMPs across specialties and providers may help to create a reliable system for pain management.

RECOMMENDED OPIOIDS

When necessary, opioids are an extremely helpful tool to mitigate postoperative pain. Opioids are a longstanding pain-relief medication dating back to Sumerian use of the poppy plant for the treatment of various medical ailments.[24] No specific regimens have been created for opioid use for sinus surgery; however, when looking at the data, postoperative pain levels following sinus surgery are generally modest. One such study evaluating patient pain over a 6-day period following sinus surgery reported mean pain scores significantly declining over the timespan.[3] Using a visual analog scale (VAS) of 1 to 10, the authors reported a decrease from 3.61 on postoperative day 1 to 1.72 on postoperative day 6.[3] Similar results have been reported across multiple studies.[1–3,25]

Opioids should be used as an adjunct medication in a multimodal system. Many physicians advocate for opioids as a "rescue" medication only prescribed once nonopioid alternatives fail to provide significant relief.[3,17,18,26] Short-acting as opposed to extended release opioids should be prescribed for acute pain. In addition, the lowest reasonable dose to adequately control pain should be provided because misuse and overdose have been shown to be linked with increasing opioid doses.[27–29] These medications should ideally be administered orally, and common side effects, such as respiratory depression, sedation, nausea, vomiting, and constipation, should be consistently monitored. Hydrocodone-acetaminophen, oxycodone-acetaminophen, and tramadol are the most commonly prescribed opioids by otolaryngologists.[7,9,30]

NONOPIOID ALTERNATIVES IN SINUS SURGERY

The APS and the ASA are both strong proponents for the use of nonopioid analgesia postoperatively.[17,18] In sinus surgery specifically, multiple studies and reviews have endorsed the efficacy of nonopioids in perioperative pain control with good evidence for nonsteroidal anti-inflammatory drugs (NSAIDs), acetaminophen, gabapentinoids, alpha agonists, and local anesthetics.[31] Dosing and adverse reactions for these nonopioid alternatives can be found in **Table 1**. **Fig. 2** illustrates an evidence-based proposed multimodal pain management algorithm for sinus surgery.

Table 1
Common dosing and adverse reactions of nonopioid alternatives

Type		Dose	Frequency	Route	Adverse Reactions
Acetaminophen		500–1000 mg	q6h	po/IV	Nausea, headache, hepatotoxicity
NSAID	Ibuprofen	400–800 mg	q6h	po	Renal dysfunction, bleeding, GI ulcers, tinnitus, allergic reactions
	Ketorolac	10–20 mg	q4-6h	po	
	Celecoxib	400 mg postoperative; 200 mg daily	qd	po	
Local anesthetics	Lidocaine	1%–2%	Intraoperative	Local infiltration	Dizziness, headache, blurred vision, twitching muscles, prolonged numbness
	Bupivacaine	0.25%–0.5%	Intraoperative	Local infiltration	
	Levobupivacaine	0.5%	Intraoperative	Local infiltration	
Alpha-2 agonists	Clonidine	2–5 μg/kg bolus, 0.3 μg/kg infusion	Varies	IV	Sedation, dry mouth, nausea, vomiting, bradycardia, hypotension, loss of smell
	Dexmedetomidine	1 μg/kg bolus, 0.2 μg/kg/h infusion	Varies	IV	
Gabapentin		600–1200 mg preoperative; 600 mg postoperative	Once preoperatively; tid postoperatively	Po	Drowsiness, unsteadiness, nausea, anxiety, confusion, dry mouth

Abbreviations: GI, gastrointestinal; h, hour; IV, intravenous; po, by mouth; q, every; qd, daily; tid, 3 times a day.

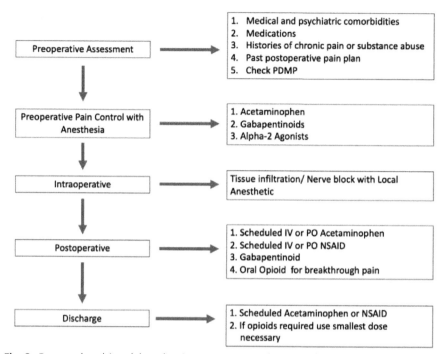

Fig. 2. Proposed multimodal analgesia management algorithm for sinus surgery.

Nonsteroidal Anti-Inflammatory Drugs

There is a plethora of evidence endorsing the use of NSAIDs for sinus surgery. NSAIDs work by reversibly inhibiting the action of cyclooxygenase enzymes (COX-1 and COX-2), thereby reducing the formation of thromboxane and the prostaglandins that mediate inflammation (**Fig. 3**). In sinus surgery, the use of NSAIDs postoperatively has been shown to effectively decrease VAS pain scores when compared with placebo controls and effective pain control (although not statistically improved) in trials

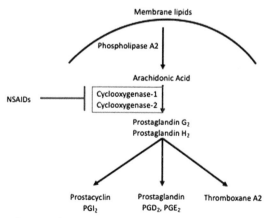

Fig. 3. Mechanism of action for NSAIDs. PGD_2, prostaglandin D_2; PGE_2, prostaglandin E_2; PGI_2, prostaglandin I_2.

against opioids.[32-37] In addition, when used in the perioperative period, NSAIDs decrease consumption of rescue analgesic medication. Both intravenous and oral routes have been studied; however, there has been no clear consensus as to which is optimal postoperatively.[38]

Traditionally, otolaryngologists have been hesitant to use NSAIDs because of the fear of bleeding and gastrointestinal complications. This fear may be unwarranted however as available evidence has shown exceedingly low levels of excessive bleeding with NSAID use after sinus surgery.[31] One such study compared ketorolac with fentanyl following endoscopic sinus surgery and reported no increased risk of hemorrhage or acute blood loss anemia.[36] COX-2 selective inhibitors may also be a suitable alternative because these drugs fail to inhibit the thromboxane and prostaglandins responsible for gastric problems and bleeding. Although there have been no sinus surgery–specific trials examining the relationship between COX-2 inhibitors and bleeding, Turan and colleagues[37] demonstrated the efficacy of preoperative rofecoxib in patients undergoing sinus surgery.

When prescribing NSAIDs, consideration should be taken for patients with histories of bleeding disorder, gastrointestinal ulcers, allergic, respiratory, or renal disease.

Acetaminophen

As with NSAIDs, acetaminophen is inexpensive, readily available, and effective. The exact mechanism of action for acetaminophen is unclear, although it is generally considered to be a weak inhibitor of prostaglandins with possible interaction of serotonergic pathways.[39] Unlike NSAIDs, acetaminophen has no anti-inflammatory action. Despite this, multiple studies have illustrated the efficacy of this medication in sinus surgery.[40-43] When compared with controls, acetaminophen given in the perioperative period significantly increased the time to analgesic rescue with concurrent significant decrease in amount of rescue analgesia required.[40,43] Interestingly, timing of administration may be of significance because preoperative administration has been shown to decrease immediate postoperative pain scores and need for additional analgesic medications.[41,42] Preoperative administration may be considered part of the pain control discussion with both the patient and the anesthesia team. When using acetaminophen postoperatively, general guidelines by the ASA and APS recommend scheduled dosing as opposed to an "as-needed" basis.[17,18] There is no clear difference between intravenous and oral administration of acetaminophen.[44] Effective dosing is 500 to 1000 mg every 4 to 6 hours. Providers should take care to adhere to daily maximum doses of 4000 mg as to prevent hepatotoxicity.

Local Anesthetics

Local anesthetic injection reduces postoperative pain and analgesic consumption in sinus surgery. Local anesthetics reversibly inhibit sodium influx through voltage-gated sodium channels, thereby preventing the conduction of action potentials (**Fig. 4**).[45] When used intraoperatively, studies have demonstrated local anesthetics to be effective in decreasing postoperative pain scores and analgesic requirements.[46-53] Levobupivacaine, lidocaine, bupivacaine, ropivacaine, and prilocaine have been studied in sinus surgery. Interestingly, although use of traditional local anesthetics has been limited by their shorter duration of action, several studies have noted decreased analgesic consumption extending up to 24 hours postoperatively.[51-53]

As compared with the other pain modalities previously mentioned, local anesthetics require some anatomic knowledge and skill to be successful. A recent systemic review reported statistically significantly improved surgical field quality with the use of a sphenopalatine local anesthetic block.[54] Infraorbital blocks have also been shown to be a

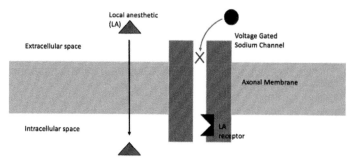

Fig. 4. Mechanism of action for local anesthetics.

valuable tool for nasal surgery.[55] Experience with performing these blocks may increase surgical field quality and decrease postoperative pain. Local pain, infection, bleeding, and changes in blood pressure should be considered when using local anesthetics.

Gabapentinoids

Gabapentinoid use in otolaryngology has been extensively studied with current guidelines recommending the use of gabapentinoid as a preoperative component to multimodal analgesia.[56] Gabapentin interacts at the binding site of the alpha-2 delta subunit of voltage-gated calcium channels (**Fig. 5**). This interaction decreases the calcium influx, thereby reducing neurotransmitter release and neuronal excitability (see **Fig. 4**). In studies comparing gabapentin to placebo controls in nasal procedures, gabapentin was shown to reduce overall postoperative pain scores as well as the amount of opioid consumption.[57–59] Optimal dosing for gabapentin is unknown, although in trials it has been dosed between 600 and 1200 mg, 1 to 2 hours before surgery with good results. Prescribers should also take into account whether the surgery is inpatient or outpatient, patient age, and mental status because this may change dosing parameters. Although higher doses may be more effective for pain control, prescribers must consider the associated increases in dizziness and sedation.

Alpha-2 Agonists

Alpha-2 agonists have sympatholytic, sedative, analgesic as well as vasoconstrictive effects. Alpha-2 agonist medications inhibit adenylyl cyclase activity, preventing

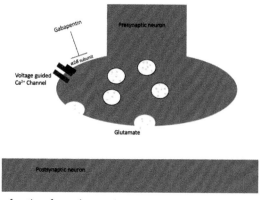

Fig. 5. Mechanism of action for gabapentin.

calcium ions from entering the nerve terminal, leading to a suppression of neural firing.[60] Therefore, when given preoperatively, these medications provide reliable postoperative pain control as well as intraoperative hemodynamic stability and improved surgical field visibility. Dexmedetomidine and clonidine have been the most frequently studied alpha-2 agonists in sinus surgery and have been shown to be reliable perioperative medications.[61–65]

NONTRADITIONAL PAIN MANAGEMENT

Cognitive behavior modalities, such as music, hypnosis, or guided imagery, have been studied as adjuvant therapies with varying results.[66–71] Physical modalities, including acupuncture, massage therapy, and cold therapy, have had inconsistent results as well.[72–75] There is currently no evidence for the support or rejection of these modalities in sinus surgery.

NONOPIOID ALTERNATIVES IN SKULL-BASE SURGERY

Technological innovations have made endoscopic and transsphenoidal approaches feasible for a significant portion of benign and malignant ventral skull-base lesions, because this technique has steadily increased at the expense of traditional approaches.[76,77] Despite the minimally invasive nature of these approaches, it is important to use the preoperative patient counseling process to reinforce that these approaches continue to harbor serious potential risks and a significant potential for postoperative pain. There have only been a few studies evaluating nonopioid alternatives for skull-base surgeries; however, ibuprofen and local anesthetics have been shown to be effective options for perioperative pain control.[78,79]

SPECIAL POPULATIONS
Geriatrics and Pediatrics

Special care must be taken when prescribing medications for geriatric and pediatric populations. Many elderly patients suffer from conditions such as arthritis or cancer that may lead to increased analgesic requirement.[80,81] Providers should be thoughtful of these comorbidities to avoid undertreatment of these patients. Medical comorbidities should also be taken into account. Patients with reduced renal clearance should have opioids dosed with caution because the therapeutic window for safe use is diminished. In addition, side effects and drug-drug interactions should be monitored closely.

In the pediatric population, analgesia should be dosed according to age and weight.[18] A multimodal approach should be taken with nonopioid alternatives and cognitive behavioral therapy where applicable.[82,83] In many states, minors must have an opioid consent form signed. Cases in which opioid consent is discussed with the patient and their family are associated with overall decreased opioid prescriptions without additional complications.[84] Families that are prescribed opioids should be educated on storing these medications in safe places to avoid accidental ingestion.

Chronic Pain

Chronic pain is traditionally described as pain persisting for at least 1 month following the usual healing time of an acute injury or pain that recurs frequently over a period of months. Clinically, chronic pain is typically defined as pain that has persisted for at least 3 months.[85] In the United States, the estimated incidence of adults with chronic pain is approximately 20%.[12,86,87] As such, it is highly likely that practicing sinus surgeons will work with chronic pain patients. In these cases, it becomes increasingly important to have a comprehensive discussion examining the pain control plan. A multidisciplinary approach using the expertise of pain specialists and pharmacists is encouraged and may even be beneficial in the preoperative period. Patients who are chronically opioid dependent may develop a tolerance, leading to higher postoperative requirements.[88] It is important to note that although tolerance to some side effects, namely, nausea, vomiting, and respiratory depression, may develop quickly, constipation and miosis remain the exception, and bowel regimen prophylaxis should be maintained.[89]

SUMMARY

Perioperative analgesic management is complex, requiring an individualized approached with each patient. Opioids are an effective analgesic option for breakthrough pain, however should not be prescribed lightly because risk for misuse and diversion is high. There is a multitude of evidence supporting the efficacy of nonopioid alternatives. A multimodal strategy encompassing acetaminophen, NSAIDs, local anesthetics, and gabapentin may decrease prescription and consumption of opioids. Special care should be taken when considering pain management plans for the geriatric, pediatric, and chronic pain populations.

REFERENCES

1. Becker SD, Becker DG. Review and update on postoperative opioid use after nasal and sinus surgery. Curr Opin Otolaryngol Head Neck Surg 2018; 26(1):41–5.
2. Pletcher SD. Rethinking pain management in endoscopic sinus surgery. JAMA Otolaryngol Head Neck Surg 2017;143(8):794–5.
3. Wise SK, Wise JC, DelGaudio JM. Evaluation of postoperative pain after sinonasal surgery. Am J Rhinol 2005;19(5):471–7.
4. Soler ZM, Smith TL. Quality of life outcomes after endoscopic sinus surgery: how long is long enough? Otolaryngol Head Neck Surg 2010;143(5):621–5.
5. Sahlstrand-Johnson P, Hopkins C, Ohlsson B, et al. The effect of endoscopic sinus surgery on quality of life and absenteeism in patients with chronic rhinosinusitis - a multi-centre study. Rhinology 2017;55(3):251–61.
6. Sommer M, Geurts JWJM, Stessel B, et al. Prevalence and predictors of postoperative pain after ear, nose, and throat surgery. Arch Otolaryngol Head Neck Surg 2009;135(2):124–30.
7. Gray ML, Fan CJ, Kappauf C, et al. Postoperative pain management after sinus surgery: a survey of the American Rhinologic Society. Int Forum Allergy Rhinol 2018;8(10):1199–203.
8. Svider PF, Arianpour K, Guo E, et al. Opioid prescribing patterns among otolaryngologists: crucial insights among the medicare population. Laryngoscope 2018;128(7):1576–81.
9. Arianpour K, Nguyen B, Yuhan B, et al. Opioid prescription among sinus surgeons. Am J Rhinol Allergy 2018;32(4):323–9.
10. Quality improvement guidelines for the treatment of acute pain and cancer pain. American Pain Society Quality of Care Committee. JAMA 1995;274(23):1874–80.
11. Opioid Overdose | Drug Overdose | CDC Injury Center. 2018. Available at: https://www.cdc.gov/drugoverdose/index.html. Accessed July 8, 2018.

12. CDC Guideline for Prescribing Opioids for Chronic Pain | Drug Overdose | CDC Injury Center. 2019. Available at: https://www.cdc.gov/drugoverdose/prescribing/guideline.html. Accessed November 30, 2019.

13. CDC WONDER. Available at: https://wonder.cdc.gov/. Accessed November 29, 2019.

14. Ahrnsbrak R. Key Substance Use and Mental Health Indicators in the United States: results from the 2016 National Survey on Drug Use and Health. 2016:86.

15. Levy B, Paulozzi L, Mack KA, et al. Trends in opioid analgesic–prescribing rates by specialty, U.S., 2007–2012. Am J Prev Med 2015;49(3):409–13.

16. Egbert LD, Battit GE, Welch CE, et al. Reduction of postoperative pain by encouragement and instruction of patients. a study of doctor-patient rapport. N Engl J Med 1964;270:825–7.

17. Chou R, Gordon DB, de Leon-Casasola OA, et al. Management of postoperative pain: a clinical practice guideline from the American Pain Society, the American Society of Regional Anesthesia and Pain Medicine, and the American Society of Anesthesiologists' Committee on Regional Anesthesia, Executive Committee, and Administrative Council. J Pain 2016;17(2):131–57.

18. Practice guidelines for acute pain management in the perioperative setting: an updated report by the American Society of Anesthesiologists Task Force on acute pain management. Anesthesiology 2012;116(2):248–73.

19. Sugai DY, Deptula PL, Parsa AA, et al. The importance of communication in the management of postoperative pain. Hawaii J Med Public Health 2013;72(6):180–4.

20. Andersson V, Otterstrom-Rydberg E, Karlsson A-K. The importance of written and verbal information on pain treatment for patients undergoing surgical interventions. Pain Manag Nurs 2015;16(5):634–41.

21. Finley EP, Garcia A, Rosen K, et al. Evaluating the impact of prescription drug monitoring program implementation: a scoping review. BMC Health Serv Res 2017;17(1):420.

22. Soelberg CD, Brown RE, Du Vivier D, et al. The US opioid crisis: current federal and state legal issues. Anesth Analg 2017;125(5):1675–81.

23. Haffajee RL, Jena AB, Weiner SG. Mandatory use of prescription drug monitoring programs. JAMA 2015;313(9):891–2.

24. Wilkerson RG, Kim HK, Windsor TA, et al. The opioid epidemic in the United States. Emerg Med Clin North Am 2016;34(2):e1–23.

25. Preoperative quality-of-life measures predict acute postoperative pain in endoscopic sinus surgery. Available at: https://www-ncbi-nlm-nih-gov.huaryu.kl.oakland.edu/pubmed/30613981. Accessed November 30, 2019.

26. Cramer JD, Wisler B, Gouveia CJ. Opioid stewardship in otolaryngology: state of the art review. Otolaryngol Head Neck Surg 2018;158(5):817–27.

27. Coyle DT, Pratt C-Y, Ocran-Appiah J, et al. Opioid analgesic dose and the risk of misuse, overdose, and death: a narrative review. Pharmacoepidemiol Drug Saf 2018;27(5):464–72.

28. Garg RK, Fulton-Kehoe D, Franklin GM. Patterns of opioid use and risk of opioid overdose death among Medicaid patients. Med Care 2017;55(7):661–8.

29. Kimmel PL, Fwu C-W, Abbott KC, et al. Opioid prescription, morbidity, and mortality in United States dialysis patients. J Am Soc Nephrol 2017;28(12):3658–70.

30. Schwartz MA, Naples JG, Kuo C-L, et al. Opioid prescribing patterns among otolaryngologists. Otolaryngol Head Neck Surg 2018;158(5):854–9.

31. Svider PF, Nguyen B, Yuhan B, et al. Perioperative analgesia for patients under-going endoscopic sinus surgery: an evidence-based review. Int Forum Allergy Rhinol 2018;8(7):837–49.
32. Church C, Stewart C, O-Lee T, et al. Rofecoxib versus hydrocodone/acetamino-phen for postoperative analgesia in functional endoscopic sinus surgery. Laryn-goscope 2006;116(4):602–6.
33. Elhakim M. A comparison of intravenous ketoprofen with pethidine for postoper-ative pain relief following nasal surgery. Acta Anaesthesiol Scand 1991;35(4):279–82.
34. Keleş G, Topçu I, Ekici Z, et al. Evaluation of piroxicam-beta-cyclodextrin as a preemptive analgesic in functional endoscopic sinus surgery. Braz J Med Biol Res 2010;43(8):806–11.
35. Leykin Y, Casati A, Rapotec A, et al. A prospective, randomized, double-blind comparison between parecoxib and ketorolac for early postoperative analgesia following nasal surgery. Minerva Anestesiol 2008;74(9):475–9.
36. Moeller C, Pawlowski J, Pappas A, et al. The safety and efficacy of intravenous ketorolac in patients undergoing primary endoscopic sinus surgery: a random-ized, double-blinded clinical trial. Int Forum Allergy Rhinol 2012;2(4):342–7.
37. Turan A, Emet S, Karamanlioğlu B, et al. Analgesic effects of rofecoxib in ear-nose-throat surgery. Anesth Analg 2002;95(5):1308–11, table of contents.
38. An update on nonopioids- ClinicalKey. Available at: https://www-clinicalkey-com.huaryu.kl.oakland.edu/#!/content/playContent/1-s2.0-S1932227517300113?scrollTo=%23hl0000183. Accessed December 1, 2019.
39. Graham GG, Scott KF. Mechanism of action of paracetamol. Am J Ther 2005;12(1):46–55.
40. Kemppainen T, Kokki H, Tuomilehto H, et al. Acetaminophen is highly effective in pain treatment after endoscopic sinus surgery. Laryngoscope 2006;116(12):2125–8.
41. Kemppainen T, Tuomilehto H, Kokki H, et al. Pain treatment and recovery after endoscopic sinus surgery. Laryngoscope 2007;117(8):1434–8.
42. Koteswara C, Sheetal D. A study on pre-emptive analgesic effect of intravenous paracetamol in functional endoscopic sinus surgeries: a randomized, double-blinded clinical study. J Clin Diagn Res 2014;8(1):108–11.
43. Tyler M, Lam K, Ashoori F, et al. Analgesic effects of intravenous acetaminophen vs placebo for endoscopic sinus surgery and postoperative pain: a randomized clinical trial. JAMA Otolaryngol Head Neck Surg 2017;143(8):788–94.
44. Jibril F, Sharaby S, Mohamed A, et al. Intravenous versus oral acetaminophen for pain: systematic review of current evidence to support clinical decision-making. Can J Hosp Pharm 2015;68(3):238–47.
45. Shandler L. Mechanism of action of local anesthetics. J Am Dent Soc Anesthesiol 1965;12(2):62–6.
46. Al-Qudah M. Endoscopic sphenopalatine ganglion blockade efficacy in pain con-trol after endoscopic sinus surgery. Int Forum Allergy Rhinol 2016;6(3):334–8.
47. Cekic B, Geze S, Erturk E, et al. A comparison of levobupivacaine and levobupivacaine-tramadol combination in bilateral infraorbital nerve block for postoperative analgesia after nasal surgery. Ann Plast Surg 2013;70(2):131–4.
48. DeMaria S, Govindaraj S, Chinosorvatana N, et al. Bilateral sphenopalatine gan-glion blockade improves postoperative analgesia after endoscopic sinus surgery. Am J Rhinol Allergy 2012;26(1):e23–7.
49. Friedman M, Venkatesan T, Lang D, et al. Bupivacaine for postoperative anal-gesia following endoscopic sinus surgery. Laryngoscope 1996;106(11):1382–5.

50. Haytoğlu S, Kuran G, Muluk NB, et al. Different anesthetic agents-soaked sinus packings on pain management after functional endoscopic sinus surgery: which is the most effective? Eur Arch Otorhinolaryngol 2016;273(7):1769–77.

51. Kesimci E, Öztürk L, Bercin S, et al. Role of sphenopalatine ganglion block for postoperative analgesia after functional endoscopic sinus surgery. Eur Arch Otorhinolaryngol 2012;269(1):165–9.

52. Mariano E, Watson D, Loland V, et al. Bilateral infraorbital nerve blocks decrease postoperative pain but do not reduce time to discharge following outpatient nasal surgery. Can J Anaesth 2009;56(8):584–9.

53. Yilmaz S, Yildizbas S, Güçlü E, et al. Topical levobupivacaine efficacy in pain control after functional endoscopic sinus surgery. Otolaryngol Head Neck Surg 2013; 149(5):777–81.

54. Shamil E, Rouhani MJ, Basetti S, et al. Role of local anaesthetic nerve block in endoscopic sinus surgery: a systematic review and meta-analysis. Clin Otolaryngol 2018;43(5):1201–8.

55. Higashizawa T, Koga Y. Effect of infraorbital nerve block under general anesthesia on consumption of isoflurane and postoperative pain in endoscopic endonasal maxillary sinus surgery. J Anesth 2001;15(3):136–8.

56. Sanders JG, Dawes PJD. Gabapentin for perioperative analgesia in otorhinolaryngology-head and neck surgery: systematic review. Otolaryngol Head Neck Surg 2016;155(6):893–903.

57. Kazak Z, Mortimer N, Sekerci S. Single dose of preoperative analgesia with gabapentin (600 mg) is safe and effective in monitored anesthesia care for nasal surgery. Eur Arch Otorhinolaryngol 2010;267(5):731–6.

58. Mohammed MH, Fahmy AM, Hakim KYK. Preoperative gabapentin augments intraoperative hypotension and reduces postoperative opioid requirements with functional endoscopic sinus surgery. Egypt J Anaesth 2012;28(3):189–92.

59. Turan A, Memiş D, Karamanlioğlu B, et al. The analgesic effects of gabapentin in monitored anesthesia care for ear-nose-throat surgery. Anesth Analg 2004;99(2): 375–8, table of contents.

60. Alpha-2 adrenergic receptor agonists: a review of current clinical applications. Available at: https://www-ncbi-nlm-nih-gov.huaryu.kl.oakland.edu/pmc/articles/PMC4389556/. Accessed December 1, 2019.

61. Balaraju T, Ramdas B, Thomas R, et al. Comparative evaluation of oral clonidine and intravenous clonidine premedication in functional endoscopic sinus surgery. Int J Pharma Bio Sci 2013;4(1):B587–91.

62. Guven DG, Demiraran Y, Sezen G, et al. Evaluation of outcomes in patients given dexmedetomidine in functional endoscopic sinus surgery. Ann Otol Rhinol Laryngol 2011;120(9):586–92.

63. Humphreys MR, Grant D, McKean SA, et al. Xylometazoline hydrochloride 0.1 per cent versus physiological saline in nasal surgical aftercare: a randomised, single-blinded, comparative clinical trial. J Laryngol Otol 2008;123(1):1–6.

64. Karabayirli S, Ugur K, Demircioglu R, et al. Surgical conditions during FESS; comparison of dexmedetomidine and remifentanil. Eur Arch Otorhinolaryngol 2017; 274(1):239–45.

65. Tang C, Huang X, Kang F, et al. Intranasal dexmedetomidine on stress hormones, inflammatory markers, and postoperative analgesia after functional endoscopic sinus surgery. Mediators Inflamm 2015;2015:939431.

66. Antall GF, Kresevic D. The use of guided imagery to manage pain in an elderly orthopaedic population. Orthop Nurs 2004;23(5):335–40.

67. Lambert SA. The effects of hypnosis/guided imagery on the postoperative course of children. J Dev Behav Pediatr 1996;17(5):307–10.
68. Tusek DL. Guided imagery: a powerful tool to decrease length of stay, pain, anxiety, and narcotic consumption. J Invasive Cardiol 1999;11(4):265–7.
69. Ebneshahidi A, Mohseni M. The effect of patient-selected music on early postoperative pain, anxiety, and hemodynamic profile in cesarean section surgery. J Altern Complement Med 2008;14(7):827–31.
70. Good M, Stanton-Hicks M, Grass JA, et al. Relief of postoperative pain with jaw relaxation, music and their combination. Pain 1999;81(1–2):163–72.
71. Ikonomidou E, Rehnström A, Naesh O. Effect of music on vital signs and postoperative pain. AORN J 2004;80(2):269–74, 277–8.
72. Sim C-K, Xu P-C, Pua H-L, et al. Effects of electroacupuncture on intraoperative and postoperative analgesic requirement. Acupunct Med 2002;20(2–3):56–65.
73. Grabow L. Controlled study of the analgetic effectivity of acupuncture. Arzneimittelforschung 1994;44(4):554–8.
74. Piotrowski MM, Paterson C, Mitchinson A, et al. Massage as adjuvant therapy in the management of acute postoperative pain: a preliminary study in men. J Am Coll Surg 2003;197(6):1037–46.
75. Mitchinson AR, Kim HM, Rosenberg JM, et al. Acute postoperative pain management using massage as an adjuvant therapy: a randomized trial. Arch Surg 2007; 142(12):1158–67 [discussion: 1167].
76. Svider PF, Setzen M, Baredes S, et al. Overview of sinonasal and ventral skull base malignancy management. Otolaryngol Clin North Am 2017;50(2):205–19.
77. Svider PF, Keeley BR, Husain Q, et al. Regional disparities and practice patterns in surgical approaches to pituitary tumors in the United States. Int Forum Allergy Rhinol 2013;3(12):1007–12.
78. Shepherd DM, Jahnke H, White WL, et al. Randomized, double-blinded, placebo-controlled trial comparing two multimodal opioid-minimizing pain management regimens following transsphenoidal surgery. J Neurosurg 2017;1–8. https://doi.org/10.3171/2016.10.JNS161355.
79. McAdam D, Muro K, Suresh S. The use of infraorbital nerve block for postoperative pain control after transsphenoidal hypophysectomy. Reg Anesth Pain Med 2005;30(6):572–3.
80. McKeown JL. Pain management issues for the geriatric surgical patient. Anesthesiol Clin 2015;33(3):563–76.
81. Naples JG, Gellad WF, Hanlon JT. The role of opioid analgesics in geriatric pain management. Clin Geriatr Med 2016;32(4):725–35.
82. Russell P, von Ungern-Sternberg BS, Schug SA. Perioperative analgesia in pediatric surgery. Curr Opin Anaesthesiol 2013;26(4):420–7.
83. Boric K, Dosenovic S, Jelicic Kadic A, et al. Interventions for postoperative pain in children: an overview of systematic reviews. Paediatr Anaesth 2017;27(9): 893–904.
84. Whelan RL, McCoy J, Mirson L, et al. Opioid prescription and postoperative outcomes in pediatric patients. Laryngoscope 2019;129(6):1477–81.
85. Rosenblum A, Marsch LA, Joseph H, et al. Opioids and the treatment of chronic pain: controversies, current status, and future directions. Exp Clin Psychopharmacol 2008;16(5):405–16.
86. Dahlhamer J. Prevalence of chronic pain and high-impact chronic pain among adults — United States, 2016. MMWR Morb Mortal Wkly Rep 2018;67. https://doi.org/10.15585/mmwr.mm6736a2.

87. Verhaak PF, Kerssens JJ, Dekker J, et al. Prevalence of chronic benign pain disorder among adults: a review of the literature. Pain 1998;77(3):231–9.

88. Yang JJ, Li WY, Jil Q, et al. Local anesthesia for functional endoscopic sinus surgery employing small volumes of epinephrine-containing solutions of lidocaine produces profound hypotension. Acta Anaesthesiol Scand 2005;49(10):1471–6.

89. Freye E, Latasch L. Development of opioid tolerance – molecular mechanisms and clinical consequences. Anasthesiol Intensivmed Notfallmed Schmerzther 2003;38(1):14–26 [in German].

Perioperative Pain Management Following Otologic Surgery

Daniel R. Morrison, MD, Lindsay S. Moore, MD,
Erika M. Walsh, MD*

KEYWORDS

- Otology • Pain • Perioperative • Nonsteroidal anti-inflammatory drug • Narcotics
- Acoustic neuroma • Skull base

KEY POINTS

- Pain in bilateral myringotomy with tubes is self-limited and best treated with acetaminophen and nonsteroidal anti-inflammatory drugs. This treatment may be performed in an in-office setting in selected patients.
- Multimodal pain therapy with emphasis on local analgesia and non-nonsteroidal anti-inflammatories anti-inflammatory drugs is critical in avoiding postoperative opioid use.
- Although opioids such as patient-controlled analgesia pumps are generally indicated postoperatively for skull base surgeries, these can be minimized with an appropriate multimodal pain regimen.

OVERVIEW

Postoperative pain control is an important and controversial issue in all surgical specialties. As a result of overprescription and subsequent overuse of narcotic medication, many providers are more conscious of the amount of narcotic pain medications they are providing at the time of surgery. Roughly 10% of all narcotic prescriptions written in the United States are written by a surgeon, and about 36% of all prescriptions written by surgeons are narcotics.[1] Data show that if opioid-naive patients are prescribed narcotics at the time of surgery, they are significantly more likely to still be prescribed narcotics a full calendar year later than patients who were not initially prescribed narcotics.[2] The onus thus lies on the surgical community to treat pain effectively while minimizing the amount of potentially addictive opioids prescribed. This article discusses pain management after various forms of otologic surgery, with a particular focus on strategies to avoid opioid overprescription.

Department of Otolaryngology, University of Alabama at Birmingham, Faculty Office Tower 1155, 1720 2nd Avenue South, Birmingham, AL 35294-3412, USA
* Corresponding author.
E-mail address: ewalsh@uabmc.edu

Otolaryngol Clin N Am 53 (2020) 803–810
https://doi.org/10.1016/j.otc.2020.05.009
0030-6665/20/© 2020 Elsevier Inc. All rights reserved.

PREOPERATIVE COUNSELING

Adequate preoperative counseling is critical to establish realistic expectations on behalf of the patient. Goals of postoperative pain control should be clear and mutually understood by both parties. The goal of pain management postoperatively is not to eliminate pain but to decrease pain to an acceptable level. As the surgeons counsel patients on the risks and benefits of the procedures, so they must discuss risks and benefits of opioid pain medication. In the case of elective outpatient surgery, many patients decline a postoperative narcotic prescription after appropriate counseling.[3] Most otologic procedures are in this category, and many patients undergoing routine middle ear or tympanomastoid surgery do not require postoperative opioid medication for optimal pain control.

MYRINGOTOMY TUBES

One of the most common procedures performed in the United States, bilateral myringotomy with tympanostomy tube placement (BMT), is not traditionally associated with high levels of postoperative pain. Almost all of these procedures are done in the pediatric population. BMT-associated pain is generally thought to be brief and self-limited; the need for any postoperative analgesics has been debated in the literature.

In adults, the procedure may be done in the office with local analgesia, traditionally phenol, although use of eutectic mixture of local anesthetics (EMLA) and tetracaine has also been reported. Although questions have been raised about the caustic nature of phenol and the risk of long-term detriment to the tympanic membrane, animal studies do not support this.[4] Adults should be counseled to take ibuprofen and acetaminophen as tolerated for discomfort.

In the pediatric population, BMT is often performed in the operating room with mask anesthesia and a volatile agent, usually eliminating the need for peripheral intravenous (IV) line placement. Administration of ketorolac preoperatively has been associated with improved pain scores postoperatively in children undergoing BMT, but there is likely a poor cost/benefit ratio.[5,6] Furthermore, although immediate postoperative pain scores with ketorolac were superior to acetaminophen and placebo, there was no difference in pain scores at the time of discharge or postdischarge analgesia requirement.[5] A recently performed randomized controlled trial (RCT) does not support the use of nonnarcotic preoperative analgesia in pediatric patients undergoing BMT.[7] A study conducted by Voronov and colleagues[8] showed efficacy of intraoperative block of Arnold nerve via injection along the posterior aspect of the tragus with 0.25% bupivacaine in controlling postoperative pain. Postoperatively, pain can be controlled with oral or rectal acetaminophen or ibuprofen. Topical anesthetic drops, such as 4% lidocaine, may also be considered in select cases and may be added to routine antibiotic drops.[9]

In pediatric patients whose caregivers are concerned about long-term effects of general anesthesia, 1 article advocated the insertion of tympanostomy tubes in the office on select children.[10] A full discussion on the developmental effects of general anesthesia on pediatric patients is beyond the scope of this article. However, there is a strong body of evidence that limited exposure to general anesthesia in children is not associated with adverse neurodevelopmental consequences.[11]

MIDDLE EAR AND MASTOID SURGERY

Tympanomastoid surgery in some form is a staple procedure for general otolaryngologists and otologists alike. The surgery may be done for chronic otologic infections, cholesteatoma, cochlear implantation, and so forth. Almost all of these procedures are done under general endotracheal anesthesia (GETA) and are outpatient surgeries. It is rare for patients, even pediatric patients, to require unplanned postoperative admission because of pain. A review of 662 patients undergoing otologic surgery found a 3.9% unplanned admission rate, which was primarily caused by refractory nausea and vomiting.[12] Transcanal middle ear surgery is not traditionally viewed as a particularly painful procedure. Many surgeons advocate for cases such as stapedectomy to be done under local anesthesia with a mild sedative administered by anesthesia.

In children, paracetamol and nonsteroidal anti-inflammatory drugs have been shown to reduce opioid requirement postoperatively.[13] In a large series of children undergoing cochlear implantation in India, no children required opioid medications after discharge from the postanesthesia care unit (PACU). These patients received scheduled IV paracetamol and IV morphine for breakthrough pain, and in the PACU and were routinely admitted postoperatively for monitoring.

A study in Turkey compared patients receiving IV infusions of dexmedetomidine during surgery versus saline infusions and found a decreased need for postoperative tramadol in the dexmedetomidine group. There was no effect on extubation times. The study did not examine narcotic use after discharge.[14] Total intravenous anesthesia with propofol and remifentanil resulted in less postoperative nausea and vomiting compared with sevoflurane and remifentanil.[15] Although pain scores were equivalent in this series between the 2 groups, postoperative nausea should also be considered in perioperative management given the significant patient discomfort it entails. Intraoperative steroids are given in many cases and are thought to improve immediate postoperative pain and nausea. An RCT conducted by Ahn and colleagues[16] examined intraoperative dexamethasone infusion and found significant improvement in postoperative dizziness and nausea but no improvement in postoperative pain. Intraoperative and postoperative steroids must be prescribed with caution because of the significant side effect profile and the patient's medical history must be thoroughly reviewed for contraindications.

Local anesthetic is routinely used in tympanomastoid surgery to assist in analgesia during the procedure and also for its hemostatic effect. Various studies have investigated different techniques and medications for local infiltration during surgery to improve postoperative analgesia. An RCT in India found that a combination of fentanyl and bupivacaine injected at the surgical site had a dose-dependent improvement in postoperative pain control in patients undergoing radical mastoidectomy.[17]

Suresh and colleagues[18] found that there was no significant improvement in postoperative pain scores in pediatric patients undergoing mastoid surgery with preincisional great auricular nerve (GAN) block (0.25% bupivacaine with 1:100,000 epinephrine) versus sham injection. However, they did theorize that the injection reduced the need for volatile anesthetics during the procedure, although there were no data to support this claim. A separate study did show decreased postoperative nausea with GAN block versus morphine injection.[19] Another RCT in India compared pain scores in adults after IV morphine (0.1 mg/kg) compared with a GAN block and an auriculotemporal nerve block with 0.25% bupivacaine and found that the nerve block group had lower pain scores and less nausea in the first 4 hours after tympanomastoidectomy.[20] One recent, small RCT in Turkey compared posttympanomastoidectomy pain scores in patients receiving ultrasonography-guided GAN or superficial cervical plexus (SCP) block with 0.25% bupivacaine. Patients were then given IV tramadol patient-controlled analgesia (PCA), and opioids were not administered. Both were effective pain control regimens up to 24 hours postoperatively without any adverse effects. There was no significant difference between the 2 groups, but there was significantly less tramadol used in the SCP group, which the investigators theorized may be caused by contributions of the lesser occipital nerve.[21] Overall, more data are needed to confirm the consistent efficacy of nerve blocks in otologic surgery, but they do offer promise as a means to reduce opioid use.

Although most otologic surgeons use high-speed drill systems for dissection, other devices are available and deserve mention. A study by Crippa and colleagues[22] examined the use of a piezoelectric device for performing intact canal-wall mastoidectomy compared with the use of a traditional drill, and found significantly improved subjective pain scores on both postoperative day 1 and postoperative day 3. The investigators theorized that the lower amount of heat generation and increased tissue selectivity lead to decreased collateral soft tissue damage compared with the high-speed drill. This technique is not widely used in the United States because of cost and lack of familiarity.[23]

Although, traditionally, otologic surgery using a postauricular incision is most commonly performed using GETA, there is precedent for performing this under local anesthetic. Sarmento and Tomita[24] performed a prospective study of 83 postauricular approaches for primarily tympanoplasty, although mastoidectomies were included. They used 2% lidocaine with 1:100,000 epinephrine for injection in the postauricular region and in a V shape around the inferior portion of the pinna. They also injected the 4 quadrants of the external auditory canal. Patients were interviewed on postoperative day 1 and generally reported good pain control. The most severe complaint was of discomfort in body position (rated as 1.5 on a 1–4 scale). Eighty-two percent of patients reported that they would undergo a second otologic surgery under local anesthetic if there was a need.[24] Yung[25] surveyed patients who underwent middle ear surgery under local anesthesia, including stapes surgery, ossiculoplasty, myringoplasty, and mastoidectomy. These patients reported that the most common discomforts with surgery were noise (29.6% of patients) and anxiety (24% of patients). Even with these discomforts, 89% of patients surveyed still preferred local anesthesia to GETA.[25]

MICROTIA REPAIR

Although most of the components of staged microtia repair surgery are similar in location and tissue manipulation to other postauricular otologic procedures, special consideration must be given to the costal cartilage donor site, which is the primary source of postoperative pain and usually necessitates overnight admission for pain control. Although a multimodal approach with anti-inflammatory agents should be considered to minimize opioid use, several RCTs have explored the efficacy of intercostal nerve blocks (ICNBs) and catheter-based continuous infusion of anesthetic to the wound.[26,27] Both studies found ICNBs with continuous catheter ropivacaine infusion to costal graft harvest site to be safe and effective, with reduced need for other analgesics[26] and superior pain control to IV analgesics alone.[27] Of note, the use of continuous catheter infusion to the wound was superior to ICNB without continuous infusion.[26]

SKULL BASE SURGERY

Postoperative pain after skull base surgery is complex, variable, and remains poorly characterized.[28] Although immediate postoperative pain is expected, persistent postoperative headache lasting weeks to months after surgery is an unpredictable but incapacitating morbidity. Data support a variable incidence of persistent postoperative headache depending on surgical approach. One study found postoperative pain to be severe in 67% of patients on whom a posterior fossa approach was used to resect acoustic neuroma, possibly caused by nuchal dissection and related traction on the dura.[29] Multiple studies have shown increased pain following the suboccipital approach compared with translabyrinthine or other lateral approaches.[28,30–32] Overall, the literature supports that postoperative pain is often undertreated with traditional analgesic regimens, likely in part because of the concern of masking neurologic changes or depressing respiratory drive.[28,33]

In general, the use of postoperative narcotic pain medications after neurotologic skull base surgery is indicated and supported. Although various protocols exist, multiple studies support the use of PCA in the immediate postoperative period. PCA has been shown to effectively control pain, including the psychological stress of pain, with overall lower total doses of opioid used.[28,34] An RCT using 1.5 mg/dose morphine PCA with 8-minute lock-out time and maximum dose of 40 mg of morphine in 4 hours supported all of these findings without any instances of respiratory depression requiring reintubation.[34]

A multimodal approach to postoperative pain is recommended to adequately control pain and minimize opioid use. Local injection of the incision site with lidocaine 2% and epinephrine 1:200,000 is common and known to prolong analgesic half-life. Given the inherent musculoskeletal trauma of many of the skull base approaches, anti-inflammatory agents such as ketorolac or indomethacin should be considered. The evidence does not support an increased risk of postoperative intracranial hemorrhage with these agents.[35,36] In addition, in patients undergoing skull base surgery, nausea and vomiting exacerbate pain and heighten its perception but may also cause increased intracranial pressures, cerebrospinal fluid leaks, and other complications. As such, diligent treatment of nausea and emesis is recommended, also with a multimodal approach.[28,37] Droperidol, ondansetron, and dexamethasone have all been shown to be effective.[38–40] However, given the potential for extrapyramidal side effects and synergistic sedation with opioids, droperidol may be used with caution,[39] and an alternative regimen of preoperative oral ondansetron with intraoperative IV ondansetron and IV dexamethasone has been shown to be effective.[40]

SUMMARY

Perioperative analgesia in otologic surgery involves a broad range of procedures, from the outpatient placement of tympanostomy tubes to extensive skull base surgery for tumor removal. In general, postoperative pain from most otologic surgeries can be managed with little to no opioids, and surgeons should make a concerted effort to minimize narcotic prescriptions in the midst of the opioid crisis. Multimodal pain regimens, local anesthesia, and alternative approaches have shown promise in accomplishing this goal, and should be considered. Preoperative counseling to appropriately manage expectations and goals is imperative to patient satisfaction and safety.

DISCLOSURE

The authors have nothing to disclose.

REFERENCES

1. Levy B, Paulozzi L, Mack KA, et al. Trends in Opioid Analgesic-Prescribing Rates by Specialty, U.S., 2007-2012. Am J Prev Med 2015;49(3):409–13.

2. Alam A, Gomes T, Zheng H, et al. Long-term analgesic use after low-risk surgery: a retrospective cohort study. Arch Intern Med 2012;172(5):425–30.

3. Sugai DY, Deptula PL, Parsa AA, et al. The importance of communication in the management of postoperative pain. Hawaii J Med Public Health 2013;72(6): 180–4.

4. Gnuechtel MM, Schenk LL, Postma GN. Late effects of topical anesthetics on the healing of guinea pig tympanic membranes after myringotomy. Arch Otolaryngol Head Neck Surg 2000;126(6):733–5.

5. Bean-Lijewski JD, Stinson JC. Acetaminophen or ketorolac for post myringotomy pain in children? A prospective, double-blinded comparison. Paediatr Anaesth 1997;7(2):131–7.

6. Watch MF, Ramirez-Ruiz M, White PF, et al. Perioperative effects of oral ketorolac and acetaminophen in children undergoing bilateral myringotomy. Can J Anaesth 1992;39(7):649–54.

7. McHale B, Badenhorst CD, Low C, et al. Do children undergoing bilateral myringotomy with placement of ventilating tubes benefit from pre-operative analgesia? A double-blinded, randomised, placebo-controlled trial. J Laryngol Otol 2018; 132(8):685–92.

8. Voronov P, Tobin MJ, Billings K, et al. Postoperative pain relief in infants undergoing myringotomy and tube placement: comparison of a novel regional anesthetic block to intranasal fentanyl–a pilot analysis. Paediatr Anaesth 2008;18(12): 1196–201.

9. Lawhorn CD, Bower CM, Brown Jr RE, et al. Topical lidocaine for postoperative analgesia following myringotomy and tube placement. Int J Pediatr Otorhinolaryngol 1996;35(1):19–24.

10. Rosenfeld RM, Sury K, Mascarinas C. Office Insertion of Tympanostomy Tubes without Anesthesia in Young Children. Otolaryngol Head Neck Surg 2015; 153(6):1067–70.

11. Graham MR. Clinical update regarding general anesthesia-associated neurotoxicity in infants and children. Curr Opin Anaesthesiol 2017;30(6):682–7.

12. Dornhoffer J, Manning L. Unplanned admissions following outpatient otologic surgery: the University of Arkansas experience. Ear Nose Throat J 2000;79(9):710, 713-7.

13. Wong I, St John-Green C, Walker SM. Opioid-sparing effects of perioperative paracetamol and nonsteroidal anti-inflammatory drugs (NSAIDs) in children. Paediatr Anaesth 2013;23(6):475–95.

14. Sitilci AT, Ozyuvaci E, Alkan Z, et al. The effect of perioperative infused dexmedetomidine on postoperative analgesic consumption in mastoidectomy operations. Agri 2010;22(3):109–16 [in Turkish].

15. Lee DW, Lee HG, Jeong CY, et al. Postoperative nausea and vomiting after mastoidectomy with tympanoplasty: a comparison between TIVA with propofol-remifentanil and balanced anesthesia with sevoflurane-remifentanil. Korean J Anesthesiol 2011;61(5):399–404.

16. Ahn JH, Kim MR, Kim KH. Effect of i.v. dexamethasone on postoperative dizziness, nausea and pain during canal wall-up mastoidectomy. Acta Otolaryngol 2005;125(11):1176–9.

17. Bhandari G, Shahi KS, Parmar NK, et al. Evaluation of analgesic effect of two different doses of fentanyl in combination with bupivacaine for surgical site infiltration in cases of modified radical mastoidectomy: A double blind randomized study. Anesth Essays Res 2013;7(2):243–7.

18. Suresh S, Barcelona SL, Young NM, et al. Does a preemptive block of the great auricular nerve improve postoperative analgesia in children undergoing tympanomastoid surgery? Anesth Analg 2004;98(2):330–3.

19. Suresh S, Barcelona SL, Young NM, et al. Postoperative pain relief in children undergoing tympanomastoid surgery: is a regional block better than opioids? Anesth Analg 2002;94(4):859–62.

20. Swain A, Nag DS, Sahu S, et al. Adjuvants to local anesthetics: Current understanding and future trends. World J Clin Cases 2017;5(8):307–23.

21. Okmen K, Metin Okmen B. Ultrasound guided superficial cervical plexus block versus greater auricular nerve block for postoperative tympanomastoid surgery pain: A prospective, randomized, single blind study. Agri 2018;30(4):171–8.

22. Crippa B, Salzano FA, Mora R, et al. Comparison of postoperative pain: piezoelectric device versus microdrill. Eur Arch Otorhinolaryngol 2011;268(9):1279–82.

23. Meller C, Havas TE. Piezoelectric technology in otolaryngology, and head and neck surgery: a review. J Laryngol Otol 2017;131(S2):S12–8.

24. Sarmento KM Jr, Tomita S. Retroauricular tympanoplasty and tympanomastoidectomy under local anesthesia and sedation. Acta Otolaryngol 2009;129(7):726–8.

25. Yung MW. Local anaesthesia in middle ear surgery: survey of patients and surgeons. Clin Otolaryngol Allied Sci 1996;21(5):404–8.

26. Niiyama Y, Yotsuyanagi T, Yamakage M. Continuous wound infiltration with 0.2% ropivacaine versus a single intercostal nerve block with 0.75% ropivacaine for postoperative pain management after reconstructive surgery for microtia. J Plast Reconstr Aesthet Surg 2016;69(10):1445–9.

27. Woo KJ, Kang BY, Min JJ, et al. Postoperative pain control by preventive intercostal nerve block under direct vision followed by catheter-based infusion of local analgesics in rib cartilage harvest for auricular reconstruction in children with microtia: A randomized controlled trial. J Plast Reconstr Aesthet Surg 2016;69(9):1203–10.

28. Jellish WS, Murdoch J, Leonetti JP. Perioperative management of complex skull base surgery: the anesthesiologist's point of view. Neurosurg Focus 2002;12(5):e5.

29. Schessel DA, Nedzelski JM, Rowed D, et al. Pain after surgery for acoustic neuroma. Otolaryngol Head Neck Surg 1992;107(3):424–9.

30. Schessel DA, Rowed DW, Nedzelski JM, et al. Postoperative pain following excision of acoustic neuroma by the suboccipital approach: observations on possible cause and potential amelioration. Am J Otol 1993;14(5):491–4.

31. De Benedittis G, Lorenzetti A, Migliore M, et al. Postoperative pain in neurosurgery: a pilot study in brain surgery. Neurosurgery 1996;38(3):466–9 [discussion: 469–70].

32. Ryzenman JM, Pensak ML, Tew JM Jr. Headache: a quality of life analysis in a cohort of 1,657 patients undergoing acoustic neuroma surgery, results from the acoustic neuroma association. Laryngoscope 2005;115(4):703–11.

33. Irefin SA, Schubert A, Bloomfield EL, et al. The effect of craniotomy location on postoperative pain and nausea. J Anesth 2003;17(4):227–31.

34. Jellish WS, Leonetti JP, Sawicki K, et al. Morphine/ondansetron PCA for postoperative pain, nausea, and vomiting after skull base surgery. Otolaryngol Head Neck Surg 2006;135(2):175–81.

35. Magni G, La Rosa I, Melillo G, et al. Intracranial hemorrhage requiring surgery in neurosurgical patients given ketorolac: a case-control study within a cohort (2001-2010). Anesth Analg 2013;116(2):443–7.

36. Richardson MD, Palmeri NO, Williams SA, et al. Routine perioperative ketorolac administration is not associated with hemorrhage in pediatric neurosurgery patients. J Neurosurg Pediatr 2016;17(1):107–15.

37. Jellish WS, Leonetti JP, Buoy CM, et al. Facial nerve electromyographic monitoring to predict movement in patients titrated to a standard anesthetic depth. Anesth Analg 2009;109(2):551–8.

38. Hartsell T, Long D, Kirsch JR. The efficacy of postoperative ondansetron (Zofran) orally disintegrating tablets for preventing nausea and vomiting after acoustic neuroma surgery. Anesth Analg 2005;101(5):1492–6.

39. Henzi I, Sonderegger J, Tramer MR. Efficacy, dose-response, and adverse effects of droperidol for prevention of postoperative nausea and vomiting. Can J Anaesth 2000;47(6):537–51.

40. Henzi I, Walder B, Tramer MR. Dexamethasone for the prevention of postoperative nausea and vomiting: a quantitative systematic review. Anesth Analg 2000; 90(1):186–94.

Acute Pain Management Following Facial Plastic Surgery

Taha S. Meraj, MD[a], Amishav Bresler, MD[b],
Giancarlo F. Zuliani, MD[c,d],*

KEYWORDS

• Opioids • Pain • Septorhinoplasty • Rhytidectomy • Blepharoplasty

KEY POINTS

- Pain control after septorhinoplasty has been extensively studied with numerous randomized control trials exploring a variety of nonopioid analgesics. Most patients require fewer than 10 to 15 opioid tablets for adequate control of pain.
- Evidence in oculoplastic procedures is limited to the use of local anesthetics. Facelift procedures have limited evidence for nonsteroidal antiinflammatory drugs (NSAIDs), although their use may be limited secondary to concern for hematoma formation.
- There is evidence that major head and neck reconstructive procedures with free tissue transfer can be managed with a limited amount of opioid pain medication, instead substituting with a multimodal analgesic protocol including acetaminophen and NSAIDs.

INTRODUCTION

Acute pain control after surgery is an important factor for patient satisfaction and clinical outcomes. Although opioids are very effective in the treatment of pain, their use has come under extreme scrutiny because of the increase in addiction and opioid-related deaths in the United States and other countries. Judicious use of opioids is appropriate; however, inadequate treatment of pain has shown negative effects on quality of life, increased hospital readmissions, and increased length of stay for patients undergoing surgery. Clinicians and researchers have used several strategies to determine the appropriate number of opioid pain pills to prescribe. These strategies include consideration of alternative analgesics and combination therapies, using analgesics in the preoperative setting, and setting appropriate expectations with the patients and families regarding the degree of postoperative pain.

[a] Department of Otolaryngology, Wayne State University, 4201 St Antoine 5E-UHC, Detroit, MI 48201, USA; [b] Department of Otolaryngology, Rutgers University, 90 Bergen Street, Suite 8100, Newark, NJ 07208, USA; [c] Department of Otolaryngology, Wayne State University, Detroit, MI, USA; [d] Zuliani Facial Aesthetics, 50 West Big Beaver, #280, Bloomfield Hills, MI 48304, USA
* Corresponding author. Zuliani Facial Aesthetics, 50 West Big Beaver, #280, Bloomfield Hills, MI 48304.
E-mail address: gfzuliani@gmail.com

Otolaryngol Clin N Am 53 (2020) 811–817
https://doi.org/10.1016/j.otc.2020.05.010
0030-6665/20/© 2020 Elsevier Inc. All rights reserved.

oto.theclinics.com

This article explores the evidence available to support these alternative modalities for the treatment of acute surgical pain in a series of common facial plastic procedures, including septorhinoplasty, oculoplastic surgery, rhytidectomy, otoplasty, and free flap reconstruction procedures (**Table 1**). It presents an evidence-based review and combines it with the authors' clinical experience.

Septorhinoplasty

Septorhinoplasty is one of the most common procedures performed by facial plastic surgeons and otolaryngologists. As such, the greatest amount of available evidence regarding perioperative analgesia is available for this procedure. The quality of evidence is strengthened by several randomized control trials and a meta-analysis. This article presents the available evidence and combines it with our own clinical experience.

Nguyen and colleagues[1] published the only systematic review on the use of nonopioid analgesia regimens following septoplasty and/or rhinoplasty. There were 37 published articles, including several randomized single-blinded and double-blinded trials evaluating evidence for the perioperative use of alpha agonists such as dexmedetomidine and xylometazoline, nonsteroidal antiinflammatory drugs (NSAIDs), gabapentinoids (pregabalin and gabapentin), local anesthetic agents, and other agents, including ketamine, magnesium, β-blockers, and acupuncture.

The strongest evidence was available for the use of local anesthetics followed by gabapentinoids. NSAIDs and alpha agonists were considerations; however, their use may be limited by their side effect profile. Fourteen articles were analyzed, all of which were randomized control trials, including several high-quality studies. Local

Table 1
Opioid alternatives following septorhinoplasty

Analgesia	Benefit	Harm	Recommendation	Dosing
Local anesthetics	Rapid onset, safe	Local irritation, toxicity with systemic absorption	Strongly recommended	Minimal amount needed to achieve analgesia up to the following: Bupivacaine 2–3 mg/kg Lidocaine 5–7 mg/kg
NSAIDs	Safe, widely used	Bleeding, GI upset, nausea	Option	Celecoxib 200 mg twice daily Ketorolac IV 30 mg once
Gabapentionoids	Neuromodulator, reduces pain scores	Potential for abuse	Option	Gabapentin 300 mg daily Pregabalin 300 mg daily
Acetaminophen	Widely used, safe	Liver toxicity with overdose	Strongly recommended	Acetaminophen 500 mg every 6 h

Abbreviations: GI, gastrointestinal; IV, intravenous; NSAIDs, nonsteroidal antiinflammatory drug.

anesthetics were found to be safe, rapid, and efficacious at decreasing other pain medication requirements in this review. The investigators recommended their use given these findings.

NSAIDs are a valuable component in the armamentarium for pain control; however, their risk profile for bleeding may limit use. NSAIDs are cyclooxygenase inhibitors, which decrease the formation of prostaglandins and thromboxane A2 and lead to pain control as well as decreased platelet function. Use has largely been limited because of the concern for bleeding. It is our practice, as well as that of other surgeons, to advise patients to avoid both preoperative and postoperative NSAIDs use because of the fear of epistaxis. This fear is compounded especially in septorhinoplasty, because the nose is a highly vascular area and the use of packing augments both pain and obstruction in the nasal cavity. The investigators reviewed 5 prospective double-blinded studies and found high-quality evidence that NSAIDs decrease postoperative rescue analgesic requirements; although no included studies specifically evaluated epistaxis, none reported significant bleeding either.

Seven prospective randomized controlled trials were included that evaluated gabapentinoids, which are medications, including gabapentin and pregabalin, that are thought to exert their effects by the inhibition of presynaptic voltage-gated calcium channels leading to decreased neurotransmitter release.[2] Although the dosage varied between studies, 6 of the 7 trials reported decreased pain scores compared with placebo. Drowsiness and dizziness limit their safety profile and their use must be carefully considered in elderly patients. These medications can be considered adjunct and are especially helpful in the first 24 hours after surgery. Recently, there has been increased concern for the potential of abuse with these medications. The state of Michigan now lists gabapentin as a schedule 5 drug. Clinicians should exercise increased caution when prescribing this medication and obtain a consent similar to that for opioid medication.

There are several other articles in the literature that further discuss how best to treat pain and set appropriate patient expectations. Gozeler and colleagues[3] explored in a randomized double-blinded study whether a single dose of 800 mg of intravenous (IV) ibuprofen given 30 minutes before septorhinoplasty would decrease perioperative opioid requirements. Fifty patients were administered either saline or ibuprofen before incision. Patients were given patient-controlled analgesia (PCA) following the procedure in their postanesthesia care unit. Patient who received IV ibuprofen reported less pain on a visual analog scale at all time points from 10 minutes to 24 hours after the procedure. They also had half the opioid consumption from their PCAs. The investigators concluded that the use of preoperative IV ibuprofen was effective as preemptive therapy to decrease postoperative opioid requirements.

Rock and colleagues[4] recently conducted a retrospective review of 64 patients that underwent septoplasty or rhinoplasty. Although an average of 42.4 tablets were prescribed, patients consumed a median of 14.7 tablets. Similarly, Patel and colleagues[5] reported a case series of 62 patients and found that patients used a median of 8.7 tablets postoperatively with 75% using less than 15 tablets. Sclafani and colleagues[6] compared septoplasty and rhinoplasty for postoperative opioid requirement and similarly found that 90% of patients required fewer than 11 tablets for optimal control.

Aulet and colleagues[7] recently reported a case-control study before and after enactment of a local state regulation requiring physicians to check a prescription monitoring system before prescribing opioids. The investigators reviewed 80 patients evenly divided between both groups and found that, although the number of tablets prescribed decreased nearly in half (18.2 pills to 9.7 pills), there was no increase in the number of complaints or additional opioid pain medication prescriptions. These studies provide important information for counseling patients on expectations regarding pain postoperatively.

It is currently our practice to prescribe 15 tablets of hydrocodone-acetaminophen 5 mg/325 mg to our patients undergoing septorhinoplasty and to have patients transition to acetaminophen alone as their pain continues to improve. A formal discussion about the untoward effects of opioid medication must be had with each patient as well. Postoperative nausea and constipation can be alleviated with prescriptions of Zofran ODT and increased consumption of water with a possible stool softener. A discussion of the functional outcomes and pain satisfaction with the procedure may also affect perception of pain and postoperative analgesic requirement, and these should also be discussed with each patient during the preoperative visit.[8]

Aging Face

In contrast with the wealth of studies addressing septorhinoplasty, considerably fewer studies are available for surgeries addressing the aging face. The available evidence for oculoplastic procedures (brow surgery and blepharoplasty) and aging face surgeries (facelift and neck lift) are discussed next.

Brow lifts are often performed under deep sedation or general anesthesia. There is a paucity of data published regarding postoperative pain control and brow lifts. There have been no investigations into the amount of opioids prescribed, the amount consumed, use of adjunct pain medications (eg, ketorolac), neuromodulators (eg, pregabalin), or long-acting local anesthetics (eg, liposomal bupivacaine). Patients who experience preoperative headaches may continue to experience headaches afterward, although the frequency may decrease.[9] These patients should continue to be treated in a similar fashion as preoperatively. Future robust studies should be initiated to identify safe and efficacious pain regimens with restrained but appropriate use of narcotics and adjunctive medications and modalities.

In general, blepharoplasty is performed under local anesthesia with sedation. Infiltration of local anesthetic can be painful and often invokes fear among patients. EMLA cream, composed of lidocaine and prilocaine with 25 mg/1 g, has been investigated as a preinjection treatment of upper lid blepharoplasty. In a surgeon-blinded randomized trial, 64% of untreated patients had moderate to severe pain during injection, which decreased to 14% in the cohort of patients treated with EMLA cream.[10] In addition, in a follow-up retrospective study by Saariniemi and colleagues,[11] EMLA cream, when used preoperatively for 15 minutes, was not associated with increased postoperative swelling or bruising, poor wound healing, unfavorable scar appearance, and need corrective procedures. Surprisingly, eye irritation was more common in the control group (EMLA, 0% vs control, 11%; $P = .03$).[11] In addition to pretreating patients with topical anesthetics, proper injection technique is of absolute importance for maximal patient comfort. In a systematic review, effective maneuvers for decreasing injection-associated pain included modifying the solution (buffering, dilution, warming), skin cooling, tactile distraction (eg, vibration), and low rate of injection.[12]

Postoperative pain associated with isolated blepharoplasty is low and patients primarily rely on acetaminophen for postoperative analgesia. However, to limit acetaminophen intake, physicians have begun investigating administering preemptive analgesics. In randomized controlled double-blinded study of 52 patients, a single dose of 150 mg of pregabalin or placebo was administered to patients 15 minutes before undergoing upper eyelid surgery (ie, blepharoplasty, ptosis repair, canthoplasty, eyelid retraction repair, pentagonal wedge resection, and Mohs reconstruction).[13] On postoperative visual analog pain scores, the pregabalin group reported pains scores on average 5.5 points lower than the control groups up to 48 hours post-operatively. In addition, the pregabalin group consumed 50% less acetaminophen (1.3 g) on average compared with the control group (2.6 g) for the first 48 hours after surgery. However, future large-scale studies are required to fully elucidate the role these neuropathic pain modulators may play in oculoplastic pain control regimens. However, no study has investigated the safety or efficacy of use of NSAIDs or opioids in oculoplastic blepharoplasty.

Evidence for acute management of pain following facelift surgery is limited in the medical literature. One of the earliest reports in the literature is by Hoefflin,[14] who in 1992 reported his practice to administer IV dexamethasone and diphenhydramine combined with a topical mist of Kenalog and bupivacaine into the surgical field to decrease surgical pain.

Aynehchi and colleagues[15] evaluated the use of celecoxib for patients undergoing deep plane facelift. In this retrospective study, 50 patients were given both preoperative and standing postoperative celecoxib, whereas 50 patients did not receive any dosing. The treatment group reported decreased pain and required almost half the number of opioid tablets compared with the nontreatment group. The study did not comment on the incidence of postoperative hematoma.

Jones and colleagues[16] investigated the use of postoperative facial cooling on 1 side of the face with the other side as the control. The use of the cooling mask increased facial swelling but did not decrease pain on that side of the face. Torgerson and colleagues[17] investigated the use of ketorolac in a prospective randomized trial of 140 patients. Ninety-five patients received locally injected therapy, 20 patients received intramuscular doses, and the remaining patients received local anesthetic alone. Patients who received locally injected ketorolac required significantly less postoperative analgesic than both the other groups.

Based on the data presented here and the theoretic risk of postoperative hematoma that can lead to flap necrosis, it is currently our practice to prescribe hydrocodone-acetaminophen and transition patients to acetaminophen as soon as their pain improves. We do not use drains in our surgery and rely on meticulous hemostasis combined with Tisseel (Baxter Healthcare) tissue adhesive spray containing sealer protein and thrombin to convert fibrinogen into a fibrin clot.

Otoplasty

The medical literature is limited regarding acute pain management with otoplasty. One case report discusses the use of a cervical plexus block with levobupivacaine resulting in the patient requiring no postoperative pain medication.[18] In another study, Cregg and colleagues[19] examined 43 children randomized to local anesthetic anterior and posterior with lidocaine to the pinna or a regional nerve blockage using levobupivacaine. Children were followed for 24 hours afterward. There were no differences in postoperative opioid requirements in these patients.

It is currently our practice to locally ring block the patient with a mixture of 0.5% lidocaine 1:200,000 epinephrine combined with an equal concentration of 0.25% Marcaine. Younger patients require liquid analgesia, whereas older patients are prescribed the standard 15 pills of opioid medications.

Free Tissue Transfer

Management of pain in complex head and neck reconstruction involving free tissue transfer can be difficult. Morbidity and pain from both the reconstruction site and donor site can amplify analgesic requirements. Patients and physicians may have different expectations regarding appropriate pain control. Despite the use of opioid PCA, patients may have inadequate control of their pain.[20]

Chiu and colleagues[21] explored the use of a single preoperative dose of gabapentin in patients undergoing anterolateral thigh free flap reconstruction for tongue defects. Fifty consecutive patients were included in this study. Half of the participants were administered 1200 mg of gabapentin preoperatively, whereas the other half did not. The investigators reported a decrease in visual analog scale pain scores and morphine PCA requirements in the first 24 hours postoperatively.

Carpenter and colleagues[22] analyzed the use of celecoxib in patients undergoing head and neck surgery with free flap reconstruction. In a retrospective review, patients who received celecoxib had decreased oral, IV, and total opioid requirements.

Eggerstedt and colleagues[23] conducted a retrospective cohort study comparing patients receiving a protocol of multimodal analgesia compared with a traditional regimen in patients undergoing head and neck free flap reconstruction. The multimodal regimen consisted of preoperative oral and IV acetaminophen and oral gabapentin. Postoperatively, patients received scheduled oral acetaminophen, gabapentin, celecoxib, and 3 days of as-needed IV ketorolac. Further requirements were satisfied with fentanyl, either IV push or PCA in opioid-tolerant patients (up to 24 hours). The control group received acetaminophen, hydrocodone-acetaminophen, and IV morphine as needed. The investigators compared morphine-equivalent doses and found a substantial decrease in the multimodal analgesia, in which patients required an average of 10.0 equivalents compared with 89.6 in the traditional analgesia group. Protocols such as this can be used to decrease opioid use even in the most complex head and neck reconstructions.

SUMMARY

Pain after facial plastic surgery procedures can vary widely based on procedure and patient factors. There are several strategies that clinicians can use to reduce the overall opioid requirements for these patients. It is incumbent on physicians to continue to educate patients on expectations regarding pain. Physicians must continue to search for novel approaches to treat pain and continue to reduce reliance on opioid pain medication to help curtail the overwhelming public health crisis.

REFERENCES

1. Nguyen BK, Yuhan BT, Folbe E, et al. Perioperative analgesia for patients undergoing septoplasty and rhinoplasty: an evidence-based review. Laryngoscope 2019;129(6):E200–12.

2. Sills GJ. The mechanisms of action of gabapentin and pregabalin. Curr Opin Pharmacol 2006;6(1):108–13.

3. Gozeler MS, Sakat MS, Kilic K, et al. Does a single-dose preemptive intravenous ibuprofen have an effect on postoperative pain relief after septorhinoplasty? Am J Otolaryngol 2018;39(6):726–30.

4. Rock AN, Akakpo K, Cheresnick C, et al. Postoperative prescriptions and corresponding opioid consumption after septoplasty or rhinoplasty. Ear Nose Throat J 2019. https://doi.org/10.1177/0145561319866824. 145561319866824.

5. Patel S, Sturm A, Bobian M, et al. Opioid use by patients after rhinoplasty. JAMA Facial Plast Surg 2018;20(1):24–30.

6. Sclafani AP, Kim M, Kjaer K, et al. Postoperative pain and analgesic requirements after septoplasty and rhinoplasty. Laryngoscope 2019;129(9):2020–5.

7. Aulet RM, Trieu V, Landrigan GP, et al. Changes in opioid prescribing habits for patients undergoing rhinoplasty and septoplasty. JAMA Facial Plast Surg 2019; 21(6):487–90.

8. Gadkaree SK, Shaye DA, Occhiogrosso J, et al. Association between pain and patient satisfaction after rhinoplasty. JAMA Facial Plast Surg 2019;21(6):475–9.

9. Panella NJ, Wallin JL, Goldman ND. Patient outcomes, satisfaction, and improvement in headaches after endoscopic brow-lift. JAMA Facial Plast Surg 2013; 15(4):263–7.

10. Henrici K, Clemens S, Tost F. Application of EMLA creme before upper lid blepharoplasty. Ophthalmologe 2005;102(8):794–7 [in German].

11. Saariniemi KM, Salmi AM, Kuokkanen HO. Can topical EMLA cream be used safely in upper blepharoplasty? Eur J Plast Surg 2013;36(8):485–8.

12. Gostimir M, Hussain A. A systematic review and meta-analysis of methods for reducing local anesthetic injection pain among patients undergoing periocular surgery. Ophthal Plast Reconstr Surg 2019;35(2):113–25.

13. Wei LA, Davies BW, Hink EM, et al. Perioperative pregabalin for attenuation of postoperative pain after eyelid surgery. Ophthal Plast Reconstr Surg 2015; 31(2):132–5.

14. Hoefflin SM. Decreasing prolonged swelling and pain associated with deep plane face lifts. Plast Reconstr Surg 1992;90(6):1125.

15. Aynehchi BB, Cerrati EW, Rosenberg DB. The efficacy of oral celecoxib for acute postoperative pain in face-lift surgery. JAMA Facial Plast Surg 2014;16(5):306–9.

16. Jones BM, Grover R, Southwell-Keely JP. Post-operative hilotherapy in SMAS-based facelift surgery: a prospective, randomised, controlled trial. J Plast Reconstr Aesthet Surg 2011;64(9):1132–7.

17. Torgerson C, Yoskovitch A, Cole AF, et al. Postoperative pain management with ketorolac in facial plastic surgery patients. J Otolaryngol Head Neck Surg 2008;37(6):888–93.

18. Ueshima H, Shimazaki A, Otake H. Cervical plexus block for perioperative analgesia during otoplasty. J Clin Anesth 2017;38:71.

19. Cregg N, Conway F, Casey W. Analgesia after otoplasty: regional nerve blockade vs local anaesthetic infiltration of the ear. Can J Anaesth 1996;43(2):141–7.

20. Hinther A, Nakoneshny SC, Chandarana SP, et al. Efficacy of postoperative pain management in head and neck cancer patients. J Otolaryngol Head Neck Surg 2018;47(1):29.

21. Chiu TW, Leung CC, Lau EY, et al. Analgesic effects of preoperative gabapentin after tongue reconstruction with the anterolateral thigh flap. Hong Kong Med J 2012;18(1):30–4.

22. Carpenter PS, Shepherd HM, McCrary H, et al. Association of celecoxib use with decreased opioid requirements after head and neck cancer surgery with free tissue reconstruction. JAMA Otolaryngol Head Neck Surg 2018;144(11):988–94.

23. Eggerstedt M, Stenson KM, Ramirez EA, et al. Association of perioperative opioid-sparing multimodal analgesia with narcotic use and pain control after head and neck free flap reconstruction. JAMA Facial Plast Surg 2019;21(5): 446–51.

Perioperative Analgesia in Pediatric Patients Undergoing Otolaryngologic Surgery

Andrew J. Maroda, MD[a,b], Kimberly K. Coca, BS[b],
Jennifer D. McLevy-Bazzanella, MD[b], Joshua W. Wood, MD[b],
Erica C. Grissom, CRNA[c], Anthony M. Sheyn, MD[a,d,e],*

KEYWORDS

- Acute pain • Analgesia • Children • Otolaryngology • Outpatient • Day surgery
- Ambulatory care • Nonopioid

KEY POINTS

- Management of peri-operative pain is an important component of surgical management of pediatric patients and affects the post-operative course.
- The best strategies for managing pain include a combination of behavioral and pharmacologic interventions.
- Very little literature exists on pain management for medically complex children such as those with head and neck cancer and sickle cell disease.

INTRODUCTION

Pediatric perioperative pain control presents a unique dilemma for medical providers, especially given the immature physiology of children and challenges in communicating about pain with the pediatric population. Historically, severe postoperative pain has been shown to be an underacknowledged surgical complication associated with increased overall morbidity and mortality in the pediatric population.[1] Some studies

[a] Department of Pediatric Otolaryngology, Le Bonheur Children's Hospital, Memphis, TN, USA; [b] Department of Otolaryngology—Head and Neck Surgery, University of Tennessee Health Science Center, Memphis, TN, USA; [c] Department of Anesthesiology, Le Bonheur Children's Hospital, Memphis, TN, USA; [d] Department of Otolaryngology—Head and Neck Surgery, University of Tennessee Health Science Center, 910 Madison Avenue, Suite 400, Memphis, TN 38163-2242, USA; [e] Department of Pediatric Otolaryngology, St. Jude Children's Research Hospital, Memphis, TN, USA
* Corresponding author. Department of Otolaryngology—Head and Neck Surgery, University of Tennessee Health Science Center, 910 Madison Avenue, Suite 400, Memphis, TN 38163-2242.
E-mail address: asheyn@uthsc.edu

Otolaryngol Clin N Am 53 (2020) 819–830
https://doi.org/10.1016/j.otc.2020.05.011
0030-6665/20/© 2020 Elsevier Inc. All rights reserved.

have also demonstrated that patients with inadequately controlled pain may become more sensitive to subsequent painful stimuli and experience decreased efficacy of future analgesics, thereby increasing risk of developing chronic pain.[2-4] In pediatric otolaryngology, uncontrolled postoperative pain is often associated with adverse events, such as airway compromise, restless sleep, behavioral changes, and difficulty tolerating oral fluids, all of which can significantly complicate the recovery period.[1,5] Recognizing the impact of perioperative pain on a patient's physical, emotional, and psychological well-being is crucial for physicians to improve surgical outcomes and reduce overall morbidity following otolaryngologic surgery.

Assessing perioperative pain in pediatric patients can often be quite challenging. Young children generally lack the verbal and cognitive abilities necessary to describe their level of pain, and certain medications have variable sedative and analgesic effects in children. Although the sensation of pain is both subjective and unique to each patient, multiple tools have been used in order to monitor and quantify a patient's pain experience. For example, these widely used tools include self-reporting (eg, faces scales), behavioral cues (eg, Parents' Postoperative Pain Measure and FLACC Pain Assessment Tool), and even tracking vital signs and physiologic reactions.[6-9] Despite these measures, a child's postoperative pain often remains inadequately recognized by both physicians and parents alike.[5,10,11] Thus, using evidence-based pain management strategies may compensate for these initial challenges.

Choice of pain medication for pediatric patients in the postoperative period has also evolved over time. Depending on the nature, location, and extent of the surgical intervention, different pain management strategies may be more effective than others. Formerly, codeine was commonly prescribed to manage a broad range of postoperative pain. However, codeine and other narcotics have now been associated with numerous adverse events in children. For example, duplication of the gene encoding cytochrome PD4502D6 (CYP2D6) is associated with ultrarapid metabolism of codeine. These patients may metabolize codeine too efficiently, leading to morphine intoxication. Furthermore, the rapid metabolism of codeine was linked to severe respiratory depression in these patients, causing multiple fatalities.[12] In 2013, the American Academy of Otolaryngology–Head and Neck Surgery adjusted clinical practice guidelines in response to the Food and Drug Administration (FDA)'s boxed warning to discontinue codeine usage in the pediatric population.[13,14] Given these catastrophic risks with narcotics, simple analgesics, such as acetaminophen and nonsteroidal anti-inflammatory drugs (NSAIDs), have become preferred alternatives to control postoperative pain with minimal adverse effects. In 2012, the World Health Organization (WHO) presented guidelines for the treatment of children with persistent pain and medical illness, which can be appropriately applied to patients in pediatric otolaryngology.[15] This article focuses on current trends in the management of perioperative pain following otolaryngologic surgery in the pediatric population.

METHODS OF PEDIATRIC PAIN ASSESSMENT

The first step in postoperative pain management is to assess the severity of pain being experienced by the patient. As mentioned previously, this task can often be difficult in children, especially in patients less than 3 years of age, because they frequently lack the cognitive development to express themselves reliably. Children with developmental disabilities may also lack the communication skills or sensory perception to effectively express associated pain and discomfort. Because uncontrolled pain impacts multiple systems, various physiologic changes may be monitored to determine the level of pain being experienced.[16]

In addition to clinical impression and monitoring, several strategies and validated tools have been developed in order to adequately assess the severity of pain in the pediatric population.[17] These tools include behavioral assessment, facial scales, self-reporting methods, projective methods, and structured interview. Behavioral assessment has been shown to be most useful in the preverbal phase. Although useful, facial analog scales have been determined to be an imprecise measure of pain when used alone, because children often have difficulty separating pain from mood when using these scales.[18] Therefore, facial analog scales are best used in combination with other self-reporting methods, such as projective methods and questionnaires. However, these methods generally require the patient to be cognitively developed enough to communicate freely and reliably with caregivers.[17]

Medication Strategies

Based on the 2012 WHO guidelines for the treatment of children with persistent pain and medical illness, a 2-step approach is recommended, using 1 type of analgesia for mild pain followed by a second type of medication for moderate to severe pain.[15] An example of this would be the utilization of NSAIDs and acetaminophen following surgery with the addition of morphine prescribed as needed for uncontrolled or breakthrough pain. However, routine rotation of opioids is not recommended.[15] In addition, these pain medications should be dosed in regular intervals in the early postoperative period even in the event of mild pain, rather than given as needed, to prevent development of moderate or severe pain. Using the appropriate route of administration is also important when considering your patient population. When administering medications in pediatric patients, the WHO recommends oral and intravenous (IV) delivery methods over intramuscular injections in order to limit any additional burden of pain.[15] Ultimately, although these guidelines are highly recommended, they are not prescriptive, and adjustments can be made so that treatment can be tailored to the specific needs of the individual child.

SURGERY SPECIFIC RECOMMENDATIONS
Otologic Surgery

Most otologic procedures in the pediatric population are generally well tolerated and do not require extensive prescription pain medication during the postoperative period. Despite an imbalance of literature discussing bilateral myringotomy and tympanostomy tube placement (BMT), many principles across otologic procedures remain consistent. Because otologic surgery is frequently performed on an outpatient basis, effective perioperative pain management may help reduce the need for excessive postoperative opioid prescriptions.[19]

BMT is one of the most common surgeries performed in pediatric otolaryngology and is generally indicated for patients with recurrent acute otitis media or chronic serous otitis media with effusion.[19–22] Effective ambulatory anesthesia for children requiring myringotomy and ventilation tubes is key to improving the child's experience and overall parental satisfaction.[20] Because tympanic membranes are primarily innervated by the auriculotemporal nerve, myringotomy incisions can be quite stimulating, and periprocedural analgesic requirements in children undergoing surgery may be variable. General anesthesia is recommended and can be maintained with either an IV or an inhalational technique. Because of the brevity of this operation and the general health of these patients, the procedure is generally performed without placement of an airway device or IV cannula.[21] Intranasal fentanyl or intranasal dexmedetomidine, both short-acting inhaled agents, are the preferred intraoperative sedatives for this procedure.[20]

Several preoperative medications and alternative therapies have been proposed for BMT over the years, but none have become formally adopted in practice because of their low comparative clinical benefit. For example, Watcha and colleagues[22] conducted a double-blinded, placebo-controlled study reporting that preoperative administration of oral ketorolac, but not acetaminophen, provided better postoperative pain control than placebo in children undergoing bilateral myringotomy ($P<.05$). However, several respondents, such as Bean-Lijewski and colleagues,[23] concluded that the slight analgesic benefit from ketorolac did not justify its cost in BMT surgery. Postoperatively, nonopioid oral analgesia should be encouraged where possible. Overall, because postoperative discomfort from BMT rarely extends beyond 48 hours, parents are advised to focus on administering simple analgesia, such as acetaminophen and NSAIDs, and regular assessment of their child's pain at home.[20]

In children undergoing tympanomastoid surgery, adequate analgesia may typically be achieved with NSAIDs or local anesthetic plus fentanyl injection at the surgical site.[19] At this time, there is still conflicting evidence for greater auricular nerve blocks in the management of postmastoidectomy pain, although these may have the largest potential to reduce the need for opiates in the perioperative period.[24,25] Other studies have reported postoperative analgesic benefit from the combination of bupivacaine and higher-dose fentanyl (100 μg vs 50 μg) for operative field infiltration.[26] However, regardless of technique, postoperative pain control is easily achieved with nonopioid medications following this procedure.[19]

Based on available literature encompassing middle ear surgeries (MES), such as stapedectomy and tympanoplasty, there are primarily data regarding systemic administration of opiates (remifentanil or fentanyl) or α-agonists (dexmedetomidine) at this time.[19] According to Mesolella and colleagues,[27] remifentanil has been found to decrease intraoperative and postoperative reactions and complications, such as dizziness, nausea, vomiting, and pain. In addition, 2 double-blinded randomized control trials by Nallam and colleagues[28] and Parrikh and colleagues,[29] respectively, found dexmedetomidine to be similarly effective to midazolam plus fentanyl in tympanoplasty and superior in combination with nalbuphine compared with nalbuphine plus propofol for MES.[19] Given the nature of these procedures and based on the available literature, it remains unclear whether nonopioid medications can provide sufficient analgesia in these patients.

Cochlear implantation surgery is another otologic surgery that is generally very well tolerated in pediatric patients. According to a prospective study of 61 patients conducted by Birman and colleagues,[30] postoperative pain in these patients was found to be minimal. In their study, 19 children required no postoperative analgesia, and 42 children used paracetamol, with an average use of 1.9 days after discharge from the hospital. In addition, children undergoing cochlear implant surgery experienced low rates of dizziness in the first 1 week postoperatively. In rare cases, infection and skin breakdown may present as postoperative complications causing patient discomfort. However, under normal circumstances, these patients require minimal pharmacologic therapy for postoperative pain management, and opioid pain medications are generally unnecessary. In general, the reported adverse events from analgesic agents used in otologic surgeries are minor and transient.

Sinonasal Surgery

Despite the wealth of literature regarding perioperative analgesia for sinonasal surgery in adults, there is a paucity of published data regarding the pediatric population.

However, some lessons learned from pain management in the adult population may also be applied to the pediatric population. In both pediatric and adult populations, there has been a focus on decreasing the use of opioid medications following sino-nasal surgery.[31] A recent review of pain control following endoscopic sinus surgery demonstrated the utility of NSAIDs, acetaminophen, and gabapentin as viable alternatives to opioids in controlling postoperative pain.[32] In the authors' experience, opioids have not been necessary in treating postoperative pain following common sinonasal procedures, including septoplasty, closed reduction of nasal fractures, or endoscopic sinus surgery. Overall, reflecting other outpatient otolaryngologic procedures, alternating acetaminophen and ibuprofen as needed has demonstrated sufficient perioperative analgesia in this pediatric population.

Airway Surgery

Balancing adequate analgesia with airway safety remains a challenge and requires attentive multidisciplinary care to achieve successful outcomes.[33] Because children have a smaller-caliber and more dynamic airway at baseline, any degree of edema increases the risk of airway compromise. Suboptimal pain control causes agitation and crying, therefore increasing the patient's risk of developing airway complications or compromise following surgery.[34] Strategies to reduce emergence agitation, optimize pain control, and avoid respiratory depression are crucial considerations for perioperative surgical airway management.

As with general pediatric postoperative pain management, the mainstay of therapy includes acetaminophen and ibuprofen. Ondansetron is also recommended to prevent nausea and vomiting in patients older than 2 years old. Retching and vomiting are potentially catastrophic events after an open airway surgery because these increase the risk of postoperative complications, such as disruption of the surgical site and aspiration of gastric contents.[35] Ondansetron is not needed in patients less than 2 years of age because of their underdeveloped chemoreceptor trigger zone. A single dose of intraoperative steroids, most commonly dexamethasone, is used to mitigate airway edema, unless there is a strong contraindication (eg, labile diabetic). Postoperatively, patients may be given 0.5 mg/kg of dexamethasone (a maximum dose of 10 mg) every 8 hours for 24 to 48 hours postoperatively Dexmedetomidine, a centrally acting alpha-2 adrenergic agonist, benefits postoperatively after airway surgery to prevent agitation, maintain pain control, and keep the patient breathing spontaneously.[36–38] Sevoflurane is an inhaled anesthetic with reduced risk of laryngospasm as compared with desflurane. It can be used in combination with propofol to provide adequate surgical sedation without paralysis in airway cases requiring spontaneous respiration.

In general, opioids suppress respiratory drive and are often avoided in airway surgery patients. If a patient requires opioids perioperatively, fentanyl is preferred over morphine. Morphine is difficult to dose and induces histamine release, risking airway spasm in patients with asthma or reactive airway disease.[39] Laryngotracheal reconstruction or high-grade laryngeal cleft repair often requires the patient to remain intubated and sedated postoperatively to allow adequate healing.[36] In these patients, opioids, such as fentanyl, are safe, appropriate, and fall within the standard of care.[39] In conclusion, effective postoperative pain management in pediatric airway patients centers on optimization of pain control, while avoiding agitation and respiratory suppression.

Sleep Surgery (Adenotonsillectomy)

Tonsillectomy is one of the most common operations in the pediatric population with more than a quarter million performed annually in the United States.[40] The operation is associated with moderate to severe postoperative pain that is often difficult to control. This pain is likely secondary to inflammation and pharyngeal spasm, and persistent discomfort can last up to 20 days postoperatively.[41] Developing strategies to obtain optimal analgesia with few adverse effects has proven challenging and is a topic of continual discussion in the literature. Tonsillectomy is indicated in the surgical management of obstructive sleep apnea, among other things, and these patients present a particular struggle in perioperative pain management because they have increased risk of opioid-induced respiratory depression and a paradoxically enhanced pain sensitivity because of chronic systemic inflammation.[42] The most recent clinical practice guidelines on pediatric tonsillectomy discuss pain management with the following recommendations: perioperative pain counseling to patients and caregivers, single dose of IV dexamethasone intraoperatively, and postoperative ibuprofen and/or acetaminophen.[40] Notably, the guidelines strongly recommended against the use of perioperative antibiotics and postoperative codeine.[13,40,43]

Operative planning may play a role in the management of postoperative pain. Studies have shown that tonsillotomy significantly reduces postoperative pain and hemorrhage but maintains a risk of future tonsillar regrowth.[44] There is also some evidence that a cold-steel tonsillectomy technique results in decreased postoperative pain when compared with a hot technique.[44]

Routine posttonsillectomy analgesia uses acetaminophen with or without ibuprofen, and opioids for severe or break-through pain.[17,40] IV acetaminophen can be given during the operation to reduce usage of morphine postoperatively.[45] There has been concern about increased bleeding risk postoperatively with use of NSAIDs. Studies have shown that there is an increased risk of bleeding with ketorolac, but other NSAIDs do not confer this increased risk.[46] NSAIDs inhibit the COX enzyme pathway and thus reduce prostaglandins and inflammation.[17] Ibuprofen is the recommended NSAID in children and successfully treats mild to moderate pain.[17] It also reduces postoperative nausea and vomiting.[46] Although not first-line analgesia, opioids prescribed at safe dosages, such as morphine (0.2–0.5 mg/kg, every 4–6 hours), oxycodone (0.05–0.15 mg/kg, every 4–6 hours), and hydrocodone (0.1–0.2 mg/kg, every 6–8 hours), as needed are an appropriate option for breakthrough or severe pain after tonsillectomy.[47] These medications are relatively safe, and most complications are preventable. The oral route is recommended for most medications, followed by IV administration, and last, the intramuscular route.[48] Most complications secondary to opiate administration are due to a miscalculation either during the initiation of opioid medication or during a change to a different drug. The most recent clinical practice guidelines recommend that if opioids are needed postoperatively, they should be used at low doses with watchful titration and continuous pulse oximetry.[40] Although NSAIDs and acetaminophen can be stopped without side effects in most cases, a prolonged course of opioid medication requires weaning to avoid withdrawal symptoms. As ideal analgesic regimens shift away from the use of opioids, numerous alternative regimens have been described to reduce the usage of opioids postoperatively.

COX-2 selective agents represent potential therapeutic opportunity in pain management because they selectively inhibit the prostaglandin pathway without having an impact on platelets. A study on rofecoxib, no longer FDA approved, showed that COX-2 agents result in improved pain scores when compared with hydrocodone-acetaminophen in postoperative pediatric patients, with no difference in adverse effects.[23] Although these agents are not widely used or studied at this time, these findings highlight a potential opportunity for growth in pediatric postoperative pain management.

Steroids have become a generally recommended and reliable method to reduce pain postoperatively. Preoperative peritonsillar infiltration with dexamethasone 0.5 mg/kg (a maximum dose of 8 mg) significantly reduces both early and late posttonsillectomy pain, allows earlier oral intake, and reduces postoperative nausea and vomiting.[14,49,50]

Usage of preoperative and intraoperative IV dexmedetomidine, an alpha-2 adrenoreceptor agonist, at a dosage of 0.2 to 0.5 μg/kg, is an effective method to reduce opioid exposure perioperatively.[51] When used in combination with 1 to 2 mL peritonsillar bupivacaine (0.25%), usage of intraoperative opioids and volatile anesthetics was significantly reduced, and patients reported lower maximum pain scores postoperatively.[51] This therapy was associated with no increase in complications.

Montelukast is a cysteinyl leukotriene receptor antagonist and reduces inflammation.[52] Although it was developed to treat bronchial asthma, some studies have also shown it has been found to reduce posttonsillectomy pain and need for rescue analgesics when given orally the night before surgery.[52]

Lidocaine spray may be useful in reducing posttonsillectomy pain.[53] Alongside pharmacologic methods, maintenance of adequate hydration and scheduling medication help keep pain under control.[17] Because most tonsillectomies occur in an ambulatory setting, much of the burden of the child's pain management falls on the parent or caregiver. Studies have shown that clear written take-home directions regarding pain medication scheduling as well as caregiver education on basic pain management in children lead to better analgesic outcomes.[48]

Nonmalignant Head and Neck Surgery

There is remarkably little literature on perioperative pain management in nontonsillectomy pediatric head and neck surgery. The few reports that do exist tend to present low- to very-low-quality evidence. In regard to surgical treatment of infantile hemangiomas (IH) of the head and neck, the use of dynamic cooling with pulsed dye laser therapy allows reduced pain associated with therapy.[54] In addition, in ulcerated cases of IH, the use of a barrier ointment between debridement procedures may alleviate pain.[54] Future studies should be performed in nonmalignant head and neck procedures to optimize specific pain management strategies for postoperative care.

ADJUNCT THERAPIES
Anesthesiology

Local nerve blocks can be used in numerous pediatric head and neck operations to help reduce pain associated with surgery. Nerve blocks are advantageous in that they provide highly effective local pain relief without the systemic side effects seen with oral or IV therapies.[55,56] As expected from the nonsystemic nature of the therapy, nerve blocks are shown to have lower incidence of postoperative bleeding, nausea, and vomiting.[55] The nerve block commonly uses a preparation of bupivacaine with epinephrine.[56] They are not without adverse effects, though, and rarely may cause hematoma and a variety of paralytic effects depending on the location of injection.[56]

Behavioral Strategies

Most studies evaluating the use of cognitive behavioral therapy (CBT) in pain management focus on forms of chronic pain, such as headaches, abdominal pain, and musculoskeletal pain. A Cochrane Review performed in 2018 focused on the utility of CBT in the management of pain associated with venipuncture, IV insertion, and vaccine management.[57] Although the quality of evidence in this review was rated low to very low, there was some support for the use of CBT, breathing interventions, and distraction as being somewhat efficacious in reducing pain associated with the above procedures. Regarding perioperative analgesia, this information may help in providing nonpharmacologic pain control for placement of preoperative or postoperative IVs and other needle sticks that may be necessary during a perioperative hospitalization. When approaching pain control with behavioral therapy, it is often most effective as an integrative, multidisciplinary approach in combination with pharmacologic treatment.[58]

SUMMARY

The primary goals of perioperative pain management in pediatric otolaryngology include controlling, preventing, and reducing acute pain while maintaining functional capacity. Management of perioperative pain is an essential component of surgical planning and plays a major role in determination of hospital stay postoperatively. With any surgical procedure, perioperative analgesic selection will depend on several factors, such as the patient's pain tolerance, safety profile of the medications to be used, and especially, the type of surgical procedure performed.[19] As it stands, adenotonsillectomy patients represent the biggest challenge in postoperative pain management of the head and neck surgeries evaluated. The low rates of pain, nausea, and vomiting reported in the days following surgery for most other procedures suggest that children can be cared for at home with simple analgesia.[59] However, discharge information, caregiver education, and prescription analgesia prescribing should be tailored to the operation performed and the patient's reasonable needs.

Pain control strategies should include a combination of behavioral modifications and pharmacologic interventions and should be managed on a case-by-case approach, evaluating the specific needs and requirements of each patient in regard to their age, type of intervention, parental anxiety about certain medications, and societal factors.[17,21] In recent years, strong emphasis has been placed on an overall reduction of opioid consumption and prescription in perioperative care and remains at the forefront of active research interest in multiple medical specialties, including otolaryngology.[19] Perioperative analgesia is one of the most common reasons that opioids are prescribed to patients, and an in-depth assessment of efficacy of alternative methods for achieving analgesia is an important step toward reducing potentially unnecessary opioid-prescribing practices.[19] As efforts have been made to optimize the use of appropriate pharmacotherapy, it remains essential for providers to recognize and anticipate pediatric pain, using techniques and regimens that allow for responsible and effective management strategies. Pain management in the pediatric population can often be a delicate balance and may also require an individualized approach for optimal patient care. By addressing the impact of perioperative pain on a patient's physical, emotional, and psychological well-being, providers will ultimately be able to reduce overall morbidity and improve surgical outcomes.

DISCLOSURE

Financial Disclosures: None.
Conflicts of Interest: None.

REFERENCES

1. Sutters KA, Miaskowski C. Inadequate pain management and associated morbidities in children at home after tonsillectomy. J Pediatr Nurs 1997;12(3):178–85.

2. Bruce J, Quinlan J. Chronic post-surgical pain. Rev Pain 2011;5(3):23–9.
3. Taddio A, Goldbach M, Ipp M, et al. Effect of neonatal circumcision on pain responses during vaccination in boys. Lancet 1995;345(8945):291–2.
4. Weisman SJ, Bernstein B, Schechter NL. Consequences of inadequate analgesia during painful procedures in children. Arch Pediatr Adolesc Med 1998;152(2): 147–9.
5. Helgadottir HL. Pain management in children after surgery. J Pediatr Nurs 2000; 15(5):334–40.
6. Hannam JA, Anderson BJ, Mahadevan M, et al. Postoperative analgesia using diclofenac and acetaminophen in children. Paediatr Anaesthesiology 2014;24: 953–61.
7. Wong I, St John-Green C, Walker SM. Opioid-sparing effects of perioperative paracetamol and nonsteroidal anti-inflammatory drugs (NSAIDs) in children. Paediatr Anaesth 2013;23(6):475–95.
8. Merkel SI, Voepel-Lewis T, Shayevitz JR, et al. The FLACC: a behavioral scale for scoring postoperative pain in young children. Pediatr Nurs 1997;23(3):293–7.
9. Kelly LE, Rieder M, van den Anker J, et al. More codeine fatalities after tonsillectomy in North American children. Pediatrics 2012;129(5):1343–7.
10. Wilson ME, Helgadottir HL. Patterns of pain and analgesic use in 3- to 7-year-old children after tonsillectomy. Pain Manag Nurs 2006;7(4):159–66.
11. Finley GA, McGrath PJ, Forward SP, et al. Parents' management of children's pain following 'minor' surgery. Pain 1996;61(1):83–7.
12. Chambers CT, Reid GJ, McGrath PJ, et al. Development and preliminary validation of a postoperative pain measure for parents. Pain 1996;68(2–3):307–13.
13. Kuehn BM. FDA: no codeine after tonsillectomy for children. JAMA 2013;309(11): 1100.
14. Baugh RF, Archer SM, Mitchell RB, et al. Clinical practice guidelines: tonsillectomy in children. Otolaryngol Head Neck Surg 2011;144(1 Suppl):S1–30.
15. WHO guidelines on the pharmacological treatment of persisting pain in children with medical illnesses. Geneva (Switzerland): World Health Organization; 2012.
16. Büttner W, Finke W. Analysis of behavioural and physiological parameters for the assessment of postoperative analgesic demand in newborns, infants and young children: a comprehensive report on seven consecutive studies. Paediatr Anaesth 2000;10(3):303–18.
17. Rodríguez MC, Villamor P, Castillo T. Assessment and management of pain in pediatric otolaryngology. Int J Pediatr Otorhinolaryngol 2016;90:138–49. Review.
18. Quinn BL, Sheldon LK, Cooley ME. Pediatric pain assessment by drawn faces scales: a review. Pain Manag Nurs 2014;15(4):909–18.
19. Campbell HT, Yuhan BT, Smith B, et al. Perioperative analgesia for patients undergoing otologic surgery: an evidence-based review. Laryngoscope 2019; 9999:1–10.
20. Robinson H, Engelhardt T. Ambulatory anesthetic care in children undergoing myringotomy and tube placement: current perspectives. Local Reg Anesth 2017;10:41–9.
21. Dewhirst E, Fedel G, Rayman V, et al. Pain management following myringotomy and tube placement: intranasal dexmedetomidine versus intranasal fentanyl. Int J Pediatr Otorhinolaryngol 2014;78(7):1090–4.
22. Watcha MF, Ramirez-Ruiz M, White PF, et al. Perioperative effects of oral ketorolac and acetaminophen in children undergoing bilateral myringotomy. Can J Anaesth 1992;39(7):649–54.

23. Bean-Lijewski JD, Kruitbosch SH, Hutchinson L, et al. Post-tonsillectomy pain management in children: can we do better? Otolaryngol Head Neck Surg 2007;137(4):545–51.

24. Suresh S, Barcelona SL, Young NM, et al. Postoperative pain relief in children undergoing tympanomastoid surgery: is a regional block better than opioids? Anesth Analg 2002;94:859–62.

25. Suresh S, Barcelona SL, Young NM, et al. Does a preemptive block of the great auricular nerve improve postoperative analgesia in children undergoing tympanomastoid surgery? Anesth Analg 2004;98:330–3.

26. Bhandari G, Shahi KS, Parmar NK, et al. Evaluation of analgesic effect of two different doses of fentanyl in combination with bupivacaine for surgical site infiltration in cases of modified radical mastoidectomy: a double-blind randomized study. Anesth Essays Res 2013;7:243–7.

27. Mesolella M, Lamarca S, Galli V, et al. Use of remifentanil for sedo-analgesia in stapedotomy: personal experience. Acta Otorhinolaryngol Ital 2004;24:315–20.

28. Nallam SR, Chiruvella S, Reddy A. Monitored anaesthesia care-comparison of nalbuphine/dexmedetomidine versus nalbuphine/propofol for middle ear surgeries: a double-blind randomised trial. Indian J Anaesth 2017;61:61–7.

29. Parikh DA, Kolli SN, Karnik HS, et al. A prospective randomized double-blind study comparing dexmedetomidine vs. combination of midazolam-fentanyl for tympanoplasty surgery under monitored anesthesia care. J Anaesthesiol Clin Pharmacol 2013;29:173–8.

30. Birman CS, Gibson WPR, Elliot EJ. Pediatric cochlear implantation: associated with minimal postoperative pain and dizziness. Otol Neurotol 2015;36:220–2.

31. Newberry CI, Casazza GC, Pruitt LC, et al. Prescription patterns and opioid usage in sinonasal surgery. Int Forum Allergy Rhinol 2019. https://doi.org/10.1002/alr.22478.

32. Svider PF, Nguyen B, Yuhan B, et al. Perioperative analgesia for patients undergoing endoscopic sinus surgery: an evidence-based review. Int Forum Allergy Rhinol 2018;8(7):837–49.

33. Kelchner LN, Brehm SB, Alarcon A, et al. Update on pediatric voice and airway disorders: assessment and care. Curr Opin Otolaryngol Head Neck Surg 2012; 20(3):160–4.

34. Faumann KR, Durgham R, Duran CI, et al. Sedation after airway reconstruction in children: a protocol to reduce withdrawal and length of stay. Laryngoscope 2015; 125:2216–9.

35. Auchincloss HG, Wright CD. Complications after tracheal resection and reconstruction: prevention and treatment. J Thorac Dis 2016;8:S160–7.

36. Silver AL, Yager P, Purohit P, et al. Dexmedetomidine use in pediatric airway reconstruction. Otolaryngol Head Neck Surg 2011;144(2):262–7.

37. Meng QT, Xia ZY, Luo T, et al. Dexmedetomidine reduces emergence agitation after tonsillectomy in children by sevoflurane anesthesia: a case-control study. Int J Pediatr Otorhinolaryngol 2012;76(7):1036–41.

38. Tobias JD. Dexmedetomidine: applications in pediatric critical care and pediatric anesthesiology. Pediatr Crit Care Med 2007;8(2):115–31.

39. Hammer GB. Sedation and analgesia in the pediatric intensive care unit following laryngotracheal reconstruction. Otolaryngol Clin North Am 2008;41:1023–44.

40. Mitchell RB, Archer SM, Ishman SL, et al. Clinical practice guideline: tonsillectomy in children (update). Otolaryngol Head Neck Surg 2019;160(1_suppl): S1–42.

41. Sampaio AL, Pinheiro TG, Furtado PL, et al. Evaluation of early postoperative morbidity in pediatric tonsillectomy with the use of sucralfate. Int J Pediatr Otorhinolaryngol 2007;71(4):645–51.

42. Yang K, Baetzel A, Chimbira WT, et al. Association of sleep disordered breathing symptoms with early postoperative analgesia requirement in pediatric ambulatory surgical patients. Int J Pediatr Otorhinolaryngol 2017;96:145–51.

43. Goldman JL, Zeigler C, Burckardt EM. Otolaryngology practice patterns in pediatric tonsillectomy: the impact of the codeine boxed warning. Laryngoscope 2018;128(1):264–8.

44. Borgström A, Nerfeldt P, Friberg D. Postoperative pain and bleeding after adenotonsillectomy versus adenotonsillectomy in obstructive sleep apnea: an RCT. Eur Arch Otorhinolaryngol 2019;276(11):3231–8.

45. Chisholm AG, Sathyamoorthy M, Seals SR, et al. Does intravenous acetaminophen reduce perioperative opioid use in pediatric tonsillectomy? Am J Otolaryngol 2019;40(6):102294.

46. Lewis SR, Nicholson A, Cardwell ME, et al. Nonsteroidal anti-inflammatory drugs and perioperative bleeding in paediatric tonsillectomy. Cochrane Database Syst Rev 2013;(7):CD003591.

47. Chidambaran V, Sadhasivam S, Mahmoud M. Codeine and opioid metabolism: implications and alternatives for pediatric pain management. Curr Opin Anaesthesiol 2017;30(3):349–56.

48. Dorkham MC, Chalkiadis GA, von Ungern Sternberg BS, et al. Effective postoperative pain management in children after ambulatory surgery, with a focus in adenotonsillectomy: barriers and possible solutions. Pediatr Anaesth 2014; 24(3):239.

49. Kilinc L, Türk B, Türk HS, et al. Peritonsillar dexamethasone—bupivacaine vs. bupivacaine infiltration for post-tonsillectomy pain relief in children: a randomized, double-blind, controlled study. Eur Arch Otorhinolaryngol 2019;276(7):2081.

50. Ahmed KA, Dreher ME, King RF, et al. Dexamethasone and postoperative bleeding risk after adenotonsillectomy in children. Laryngoscope 2011;121(5): 1060–1.

51. DeHart AN, Potter J, Anderson J, et al. Perioperative interdisciplinary approach for reduction of opioid use in pediatric tonsillectomy: protocol using dexmedetomidine and bupivacaine as adjunct agents. Am J Otolaryngol 2019;40(3):382–8.

52. Ince I, Ahiskalioglu A, Aksoy M, et al. Does montelukast have an effect on post-tonsillectomy pain control in children? A randomized trial study. Otolaryngol Head Neck Surg 2015;153(2):269–74.

53. Fedorowicz Z, Al-Muharraqi MA, Nasser M, et al. Oral rinses, mouthwashes and sprays for improving recovery following tonsillectomy. Cochrane Database Syst Rev 2013;(9):CD007806.

54. Harter N, Mancini AJ. Diagnosis and management of infantile hemangiomas in the neonate. Pediatr Clin North Am 2019;66(2):437–59.

55. Peutrell JM, McIlveney S. Peripheral local anaesthetic techniques for pediatric surgery. Anaesth Intensive Care Med 2003;4(12):407–11.

56. Voronov P, Suresh S. Head and neck blocks in children. Curr Opin Anaesthesiol 2008;21(3):317–22.

57. Birnie KA, Noel M, Chambers CT, et al. Psychological interventions for needle-related procedural pain and distress in children and adolescents. Cochrane Database Syst Rev 2018;(10):CD005179.

58. Wren AA, Ross AC, D'Souza G, et al. Multidisciplinary pain management for pediatric patients with acute and chronic pain: a foundational treatment approach when prescribing opioids. Children 2019;6(33):1–22.

59. Wilson CA, Sommerfield D, Drake-Brockman TFE, et al. Pain after discharge following head and neck surgery in children. Paediatr Anaesth 2016;26: 992–1001.

Nonopioid Adjuncts and Alternatives

Qasim Husain, MD[a],*, Catherine Banks, MD[b], Stacey T. Gray, MD[c]

KEYWORDS

- Nonopioid • Pain control • Postoperative care

KEY POINTS

- Multi-modality non-opioid analgesia can be effective for pain control.
- Otolaryngologists should be well versed in the role of non-opioid analgesia based on surgical subsite.
- Balancing risks and benefits of treatment can help cater to the appropriateness of opioid versus non-opioid pain control.

INTRODUCTION

Opioid use in the United States of America has become an epidemic, affecting approximately 2.5 million adults and resulting in close to 50,000 deaths in 2017 alone.[1] The opioid crisis has garnered significant attention in the past decade, leading to increased oversight and monitoring of physician prescribing patterns in an attempt to quell the surge of prescription opioid drug addiction and abuse. This escalating health crisis and the increased attention to prescribing patterns have led to the need for otolaryngology providers to consider nonopioid adjuncts and alternatives for pain management. Otolaryngologists frequently employ the use of medication for pain control after surgical intervention, and adjunctive treatment options for these patients potentially can decrease opioid prescriptions provided while optimizing patient analgesia.

The concept of perioperative multimodal opioid-sparing pain control starts in the preoperative period, includes intraoperative pain management, and extends to the acute postoperative period. Effective adoption of these methods requires communication and collaboration with the anesthesiologist providing care during the surgical period. Administration of therapy prior to the start of surgery, preemptive analgesia, is intended to prevent sensitization of the nervous system to the subsequent noxious

[a] Hackensack Meridian School of Medicine at Seton Hall University, Coastal Ear, Nose, and Throat, 100 Commons Way, Suite 210, Holmdel, NJ 07733, USA; [b] Department of Otolaryngology–Head and Neck Surgery, Prince of Wales Hospital, University of New South Wales, Sydney, Australia; [c] Department of Otolaryngology–Head and Neck Surgery, Massachusetts Eye and Ear, Harvard Medical School, 243 Charles Street, Boston, MA 02114, USA
* Corresponding author.
E-mail address: qhusain@coastalhearing.com

Otolaryngol Clin N Am 53 (2020) 831–842
https://doi.org/10.1016/j.otc.2020.05.012
0030-6665/20/© 2020 Elsevier Inc. All rights reserved.

stimuli during surgery that can amplify pain. Commonly employed nonopioid pre-emptive analgesic drugs that have been investigated in otolaryngologic procedures include acetaminophen, nonsteroidal anti-inflammatory drugs (NSAIDs), gabapentinoids, ketamine, corticosteroids, and dexmedetomidine. Intraoperative use of topical and infiltrated local anesthetic medications has been employed in several otolaryngologic procedures to decrease the need for postoperative pain control. Finally, postoperative use of gabapentinoids, acetaminophen, and NSAIDs has been reported in multiple otolaryngologic procedures. **Table 1** summarizes the types of drug classes and their mechanisms of actions discussed throughout this article. This article highlights the role of nonopioid pain management throughout the different subspecialties of otolaryngology–head and neck surgery.

HEAD AND NECK SURGERY

Head and neck surgery comprises the largest and most extensive array of surgical procedures performed in the field of otolaryngology. Pain management, however, is not isolated to postsurgical patients with head and neck cancer but also is an issue for those patients who receive radiation and chemotherapy as well as patients with chronic pain after completion of treatment. One study demonstrated that 13% of patients with head and neck malignancies who received radiation treatment of curative intent had prolonged opioid use 6 months after treatment.[2] Another study demonstrated that more than 50% of oropharyngeal squamous cell carcinoma patients treated with radiation became chronic users of opioid medications.[3]

Immediately after surgical intervention, many patients receive scheduled opioids but also are treated with patient-controlled analgesia (PCA) devices to give low dose boluses of opioids on demand. In this group of patients, the current management goals are to provide opioid-sparing multimodal analgesia and to focus on reducing opioid use with nonopioid adjuncts while preserving patient analgesia.[4] Smith and colleagues[5] examined the utility of regularly scheduled intravenous (IV) acetaminophen in addition to the standard PCAs given to head and neck cancer patients in the first 24 hours after surgery. This study found significantly decreased total narcotic requirement, a reduction in the need for PCA, and a significantly decreased length of stay. Another study examined the use of the NSAID celecoxib, a selective cyclooxygenase (COX)-2 inhibitor, for the treatment of postoperative pain management in head and neck cancer patients undergoing surgical resection and free flap reconstruction. NSAIDs that are nonselective inhibit COX-1 and COX-2, whereas selective COX-2 inhibitors do not affect platelets in the same manner, and this theoretically reduces the risk of bleeding. This study determined that there was a significant decrease in oral, IV, and total opioid requirements without increasing surgical-related or flap-related complications.[6] Currently, there are open trials examining the utility of IV lidocaine administration as a means to reduce opioid consumption postoperatively after major head and neck cancer surgery.[7]

Mucositis is a common side effect after treatment of head and neck cancer patients with chemotherapy and/or radiation therapy and results in tremendous discomfort. A recent systematic review examining treatment of mucositis pain with nonopioid adjuncts demonstrated significant pain relief compared with placebo with topical doxepin, amitriptyline, diclofenac, and benzydamine.[8]

SLEEP SURGERY

An additional area of concern with postoperative opioid use in the field of otolaryngology is the potential acute complications of narcotics. Opioids can cause respiratory

Table 1
Nonopioid drug classes used for pain in otolaryngology

Drug Class	Examples	Mechanism of Action	Common Side Effects
NSAID	Aspirin Ibuprofen Naproxen Ketorolac Diclofenac Celecoxib	COX-1 inhibitor → inhibits prostaglandin production COX-2 inhibitor → inhibits prostaglandin production	Gastric ulcers, platelet dysfunction, nephrotoxicity, cardiovascular events Fewer gastric side effects
	Acetaminophen	Exact mechanism unclear, prevents central prostaglandin synthesis	Liver toxicity
Muscle relaxants	Cyclobenzaprine Tizanidine Baclofen Diazepam	Centrally acting, mechanism varies by drug	Drowsiness, dizziness, drug-drug interactions, respiratory depression
Antidepressants	Amitriptyline Nortriptyline Duloxetine	Tricyclic antidepressant SNRI	Blurred vision, dry mouth, orthostatic hypotension, urinary retention, prolonged QTc, drug-drug interactions
α-Agonists	Dexmedetomidine Clonidine	α_2-Aadrenergic receptor agonist	Hypotension, bradycardia, sedation
Gabapentinoids	Gabapentin Pregabalin	Calcium channel blockade	Dizziness, somnolence, peripheral edema, blurred vision Pregabalin is a controlled substance
Corticosteroids	Prednisone Methylprednisolone Triamcinolone Cortisone	Inhibition of phospholipase	Mood changes, hypertension, increase in glucose, adrenal suppression, osteoporosis

(continued on next page)

Drug Class	Examples	Mechanism of Action	Common Side Effects
Local anesthetics	Lidocaine Bupivacaine Ropivacaine	Sodium channel blockade	Local anesthetic system toxicity, including tinnitus, perioral numbness/tingling, altered mental status, seizures, cardiac arrhythmias, and cardiac arrest
Other anesthetics	Ketamine	NMDA receptor antagonist	Hallucinations, increased oral secretions, sympathomimetic effects, direct myocardial depression, increased intracranial pressure, increased pulmonary hypertension

Table 1 (*continued*)

Abbreviations: NMDA, *N*-methyl-ᴅ-aspartate; SNRI, serotonin norepinephrine reuptake inhibitor.

depression and increased upper airway collapse. Patients with severe obstructive sleep apnea undergoing sleep surgery, therefore, are particularly vulnerable to this potential complication. Surgeries for obstructive sleep apnea, such as uvulopalatopharyngoplasty, are known to be painful, with reported 20% of postoperative return visits to the hospital for inadequate pain control. Additionally, there is a high rate of postoperative bleeding, accounting for up to 40% of unplanned revisits.[9] Therefore, it is important to develop analgesic protocols that provide adequate pain relief while minimizing opioid use and risk of bleeding in this population of surgical patients. There have been numerous studies demonstrating the effectiveness of perioperative regional anesthesia in the form submucosal infiltration of long-acting local anesthetic in the oropharyngeal region prior to incision. These interventions at the time of surgery can provide effective postoperative analgesia in the immediate postoperative period.[10,11] Ayatollahi and colleagues[12] found that the administration of IV vitamin C intraoperatively during uvulopalatopharyngoplasty reduced postoperative pain, both in overall severity and duration, prior to requesting analgesic, without side effects.

THYROID AND PARATHYROID SURGERY

Sensitivity of the anterior neck from thyroid and parathyroid surgery can result in significant postoperative pain. A national survey examining trends in pain management after thyroid and parathyroid surgery demonstrates that there is significant variability in practice patterns and that only 35% of practitioners do not utilize opioids.[13] There have been several studies that sought to reduce postoperative opioid consumption with the use of various perioperative adjuncts. In a metanalysis of 14 randomized controlled trials (RCTs), Mayhew and colleagues[14] demonstrated the analgesic efficacy of bilateral cervical plexus block in the early postoperative period with significant reduction in analgesic requirements and decreased length of hospital stay. Another study examined the use of preemptive IV ibuprofen preoperatively and found there was a significant reduction in visual analog scale (VAS) for pain as well as reduced opioid consumption and use of rescue analgesia.[15] Preoperative administration of gabapentin also has been shown to have similar effects in decreasing pain scores and opioid consumption postoperatively.[16] One of the arguments against using NSAIDs in thyroid and parathyroid surgery is the risk of postoperative hematoma. A study by Chin and colleagues,[17] demonstrated an increased incidence of hematoma in patients who received ketorolac perioperatively (2.7% vs 1.3%); however, there were low number of hematomas and these findings were not statistically significant. Studies have demonstrated that the implementation of protocols utilizing multimodality analgesia (preoperative acetaminophen, NSAIDs, and gabapentin with postoperative acetaminophen and ibuprofen) can help decrease prescriptions for postoperative opioid analgesics for patients undergoing thyroid and parathyroid surgery.[18]

SINONASAL SURGERY

Postoperative opioid analgesics are prescribed by up to 95% of providers after sinonasal surgery, according to a recent national survey.[19] Some studies, however, have demonstrated that patients utilize only a small number of pills and a majority of the medication remains unused.[20,21] Therefore, the judicious prescribing of opioids after rhinologic surgery coupled with adjunctive nonopioid use represents a practical opportunity for otolaryngologists to reduce the possibility for abuse by patients and opioid diversion. Acetaminophen is a mainstay for analgesia after sinonasal surgery, but there also have been several RCTs examining perioperative IV acetaminophen dosing prior to the start of surgery, which led to reduction of immediate postoperative pain and decreased opioid requirements.[22-24]

There have been several double-blind RCTs for NSAID use for septoplasty, rhinoplasty, and endoscopic sinus surgery.[25-30] Moeller and colleagues[27] demonstrated that IV ketorolac is a safe analgesic in the setting of septoplasty and sinus surgery. Ozer and colleagues[28] determined that administration of IV dexketoprofen provides good postoperative analgesia in septorhinoplasty patients irrespective of intraoperative versus postoperative administration. Turan and colleagues,[25] meanwhile, showed that rofecoxib, a COX-2 inhibitor, demonstrated decreased pain scores, reduced rescue analgesia, and prolonged times to first analgesic requirement. Rofecoxib was pulled from the market due to adverse cardiovascular events. Celecoxib currently is an available COX-2 inhibitor with safer side-effect profile.

Pregabalin and gabapentin are new-generation anticonvulsants with antihyperalgesic and antinociceptive properties. These drugs were initially used for the treatment of neuropathic pain, but their use has been expanded to treat multiple types of acute and chronic pain. The use of preemptive gabapentinoids in nasal surgery has also been well documented in several RCTs, with a majority reporting significantly lower VAS pain scores compared with placebo.[31-36]

Local anesthestic agents also have been explored as a means to provide analgesia after sinonasal surgery. Several studies reported that the use of local anesthetics, including lidocaine and bupivacaine, either as injection or infusion in postoperative nasal packing, led to decreased VAS scores and lower analgesic requirements.[30,37] Other studies have utilized a sphenopalatine ganglion block or infraorbital nerve block to provide analgesia by targeting the sensory innervation of the nasal mucosa.[38,39]

Dexmedetomidine, a highly selective α_2-adrenergic receptor agonist, has been utilized more frequently in the practice of anesthesia because it produces sedation, anxiolysis, and analgesia without causing respiratory depression. Administration prior to sinonasal surgery was found to result in significant reductions in VAS pain scores compared with placebo-saline solutions in 1 study.[40]

FACIAL PLASTIC SURGERY

Distinct from septorhinoplasty surgery, there are a variety of procedures in facial plastic surgery that require consideration with respect to the type of analgesia utilized, including rhytidectomy, brow-lift, and blepharoplasty. Studies have reported the use of a multimodality approach to pain control for facial rejuvenation procedures, balancing the use of intraoperative tumescence with dilute local anesthesia and nerve blocks at the completion of surgery as well as supportive wraps and cold compresses postoperatively.[41] Rhytidectomy is an important procedure in facial rejuvenation, and hematoma is considered the most dreaded complication, which has limited the study of postoperative pain control that increases the risk of bleeding. One study demonstrated that perioperative celecoxib use was associated with reduced opioid use, nausea, and later sedation without any adverse side effects, including bleeding.[42]

OTOLOGIC SURGERY

Otologic surgery can be divided into myringotomy and tube (MT) surgery versus more involved ear surgery, such as middle ear or transmastoid surgery in regard to perioperative pain control. MT surgery has been studied extensively, with a majority of studies reporting acetaminophen, NSAIDs, or both for effective analgesia.[43] The addition of ketorolac or codeine, while providing superior analgesia, were not found cost effective or necessary for this limited surgery.[44–46] Nonpharmacologic adjuncts also have been examined, with acupuncture therapy diminishing pain and emergence agitation after MT placement.[47] For more extensive otologic surgery, Suresh and colleagues[48] showed the benefit of a greater auricular nerve block performed intraoperatively during transmastoid surgery to provide superior analgesia and a reduction in overall postoperative opioid requirement. Another analysis examined intramuscular NSAID injection after mastoidectomy, which did not lead to any major adverse events, such as hematoma.[49] These findings taken together indicate that the use of postoperative opioid analgesia likely can be reduced with judicious local anesthetic infiltrate at the time of surgery and the use of NSAID and acetaminophen in the postoperative period.

PEDIATRIC SURGERY

Some of the most common procedures performed in pediatric otolaryngology practices include MT surgery and adenotonsillectomy. Although these procedures also are performed in adult patients, pain management in the pediatric population requires separate evaluation for several reasons. The assessment of postoperative pain is challenging in children due to their lack of understanding and of ability to verbalize the degree of pain being experienced. VAS systems have been validated for children to help explain their experience and this can be utilized to improve their ability to communicate with practitioners.[50] One of the most basic steps in the management of pain and anxiety in children is to utilize cognitive behavioral strategies, such as distraction (music or video), positive reinforcement, and environment optimization (not performing procedures inside a hospitalized patient's bedroom).[51] These steps, when combined with topical anesthetic, allowed for the placement of tympanostomy tubes in awake pediatric patients ranging from age 8 months to 17 years.[52] Local anesthetics also can be used to perform blocks of the auricular branch of the vagus nerve to facilitate tolerance of MT placement in children.[53] Infiltration of local anesthetic after tonsillectomy also has been studied extensively, with a metanalysis demonstrating it to be a safe and effective method to treat pediatric post-adenotonsillectomy pain.[54]

Given the potentially significantly morbid side effects of respiratory depression associated with narcotic use in pediatric patients undergoing tonsillectomy, the use of nonopioid adjuncts has received significant attention. Evidence has demonstrated the most effective first step in management for pain control after tonsillectomy includes the use of acetaminophen with or without ibuprofen. This treatment regimen has demonstrated similar efficacy to opioid analgesics without the added risk of oxygen desaturations from respiratory depression.[55] Although many practitioners worry that the use of NSAIDs could lead to increased post-tonsillectomy hemorrhage, a Cochrane review demonstrated postoperative ibuprofen was not associated with increased bleeding risk.[56] Literature on the usage of ketorolac in the setting of tonsillectomy has been less clear with respect to its effect on bleeding. Some studies suggest that post-tonsillectomy ketorolac is safe in children but can increase the bleeding up to 5-fold in adults.[57] Other reviews have concluded that risks and benefits should be considered before routinely using ketorolac for tonsillectomy.[58]

The intraoperative usage of dexamethasone during tonsillectomy has been endorsed by the American Academy of Otolaryngology–Head and Neck Surgery guidelines for its analgesic and antinausea properties.[59] Postoperative dosing also has shown improved outcomes, with recent literature demonstrating the effectiveness of oral steroids for improvement in pain, diet, activity, re-epithelialization of tonsillar bed, and sleep disturbance.[60] Another study examined the utility of a short course of steroid, 3 doses of dexamethasone, which decreased pain-related postoperative phone calls as well as hemorrhage rate.[60,61] In addition to steroids, a low dose of IV ketamine after tonsillectomy also has been reported to effectively reduce pain without side effects, such as nausea, vomiting, and agitation.[50,62]

EMERGING TECHNOLOGY

Some of the most difficult patients to treat are those with chronic pain. A specific category that can be encountered in otolaryngology practice is atypical facial pain. These patients often are comanaged with neurology or pain medicine specialists, and newer options for nonmedical therapy are being developed in the field of chronic pain. When medical management with neuromodulating agents (amitriptyline, gabapentin, and pregabalin) fails, additional adjunct interventions, such as botulinum toxin injections, can be attempted. Nonpharmacologic approaches, such as acupuncture and biofeedback, have been shown to have mixed results in this patient population.[63] Transcutaneous electrical nerve stimulation (TENS) has been shown to relieve chronic pain from facial myalgias.[64] This technology has recently been applied to patients with sinus pain—with an RCT indicating that microcurrent-treated patients had a significantly greater reduction in pain compared with placebo controls.[65] Future studies will investigate the reliability and durability of these findings, but TENS does show promise in alternative nonopioid therapies for patients with chronic pain in the head and neck.

The continued expansion of app development for smartphones has spilled over into assessment of postoperative pain. The utilization of patient-reported outcome measures has become an important tool for clinical research, quality improvement, and optimization of patient care. A recent study examined the use of a mobile health platform to assess functional outcomes and pain after endoscopic sinus surgery and rhinoplasty. The study found that there were high response rates with this digital engagement platform, demonstrating that it can be an effective approach to assess postoperative outcomes, including pain control.[66] The implementation of these platforms has been useful particularly in the pediatric population, where the ability to communicate pain control may be difficult.[67]

SUMMARY

Across all subspecialties of otolaryngology–head and neck surgery, multimodality nonopioid analgesia is an effective way to control postoperative pain without causing increased morbidity. Pain is multifactorial, and clinical judgment should be made when choosing between opioid versus nonopioid adjuncts.

DISCLOSURE

Financial Disclosures: None.
Conflicts of Interest: None.

REFERENCES

1. National Institute on Drug Abuse: Trends and Statistics, Overdose death rates. Available at: https://www.drugabuse.gov/related-topics/trends-statistics/overdose-death-rates. Accessed May 5, 2019.
2. Smith WH, Luskin I, Salgado RL, et al. Risk of prolonged opioid use among cancer patients undergoing curative intent radiation therapy for head and neck malignancies. Oral Oncol 2019;92:1–5.
3. Silver N, Dourado J, Hitchcock K, et al. Chronic opioid use in patients undergoing treatment for oropharyngeal cancer. Laryngoscope 2019;129(9):2087–93.
4. Dort JC, Farwell DG, Findlay M, et al. Optimal Perioperative Care in Major Head and Neck Cancer Surgery With Free Flap Reconstruction: A Consensus Review and Recommendations From the Enhanced Recovery After Surgery Society. JAMA Otolaryngol Head Neck Surg 2017;143:292–303.
5. Smith E, Lange J, Moore C, et al. The role of intravenous acetaminophen in postoperative pain control in head and neck cancer patients. Laryngoscope Investig Otolaryngol 2019;4:250–4.
6. Carpenter PS, Shepherd HM, McCrary H, et al. Association of Celecoxib Use With Decreased Opioid Requirements After Head and Neck Cancer Surgery With Free Tissue Reconstruction. JAMA Otolaryngol Head Neck Surg 2018;144:988–94.
7. Omar E, Wallon G, Bauer C, et al. Evaluation of intravenous lidocaine in head and neck cancer surgery: study protocol for a randomized controlled trial. Trials 2019; 20:220.
8. Christoforou J, Karasneh J, Manfredi M, et al. Non-opioid pain management of head and neck chemo/radiation-induced mucositis: A systematic review. Oral Dis 2019;25(S1):182–92.
9. Bhattacharyya N. Revisits and readmissions following ambulatory uvulopalatopharyngoplasty. Laryngoscope 2015;125:754–7.
10. Li L, Feng J, Xie SH, et al. Preemptive submucosal infiltration with ropivacaine for uvulopalatopharyngoplasty. Otolaryngol Head Neck Surg 2014;151:874–9.

11. Haytoglu S, Arikan OK, Muluk NB, et al. Relief of pain at rest and during swallowing after modified cautery-assisted uvulopalatopharyngoplasty: bupivacaine versus lidocaine. J Craniofac Surg 2015;26:e216–23.

12. Ayatollahi V, Dehghanpour Farashah S, Behdad S, et al. Effect of intravenous vitamin C on postoperative pain in uvulopalatopharyngoplasty with tonsillectomy. Clin Otolaryngol 2017;42:139–43.

13. Ferrell JK, Singer MC, Farwell DG, et al. Evaluating contemporary pain management practices in thyroid and parathyroid surgery: A national survey of head and neck endocrine surgeons. Head Neck 2019;41(7):2315–23.

14. Mayhew D, Sahgal N, Khirwadkar R, et al. Analgesic efficacy of bilateral superficial cervical plexus block for thyroid surgery: meta-analysis and systematic review. Br J Anaesth 2018;120:241–51.

15. Mutlu V, Ince I. Preemptive intravenous ibuprofen application reduces pain and opioid consumption following thyroid surgery. Am J Otolaryngol 2019;40:70–3.

16. Al-Mujadi H, A-Refai AR, Katzarov MG, et al. Preemptive gabapentin reduces postoperative pain and opioid demand following thyroid surgery. Can J Anaesth 2006;53:268–73.

17. Chin CJ, Franklin JH, Turner B, et al. Ketorolac in thyroid surgery: quantifying the risk of hematoma. J Otolaryngol Head Neck Surg 2011;40:196–9.

18. Militsakh O, Lydiatt W, Lydiatt D, et al. Development of Multimodal Analgesia Pathways in Outpatient Thyroid and Parathyroid Surgery and Association With Postoperative Opioid Prescription Patterns. JAMA Otolaryngol Head Neck Surg 2018;144:1023–9.

19. Gray ML, Fan CJ, Kappauf C, et al. Postoperative pain management after sinus surgery: a survey of the American Rhinologic Society. Int Forum Allergy Rhinol 2018;8:1199–203.

20. Riley CA, Kim M, Sclafani AP, et al. Opioid analgesic use and patient-reported pain outcomes after rhinologic surgery. Int Forum Allergy Rhinol 2019;9:339–44.

21. Sethi RKV, Miller AL, Bartholomew RA, et al. Opioid prescription patterns and use among patients undergoing endoscopic sinus surgery. Laryngoscope 2019;129:1046–52.

22. Kemppainen T, Kokki H, Tuomilehto H, et al. Acetaminophen is highly effective in pain treatment after endoscopic sinus surgery. Laryngoscope 2006;116:2125–8.

23. Koteswara CM, Sheetal D. A Study on pre-emptive analgesic effect of intravenous paracetamol in functional endoscopic sinus surgeries (FESSs): a randomized, double-blinded clinical study. J Clin Diagn Res 2014;8:108–11.

24. Tyler MA, Lam K, Ashoori F, et al. Analgesic effects of intravenous acetaminophen vs placebo for endoscopic sinus surgery and postoperative pain: a randomized clinical trial. JAMA Otolaryngol Head Neck Surg 2017;143:788–94.

25. Turan A, Emet S, Karamanlioglu B, et al. Analgesic effects of rofecoxib in ear-nose-throat surgery. Anesth Analg 2002;95:1308–11, table of contents.

26. Sener M, Yilmazer C, Yilmaz I, et al. Efficacy of lornoxicam for acute postoperative pain relief after septoplasty: a comparison with diclofenac, ketoprofen, and dipyrone. J Clin Anesth 2008;20:103–8.

27. Moeller C, Pawlowski J, Pappas AL, et al. The safety and efficacy of intravenous ketorolac in patients undergoing primary endoscopic sinus surgery: a randomized, double-blinded clinical trial. Int Forum Allergy Rhinol 2012;2:342–7.

28. Ozer AB, Erhan OL, Keles E, et al. Comparison of the effects of preoperative and intraoperative intravenous application of dexketoprofen on postoperative analgesia in septorhinoplasty patients: randomised double blind clinical trial. Eur Rev Med Pharmacol Sci 2012;16:1828–33.

29. Nguyen BK, Yuhan BT, Folbe E, et al. Perioperative Analgesia for Patients Undergoing Septoplasty and Rhinoplasty: An Evidence-Based Review. Laryngoscope 2019;129(6):E200–12.

30. Svider PF, Nguyen B, Yuhan B, et al. Perioperative analgesia for patients undergoing endoscopic sinus surgery: an evidence-based review. Int Forum Allergy Rhinol 2018;8:837–49.

31. Kim JH, Seo MY, Hong SD, et al. The efficacy of preemptive analgesia with pregabalin in septoplasty. Clin Exp Otorhinolaryngol 2014;7:102–5.

32. Demirhan A, Akkaya A, Tekelioglu UY, et al. Effect of pregabalin and dexamethasone on postoperative analgesia after septoplasty. Pain Res Treat 2014;2014: 850794.

33. Demirhan A, Tekelioglu UY, Akkaya A, et al. Effect of pregabalin and dexamethasone addition to multimodal analgesia on postoperative analgesia following rhinoplasty surgery. Aesthetic Plast Surg 2013;37:1100–6.

34. Kazak Z, Meltem Mortimer N, Sekerci S. Single dose of preoperative analgesia with gabapentin (600 mg) is safe and effective in monitored anesthesia care for nasal surgery. Eur Arch Otorhinolaryngol 2010;267:731–6.

35. Turan A, Memis D, Karamanlioglu B, et al. The analgesic effects of gabapentin in monitored anesthesia care for ear-nose-throat surgery. Anesth Analg 2004;99: 375–8, table of contents.

36. Salama ER, Amer AF. The effect of pre-emptive gabapentin on anaesthetic and analgesic requirements in patients undergoing rhinoplasty: A prospective randomised study. Indian J Anaesth 2018;62:197–201.

37. Yilmaz S, Yildizbas S, Guclu E, et al. Topical levobupivacaine efficacy in pain control after functional endoscopic sinus surgery. Otolaryngol Head Neck Surg 2013; 149:777–81.

38. Al-Qudah M. Endoscopic sphenopalatine ganglion blockade efficacy in pain control after endoscopic sinus surgery. Int Forum Allergy Rhinol 2016;6: 334–8.

39. Cekic B, Geze S, Erturk E, et al. A comparison of levobupivacaine and levobupivacaine-tramadol combination in bilateral infraorbital nerve block for postoperative analgesia after nasal surgery. Ann Plast Surg 2013;70:131–4.

40. Guven DG, Demiraran Y, Sezen G, et al. Evaluation of outcomes in patients given dexmedetomidine in functional endoscopic sinus surgery. Ann Otol Rhinol Laryngol 2011;120:586–92.

41. Richards BG, Schleicher WF, Zins JE. Putting it all together: recommendations for improving pain management in plastic surgical procedures-surgical facial rejuvenation. Plast Reconstr Surg 2014;134:108S–12S.

42. Aynehchi BB, Cerrati EW, Rosenberg DB. The efficacy of oral celecoxib for acute postoperative pain in face-lift surgery. JAMA Facial Plast Surg 2014;16: 306–9.

43. Campbell HT, Yuhan BT, Smith B, et al. Perioperative analgesia for patients undergoing otologic surgery: An evidence-based review. Laryngoscope 2019;130(1): 190–9.

44. Watcha MF, Ramirez-Ruiz M, White PF, et al. Perioperative effects of oral ketorolac and acetaminophen in children undergoing bilateral myringotomy. Can J Anaesth 1992;39:649–54.

45. Bean-Lijewski JD, Stinson JC. Acetaminophen or ketorolac for post myringotomy pain in children? A prospective, double-blinded comparison. Paediatr Anaesth 1997;7:131–7.

46. Tobias JD, Lowe S, Hersey S, et al. Analgesia after bilateral myringotomy and placement of pressure equalization tubes in children: acetaminophen versus acetaminophen with codeine. Anesth Analg 1995;81:496–500.
47. Lin YC, Tassone RF, Jahng S, et al. Acupuncture management of pain and emergence agitation in children after bilateral myringotomy and tympanostomy tube insertion. Paediatr Anaesth 2009;19:1096–101.
48. Suresh S, Barcelona SL, Young NM, et al. Postoperative pain relief in children undergoing tympanomastoid surgery: is a regional block better than opioids? Anesth Analg 2002;94:859–62, table of contents.
49. Nalini R, Ezhilramya J. A Comparative Study of Efficacy and Safety of Lornoxicam and Diclofenac as Postoperative Analgesics after Mastoidectomy Surgery. Int J Pharm Pharm Sci 2017;9:77–83.
50. Rodriguez MC, Villamor P, Castillo T. Assessment and management of pain in pediatric otolaryngology. Int J Pediatr Otorhinolaryngol 2016;90:138–49.
51. Uman LS, Birnie KA, Noel M, et al. Psychological interventions for needle-related procedural pain and distress in children and adolescents. Cochrane Database Syst Rev 2013;(10):CD005179.
52. Cohen LL, Martin SR, Gamwell KL, et al. Behavioral techniques to optimize success of in-office pediatric tympanostomy tube placement without sedation. Int J Pediatr Otorhinolaryngol 2015;79:2170–3.
53. Voronov P, Tobin MJ, Billings K, et al. Postoperative pain relief in infants undergoing myringotomy and tube placement: comparison of a novel regional anesthetic block to intranasal fentanyl–a pilot analysis. Paediatr Anaesth 2008;18:1196–201.
54. Sun J, Wu X, Meng Y, et al. Bupivacaine versus normal saline for relief of post-adenotonsillectomy pain in children: a meta-analysis. Int J Pediatr Otorhinolaryngol 2010;74:369–73.
55. Kelly LE, Sommer DD, Ramakrishna J, et al. Morphine or Ibuprofen for post-tonsillectomy analgesia: a randomized trial. Pediatrics 2015;135:307–13.
56. Lewis SR, Nicholson A, Cardwell ME, et al. Nonsteroidal anti-inflammatory drugs and perioperative bleeding in paediatric tonsillectomy. Cochrane Database Syst Rev 2013;(7):CD003591.
57. Chan DK, Parikh SR. Perioperative ketorolac increases post-tonsillectomy hemorrhage in adults but not children. Laryngoscope 2014;124:1789–93.
58. Phillips-Reed LD, Austin PN, Rodriguez RE. Pediatric Tonsillectomy and Ketorolac. J Perianesth Nurs 2016;31:485–94.
59. Baugh RF, Archer SM, Mitchell RB, et al. Clinical practice guideline: tonsillectomy in children. Otolaryngol Head Neck Surg 2011;144:S1–30.
60. Park SK, Kim J, Kim JM, et al. Effects of oral prednisolone on recovery after tonsillectomy. Laryngoscope 2015;125:111–7.
61. Redmann AJ, Maksimoski M, Brumbaugh C, et al. The effect of postoperative steroids on post-tonsillectomy pain and need for postoperative physician contact. Laryngoscope 2018;128:2187–92.
62. Kimiaei Asadi H, Nikooseresht M, Noori L, et al. The Effect of Administration of Ketamine and Paracetamol Versus Paracetamol Singly on Postoperative Pain, Nausea and Vomiting After Pediatric Adenotonsillectomy. Anesth Pain Med 2016;6:e31210.
63. Weiss AL, Ehrhardt KP, Tolba R. Atypical Facial Pain: a Comprehensive, Evidence-Based Review. Curr Pain Headache Rep 2017;21:8.
64. De Giorgi I, Castroflorio T, Sartoris B, et al. The use of conventional transcutaneous electrical nerve stimulation in chronic facial myalgia patients. Clin Oral Investig 2017;21:275–80.

65. Maul XA, Borchard NA, Hwang PH, et al. Microcurrent technology for rapid relief of sinus pain: a randomized, placebo-controlled, double-blinded clinical trial. Int Forum Allergy Rhinol 2019;9:352–6.

66. Khanwalkar AR, Shen J, Kern RC, et al. Utilization of a novel interactive mobile health platform to evaluate functional outcomes and pain following septoplasty and functional endoscopic sinus surgery. Int Forum Allergy Rhinol 2019;9: 345–51.

67. Birnie KA, Campbell F, Nguyen C, et al. iCanCope PostOp: user-centered design of a smartphone-based app for self-management of postoperative pain in children and adolescents. JMIR Form Res 2019;3:e12028.

Postoperative Analgesia in the Chronic Pain Patient

Natasa Grancaric, MD*, Woojin Lee, MD, Madeline Scanlon, MD, MPH

KEYWORDS

- Chronic pain • Opioid management • Postoperative pain • Opioids

KEY POINTS

- An increasing number of chronic pain patients are on long-term opioid therapy.
- Chronic opioid users may have increased analgesic requirements postoperatively due to tolerance, dependence, and opioid-induced hyperalgesia.
- Chronic pain patients are at risk of inadequate pain management in the perioperative setting.
- Undertreated acute pain may lead to the development of chronic pain syndromes in several patients.
- The use of multimodal analgesia is essential to reducing opioid consumption.

INTRODUCTION

The chronic pain patient poses a variety of challenges to the clinician. These often are attributed to psychosocial implications and physiologic changes that occur as a result of long-term opioid use. It is important to be aware of several pharmacologic phenomena that are typical of chronic opioid users.

Tolerance refers to the decreased responsiveness to the effect of opioids as a result of chronic use. Closely related to tolerance is physical *dependence*, which is characterized by withdrawal symptoms precipitated by the abrupt cessation or drastic dose reduction of opioids.[1]

Addiction, on the other hand, is a chronic disease that is characterized by craving, impaired control, and compulsive substance use, which is continued despite negative consequences. In contrast, the term, *pseudoaddiction*, refers to behaviors engaged by those whose pain conditions are undertreated.[1]

Chronic pain syndromes and addiction are not mutually exclusive. A majority of patients taking opioids for chronic pain, however, do not demonstrate the behaviors associated with addiction, such as craving, compulsive use, and loss of control.

Department of Anesthesiology, Columbia University Irving Medical Center, 622 W 168 Street PH5-505, New York, NY 10032, USA
* Corresponding author.
E-mail address: ng2688@cumc.columbia.edu

Otolaryngol Clin N Am 53 (2020) 843–852
https://doi.org/10.1016/j.otc.2020.05.013
0030-6665/20/© 2020 Elsevier Inc. All rights reserved.

Opioid-induced hyperalgesia (OIH) occurs when opioid exposure results in nociceptive sensitization, rendering patients more responsive to painful stimuli. The exact mechanism of the development of OIH is not yet understood. In addition to genetic factors, proposed mechanisms involve enhanced nociceptive response as a result of sensitization of spinal neurons as well as the decreased reuptake of neurotransmitters from primary afferent nociceptive fibers. OIH is thought to explain the loss of efficacy of opioid medications in some patients, especially in the absence of known pathology or existing disease progression.[1]

FROM ACUTE TO CHRONIC PAIN: THE WIND-UP PHENOMENON AND SENSITIZATION

Several patients recovering from surgery develop chronic pain syndromes beyond what is expected in the immediate postoperative setting. The *wind-up phenomenon* refers to peripheral and central nociceptive sensitization that is a result of neurochemical changes after repeated noxious stimuli. Initial *primary sensitization* refers to a hyperexcitable neuronal state following neurogenic inflammation.[2] *Secondary sensitization* occurs in the central nervous system (CNS) and leads to increased sensitivity to noxious stimuli of the area surrounding injured tissue. This occurs as a result of the conversion of nociceptive-specific neurons to nonspecific wide dynamic range neurons, which respond to both noxious and non-noxious stimuli.[2] Central sensitization is thought to be responsible for the development of hyperalgesia and allodynia. *Allodynia* refers to the perceived sensation of pain in response to a non-noxious stimulus, such as light touch.[3]

Risk factors for the development of chronic pain after surgery include type and location of surgery (mastectomy, thoracotomy, and inguinal hernia repair being the most common), duration of procedure greater than 3 hours, intraoperative nerve damage, surgical techniques, and preoperative pain levels.[2] In addition, genetic and psychosocial factors—such as fear of pain, posttraumatic stress disorder, and catastrophizing—are important predisposing factors.

There are several important strategies clinicians may employ for the prevention of chronic pain developing after surgical intervention. These include the early identification of high-risk patients, multimodal analgesic techniques, communication between members of the care team, and setting realistic patient expectations.

To develop an effective perioperative pain management plan, a thorough pain assessment is necessary starting in the preoperative period. This includes determining previous exposure to opioid medications. It is useful to categorize the proposed procedure as minor, intermediate, or major. In general, the pain related to minor interventions may be managed with local anesthetic infiltration and oral analgesic medications postoperatively. Where applicable, regional anesthetic techniques should be employed to decrease opioid requirements. Intermediate and major surgical procedures may require intravenous analgesics postoperatively as well as consultation of the pain management service.

Opioid Management

The risk of the undertreatment of postoperative pain in chronic opioid users is high due to common prejudices and misconceptions regarding patients receiving opioids for chronic pain syndrome and those with addiction. Adequate postoperative analgesia is important for reducing patient anxiety and decreasing pulmonary and vascular complications related to undertreated pain.[4] Preoperatively, the surgeon should obtain a medication history that includes any opioid medications and doses. Generally, patients should continue their usual oral opioid dose on the day of surgery, with additional administration prior to induction of anesthesia. It is important to maintain baseline opioid requirements to reduce the risk of withdrawal. Postoperatively, the patient requires at least the preoperative opioid requirement (for surgeries causing little to no postoperative pain) and possibly supplemental opioids (for surgeries causing moderate–severe pain). If high-dose opioid needs are anticipated, it is reasonable to use a patient-controlled analgesia system to provide patients with adequate analgesia according to their needs. Multimodal analgesia, including regional anesthesia and nonopioid medications (**Table 1**), is essential to reduce opioid consumption. Close co-ordination with a patient's outpatient provider is helpful prior to discharge.

Nonopioid Adjuvants

Since the recognition of current opioid epidemic, there has been growing emphasis on nonopioid adjuvants in chronic pain management.[5] The most commonly utilized non-opioid medications are nonsteroidal anti-inflammatory drugs (NSAIDs), acetaminophen, anticonvulsants, antidepressants, anxiolytics, musculoskeletal agents, and topical anesthetics.[6] Employing these medications with differing target receptors provides multimodal analgesia that leads to reduction in opioid consumption in chronic pain patients.[1] Because these medications have mutually exclusive mechanisms of action, they often complement one another in efficacy.

Nonsteroidal anti-inflammatory drugs

Readily available as over-the-counter medications, NSAIDs are best used for treating inflammatory pain. Nonselective NSAIDs, notably aspirin, ibuprofen, and naproxen, inhibit both cyclooxygenase (COX)-1 and COX-2 enzymes, which are involved in synthesis of biological substrates responsible for inflammation and blood clotting. Therefore, nonselective NSAIDs can put patients at increased risk for gastrointestinal (GI) ulcers or bleeds. More selective NSAIDs, notably celecoxib, inhibit COX-2 selectively, resulting in fewer GI adverse effects. All NSAIDs are associated with decreased kidney function and increased risk of adverse cardiac events, including myocardial infarction; thus, caution is recommended in patients with chronic cardiac or renal disease.[7]

Acetaminophen

Readily available over the counter, acetaminophen is best for treating generalized, nonspecific mild to moderate pain. The mechanism of action for acetaminophen is not understood completely but it appears to inhibit the reuptake of endogenous cannabinoids resulting in generalized analgesia. The most common and serious adverse effect is hepatic injury, because large intake of acetaminophen can lead to accumulation of hepatotoxic metabolites. Due to wide availability of acetaminophen, patients with acute or chronic liver disease, history of alcohol use disorder, or concomitant use of other hepatotoxic medications must be educated in avoiding acetaminophen. Historically and by current Food and Drug Administration standards, the maximum recommended daily dose for acetaminophen in adult is 4 g.[8] In 2011, however, McNeil Consumer Healthcare, a major manufacturer of acetaminophen, lowered the recommended maximum daily dose to 3 g, in advocate of lowering the risk for liver toxicity.[9]

Anticonvulsants

Although most anticonvulsants are used primarily as antiepileptic medications, some anticonvulsants, such as gabapentin and pregabalin, also are effective in treating neuropathic pain. Their main mechanism of action involves blocking $\alpha_2\delta$ subunit of voltage-dependent calcium channels, resulting in decreased neuronal firing. Clinically, this is exhibited as decrease in neuropathic pain and anxiety. In chronic pain medicine,

Table 1
An overview of the most common nonopioid adjuvants used in chronic pain practice

Drug	Mechanism of Action	Uses	Adverse Effects	Special Consideration
NSAIDs (nonselective: aspirin, ibuprofen, naproxen; selective: celecoxib)	Inhibits COX-1 and COX-2 (nonselective) or COX-2 only (selective) = decreased inflammatory mediators	Best for inflammatory pain	GI bleeds/ulcers (nonselective), thrombosis, worsening kidney function (all), increased risk of cardiac events (all)	Avoid in patients with cardiac history, acute or chronic kidney disease, history of stroke, peptic ulcer disease, or active bleeding
Acetaminophen	Modulation of endogenous cannabinoid system = increased analgesia	Best used for generalized mild to moderate pain	Liver damage/toxicity	Avoid in patients with acute or chronic liver disease, history of alcohol use disorder or concomitant use of other hepatotoxic medications. Maximum recommended daily dose: 3 g/d, or 2 g/d for patients with stable liver disease
Anticonvulsants (gabapentin, pregabalin)	Blocks $\alpha_2\delta$ subunit of voltage-dependent calcium channel (gabapentin, pregabalin) = anticonvulsant, analgesic, and anxiolytic effects	Best used for neuropathic pain, migraine	Sedation, increased suicidal ideation, lower extremity edema	Must be dosed 2–3 times a day to maintain therapeutic level; decreased dosage in patients with kidney disease
Antidepressants (SSRI: fluoxetine, sertraline. SNRI: duloxetine, venlafaxine. TCA: nortriptyline, amitriptyline)	Inhibits reuptake of serotonin (SSRI), inhibits reuptake of serotonin and norepinephrine (SNRI, TCA) = endogenous opioid modulation	Best used for neuropathic pain, fibromyalgia (SNRI), musculoskeletal pain (SNRI), and associated depression (SSRI)	Convulsion, cardiac arrhythmia, urinary retention, dry mouth, postural hypotension (TCA), sedation (TCA, SNRI), GI distress, sexual dysfunction (SSRI)	Careful risk-benefit analysis is warranted, especially when prescribing TCA due to serious side-effect profile. Effective in treating depression associated with chronic pain

Drug class	Mechanism	Best used for	Side effects	Warnings/cautions
Anxiolytics (benzodiazepines, buspirone)	Increases effectiveness of GABA at $GABA_A$ receptors = decreases neuronal excitability (benzodiazepines); serotonin agonist (buspirone)	Best used for muscle spasms (benzodiazepine), associated anxiety (benzodiazepine, buspirone)	Sedation, respiratory depression, anterograde amnesia, sexual dysfunction (benzodiazepine), dizziness, headache (buspirone)	Potential for addiction and overdose (benzodiazepine). Avoid taking with other serotoninergic medications (buspirone)
Musculoskeletal agents (baclofen, tizanidine, cyclobenzaprine)	Activates $GABA_B$ receptors (baclofen), $\alpha2$-receptors (tizanidine), serotonin receptor antagonist (cyclobenzaprine)	Best used for muscle spasms	Drowsiness, dizziness, dry mouth	Avoid taking with alcohol/benzodiazepines (all). Must be aware of numerous drug-drug interactions. Avoid taking with serotonergic drugs (cyclobenzaprine).
Topical anesthetics (lidocaine patch, capsaicin)	Blocks voltage-gated sodium channels in sensory neurons (lidocaine). Activates TRPV 1 = depletion of substance P (capsaicin)	Best used for peripheral neuropathy (all), musculoskeletal pain (capsaicin)	Burning, redness, skin discomfort	No more than 3 lidocaine patches at a time, because local anesthetic toxicity is possible

these medications are used most commonly in treating postherpetic neuralgia, central and peripheral neuoropathy, and migraine.[10] Gabapentin and pregabalin both have a short elimination half-life (approximately 6 hours), thus require redosing 2 times to 3 times a day to remain therapeutic. Because these medications are excreted renally, patients with acute or chronic kidney disease are prone to increased adverse effects, most commonly sedation.[11] Caution should be used in patients with renal disease and the medication dose should be adjusted.

Antidepressants

Two classes of antidepressants, tricyclic antidepressants (TCAs) and serotonin-norepinephrine reuptake inhibitors (SNRIs), commonly are used to treat pain. Numerous studies have shown that TCAs, such as amitriptyline and nortriptyline, and SNRIs, including duloxetine and venlafaxine, are effective in treating different types of chronic pain, notably neuropathic pain and fibromyalgia.[10] Although the direct mechanism of action in which these medications provide analgesia is unknown, it is thought that their inhibition against serotonin and norepinephrine reuptake leads to endogenous opioid modulation resulting in analgesia.[12,13] TCAs must be prescribed with caution, because they have deleterious effects, notably cardiac arrhythmias, orthostatic hypotension, and convulsions. The most common side effects include sedation, dry mouth, urinary retention, and tachycardia. TCAs often are started at a low dose and titrated until maximum efficacy can be seen with minimal side effects. SNRIs have less notable side-effect profile, the most common being sedation.

Anxiolytics

Among the most common comorbidities that many chronic pain patients suffer are depression and anxiety.[14] Although anxiolytics, such as benzodiazepines and buspirone, do not have direct analgesic effects, these medications provide benefits to patients' perception of pain by alleviating their anxiety. Benzodiazepines also provide muscle relaxation, which can indirectly alleviate pain secondary to muscle spasms.[15,16] The main mechanism of action of benzodiazepines is allosteric binding to γ-aminobutyric acid (GABA) receptor, resulting in increased effectiveness of endogenous GABA. This leads to depression in neuronal activity. Along with anxiolysis, patients also may experience sedation, respiratory depression, anterograde amnesia, and sexual dysfunction. Some experience euphoria with benzodiazepine use, which puts patients at risk for addiction, abuse, and possible overdose. Because of their relatively safer side effect profiles and low potential for abuse compared with benzodiazepines, SSRIs and SNRIs are often considered more favorable adjuvants. Caution must be exercised when prescribing benzodiazepines, as concurrent use with opioids increase risk of respiratory depression and death.

Musculoskeletal agents

Among musculoskeletal agents, the most commonly used are baclofen, tizanidine, and cyclobenzaprine. They are most effective in treating painful muscle spasms accompanied by spastic movement disorders, such as cerebral palsy and multiple sclerosis. Each medication has different mechanism of action but all 3 medications achieve the goal of CNS depression, leading to the relaxation of skeletal muscles. Although these medications have relatively safe side-effect profiles, they have many drug-drug interactions that physicians must be aware of. All musculoskeletal agents must be prescribed with caution in patients who use alcohol, benzodiazepine, or any other CNS depressants due to synergistic CNS depression.[17] Tizanidine and concomitant use of cytochrome P450 1A2 inhibitors should be avoided because this combination may impair the metabolism of tizanidine.[18] Cyclobenzaprine should be avoided in patients taking serotonergic medications because it could put patients at risk for serotonin syndrome.[19]

Topical anesthetics

Topical agents can be useful to target specific painful areas with decreased systemic effects compared with oral medications. Some of the most commonly used topical analgesics are lidocaine and capsaicin. Lidocaine targets voltage-gated sodium channels of sensory neurons. By blocking these channels, lidocaine inhibits neural conduction along the sensory neurons. Capsaicin works by activating transient receptor potential vanilloid (TRPV 1), which ultimately results in depletion of substance P, one of the major pain transmission neuropeptides. Capsaicin is effective in treating both peripheral neuropathy and musculoskeletal pain, such as osteoarthritis.[20] Outside of skin irritation and burning sensation, patients rarely experience adverse effects from these medications. Although local anesthetic toxicity is still a possibility with the use of lidocaine patches, it is rare even when applied above the recommended maximum dose of 3 patches daily.[21] If a patient's insurance does not cover prescription 5% lidocaine patches, over-the-counter 4% lidocaine patches or lidocaine cream may be offered to the patient as an alternative.

RECOMMENDATIONS FOR PATIENTS ON MAINTENANCE THERAPY

Patients on maintenance opioid therapy are a unique subset of patients who require particular attention in the postoperative period. Specific recommendations for patients on methadone, suboxone, or naloxone maintenance therapy are described.

Methadone

Methadone is a long-acting opioid that is used to treat chronic pain as well as opioid dependence. The drug binds and occupies μ-opioid receptors and effectively reduces pain, decreases opioid craving, and reduces the euphoric effects of subsequent illicit opioid use.

Patients on methadone maintenance therapy (MMT) should continue to receive their daily methadone maintenance dose in the perioperative period.[22] In the event that a patient is not receiving oral intake, the methadone may be dosed parenterally at half the oral dose, as noted in the manufacturer's labeling (ie, a patient receiving methadone, 10 mg orally, daily may receive methadone, 5 mg intravenously, daily). It is important to recognize that patients receiving methadone for maintenance therapy do not receive adequate analgesia from their maintenance dose. Although the duration of action of methadone for prevention of withdrawal is 24 hours to 48 hours, the duration of action for analgesia is only 4 hours to 8 hours. Thus, patients on MMT likely require additional opioid for treatment of acute postsurgical pain. The total methadone dose may be split into 3 doses, 8 hours apart, to improve analgesia. For example, a patient on methadone, 30 mg daily, may be given methadone, 10 mg every 8 hours, only while the patient is inpatient. The total daily dose of methadone should not be adjusted without consultation of the patient's MMT provider.

In the postoperative period, it is recommended that patients on MMT be treated aggressively with nonopioid analgesics. If patients require opioids, it is recommended to start short-acting opioids in addition to the methadone dosing. Long-term opioid use causes opioid tolerance and OIH. Thus, patients on MMT often have an increased short-acting opioid dose requirement in comparison to patients not on opioid maintenance therapy and often need higher and more frequent doses of opioid analgesics to achieve adequate pain control. If a patient requires ongoing short-acting opioids on discharge, the dose and duration of therapy should be communicated to the patient's methadone clinic. If the patient is discharged home postoperatively, a methadone prescription should not be provided, because the patient should instead return to the methadone clinic.

Suboxone is a combination of 2 opioid medications: buprenorphine and naloxone. Buprenorphine is a partial μ-opioid agonist that has high affinity and low intrinsic activity at the μ-receptor. The drug's partial agonist properties make it effective in treating opioid dependence while its high affinity for the μ-opioid receptor blocks the effects of illicit opioids.[23–26] In suboxone, naloxone is only present to discourage misuse because it has low bioavailability when administered sublingually. Similar to methadone, suboxone has a duration of action for analgesia that is substantially shorter than its duration of action for suppression of opioid withdrawal.

The decision of whether to continue or discontinue suboxone prior to surgery is based on many factors. The type and urgency of the surgery, expected postoperative opioid requirement, and patient characteristics must be considered.[27] This decision should be discussed and agreed on between the patient, surgeon, and buprenorphine provider. If suboxone is discontinued prior to surgery, the drug should be restarted only once the patient no longer has acute pain requiring narcotic analgesics because suboxone can precipitate withdrawal.[28] If, however, suboxone is continued during the perioperative period, it is recommended that the patient's acute pain be treated with short-acting opioids. In this case, the patient likely requires significantly higher doses of opioids to achieve adequate pain control. Managing patients on suboxone is best achieved in consultation with the acute or chronic pain service.[29] For further discussion, the reader is referred to the chapter on Pre-Operative Optimization.

Naltrexone

Naltrexone is a long-acting competitive antagonist that has a high affinity for the μ-opioid receptor.[30] When taken prior to other opioids, naltrexone blocks the euphoric, sedative, and analgesic effects of opioids. Naltrexone may be prescribed for patients with mild opioid use disorder who do not demonstrate withdrawal symptoms.[31]

Oral naltrexone should be discontinued 2 days to 3 days prior to surgery to allow for intraoperative or postoperative opioids to effectively provide analgesia.[32] Extended-release naltrexone intramuscular injection is administered every 28 days, and elective surgeries should be postponed 4 weeks after administration.[33] The abrupt discontinuation of naltrexone may cause an increase in μ-opioid receptors, making patients more sensitive to perioperative opioids. Thus, patients previously taking naltrexone should be monitored closely and perioperative opioids should be titrated carefully to avoid sedation and respiratory depression.[34]

SUMMARY

The management of pain in patients with chronic pain syndromes who are on chronic opioid therapy or maintenance opioid therapy can be challenging for clinicians. Inadequate postoperative pain management in this population can have several adverse outcomes, such as increase hospital length of stay, precipitation of withdrawal in some cases, and overall increase in health care costs. In these patients, it is recommended to employ multimodal analgesic therapies whenever possible and to ensure baseline opioid requirements are met, while avoiding restricting opioid treatment of acute pain.

REFERENCES

1. Coluzzi F, Bifulco F, Cuomo A, et al. The challenge of perioperative pain management in opioid-tolerant patients. Ther Clin Risk Manag 2017;13:1163–73.
2. Feizerfan A, Sheh G. Transition from acute to chronic pain. Cont Educ Anaesth Crit Care Pain 2014;15(2):98–102.
3. Latremoliere A, Woolf CJ. Central sensitization: a generator of pain hypersensitivity by central neural plasticity. J Pain 2009;10(9):895–926.
4. Leung E. Physiology of pain. In: Sackheim K, editor. Pain management and palliative care. New York: Springer; 2015. p. 253–63.
5. Woolf CJ. Central sensitization: implications for the diagnosis and treatment of pain. Pain 2011;152(3, Supplement):S2–15.
6. Daubresse M, Chang HY, Yu Y, et al. Ambulatory diagnosis and treatment of nonmalignant pain in the United States, 2000-2010. Med Care 2013;51(10):870–8.
7. Pyati S, Gan TJ. Perioperative pain management. CNS Drugs 2007;21(3):185–211.
8. Day R, Graham GG. The vascular effects of COX-2 selective inhibitors. Aust Prescr 2004;27(6):142–5.
9. Bleumink GS, Feenstra J, Sturkenboom M, et al. Nonsteroidal anti-inflammatory drugs and heart failure. Drugs 2003;63(6):525–34.
10. Major JM, Zhou EH, Wong HL, et al. Trends in rates of acetaminophen-related adverse events in the United States. Pharmacoepidemiol Drug Saf 2016;25(5):590–8.
11. Prescription acetaminophen products to be limited to 325 Mg per dosage. In: U.S. Food and Drug Administration. 2018. Available at: https://www.fda.gov/drugs/drug-safety-and-availability/fda-drug-safety-communication-prescription-acetaminophen-products-be-limited-325-mg-dosage-unit. Accessed December 1, 2019.
12. Tylenol dosage for adults. In: Tylenol. 2019. Available at: https://www.tylenol.com/safety-dosing/usage/dosage-for-adults. Accessed December 1, 2019.
13. Wiffen PJ, Derry S, Moore RA, et al. Antiepileptic drugs for neuropathic pain and fibromyalgia – an overview of Cochrane reviews. Cochrane Database Syst Rev 2013;(11):CD010567.
14. Evoy KE, Morrison MD, Saklad SR. Abuse and misuse of pregabalin and gabapentin. Drugs 2017;77(4):403–26.
15. Beal BR, Wallace MS. An overview of pharmacologic management of chronic pain. Med Clin North Am 2016;100(1):65–79.
16. Lunn MPT, Hughes RAC, Wiffen PJ. Duloxetine for treating painful neuropathy, chronic pain or fibromyalgia. Cochrane Database Syst Rev 2014;(1):CD007115.
17. Benbouzid M, Gaveriaux-Ruff C, Yalcin I, et al. Delta-opioid receptors are critical for tricyclic antidepressant treatment of neuropathic allodynia. Biol Psychiatry 2008;63(6):633–6.
18. Furukawa T, McGuire H, Barbui C. Meta-analysis of effects and side effects of low dosage tricyclic antidepressants in depression: systematic review. Br Med J 2002;325:991.
19. Van Korff M, Crane P, Lane M, et al. Chronic spinal pain and physical-mental comorbidity in the United States: results from the national comorbidity survey replication. Pain 2005;113(3):331–9.
20. Reddy S, Patt RB. The benzodiazepines as adjuvant analgesics. J Pain Symptom Manage 1994;9(8):510–4.

21. Ballenger JC. Benzodiazepine receptors agonists and antagonists. Kaplan and Sadock's Comprehensive Textbook of Psychiatry 2000;7:2317–23.
22. Agabio R, Preti A, Gessa GL. Efficacy and tolerability of baclofen in substance use disorders: a systematic review. Eur Addict Res 2013;19(6):325–45.
23. Granfors MT, Backman JT, Laitila J, et al. Tizanidine is mainly metabolized by cytochrome P450 1A2 in vitro. Br J Clin Pharmacol 2004;57(3):349–53.
24. Keegan MT, Brown DR, Rabinstein AA. Serotonin syndrome from the interaction of cyclobenzaprine with other serotoninergic drugs. Anesth Analg 2006;103(6): 1466–8.
25. Anand P, Bley K. Topical capsaicin for pain management: therapeutic potential and mechanisms of action of the new high-concentration capsaicin 8% patch. Br J Anaesth 2011;107(4):490–502.
26. Gammaitoni A, Ford C, Alvared N. 24-hour application of the lidocaine patch 5% for 3 consecutive days is safe and well tolerated in healthy adult men and women. Pain Med 2002;3(2):172.
27. Alford DP, Compton P, Samet JH. Acute pain management for patients receiving maintenance methadone or buprenorphine therapy. Ann Intern Med 2006;144(2): 127–34.
28. White JM. Pleasure into pain: the consequences of long-term opioid use. Addict Behav 2004;29(7):1311–24.
29. Johnson RE, Strain EC, Amass L. Buprenorphine: how to use it right. Drug Alcohol Depend 2003;70(2 Suppl):S59–77.
30. Nelson EE, Guyer AE, Stern E, et al. Buprenorphine: clinical best practices for periop management. Casp J Intern Med 2015;1(3):280–5.
31. Bryson EO. The perioperative management of patients maintained on medications used to manage opioid addiction. Curr Opin Anaesthesiol 2014;27(3): 359–64.
32. Warltier DC. Perioperative management of acute pain in the opioid-dependent patient. Anesthesiology 2004;101(1):212–27.
33. Prescribing Information. In: Vivitrol. 2019. Available at: https://www.vivitrol.com/content/pdfs/prescribing-information.pdf. Accessed March 1, 2019.
34. Harrison TK, Kornfeld H, Aggarwal AK, et al. Perioperative considerations for the patient with opioid use disorder on buprenorphine, methadone, or naltrexone maintenance therapy. Anesthesiol Clin 2018;36(3):345–59.

Nonenteral Pain Management

Katherine Tinkey, MD[a], Sai Alla, MD[a], Nan Xiang, MD[b],*

KEYWORDS

- Nonenteral • Analgesia • Pain • Adjuncts • Otolaryngology

KEY POINTS

- Otolaryngologic surgeries provide unique challenges to postoperative pain management as the location and nature of the surgeries may make enteral medication administration difficult or impossible.
- Several nonenteral routes of administration exist, including intravenous, transdermal, subcutaneous, and rectal.
- There are a multitude of medications that are available in nonenteral formulations, including acetaminophen, nonsteroidal anti-inflammatory drugs, opioids, and ketamine.
- Nonenteral opioids can be delivered as intermittent intravenous boluses, patient-controlled analgesia, or transdermal patches.
- Even when limited to nonenteral medications, a multimodal approach with opioids and adjuncts can provide appropriate analgesia for the otolaryngologic patient.

INTRODUCTION

Adequate postoperative pain control in patients undergoing otolaryngologic (ENT) surgeries is a key component of their postoperative care. However, pain management in these patients poses unique challenges to their physicians given the location of the surgical site and the nature of the procedures. Postoperatively, many ENT procedures may impose certain anatomic limitations that make oral intake impossible or contraindicated, often requiring prolonged nil per os (NPO) status to protect against postsurgical bleeding or aspiration events. Given these barriers to enteral access, these patients are at greater risks for poor postoperative pain control, which could have short-term and long-term consequences. Effectively managing pain can have significant benefits in avoiding postoperative complications, such as infections, deep vein thrombosis, poor wound healing, and prolonged hospitalization,[1] while expediting successful functional recovery. The key to achieving adequate postoperative pain

[a] Department of Anesthesiology, Emory University, 1440 Clifton Road Northeast, Suite 400, Atlanta, GA 30322, USA; [b] Department of Anesthesiology, Emory University, 550 Peachtree Street Northeast, 7th Floor, Atlanta, GA 30308, USA
* Corresponding author.
E-mail address: Nan.xiang@emory.edu

Otolaryngol Clin N Am 53 (2020) 853–863
https://doi.org/10.1016/j.otc.2020.05.014
0030-6665/20/© 2020 Elsevier Inc. All rights reserved.

lies in understanding and using various medications with nonenteral routes of administration. This article aims to review different nonenteral routes and medication groups that could be used via these routes in patients after ENT surgery with restricted enteral access to improve postoperative pain management.

ROUTES OF NONENTERAL DRUG ADMINISTRATION

Enteral drugs use the gastrointestinal (GI) tract as the primary site of absorption and is the most commonly used route for drug administration. Nonenteral routes of administration avoid the GI tract completely, often owing to limitations on oral intake, lack of enteral drug formations, or lack of a functioning GI system. Safety, efficacy, pharmacodynamics, and patient preference must be taken into account before choosing the most appropriate route of administration. In this article, we review the intravenous, subcutaneous, transdermal, and rectal routes of administration and highlight the advantages and disadvantages of each route.[2]

Intravenous

The intravenous method of administration involves injecting drugs directly into the systemic venous circulation. Many drugs have formulations that allow them to be given intravenously. It is an effective and rapid method to achieve adequate analgesic concentrations in the systemic circulation. Drugs given intravenously also have 100% bioavailability because they bypass many of the metabolic and absorptive barriers encountered through the enteral route, also known as first-pass metabolism. Patients can also be placed on infusions that allow short-term, long-term, and titratable pain control. Other advantages include decreased irritation at the site of injection, decreased cost, lower volumes needed to achieve proper analgesia, and rapid exposure of the drug to its target organs. However, clinicians should also weigh the potential disadvantages. The intravenous route of administration requires an adequate functioning cannula for access, can be labor intensive compared with other routes, is unforgiving to dosing errors, and is also prone to line infections with long-term use. Certain medications can irritate the veins and lead to phlebitis. Lastly, although intravenous medications can be an excellent option while the patient is admitted, the logistics of outpatient use make it a poor long-term option in most cases.

Subcutaneous

Subcutaneous injection is another mode of administration of analgesic medications that can be used for patients with limited enteral access. The drug is injected or implanted beneath the surface of the skin known as the cutis, a layer of skin directly below the dermis and epidermis. Subcutaneous tissue absorption is slower than intravenous owing to the reduced vasculature surface area supplying this region, while still able to obtain 100% bioavailability. Typically, 25- to 31-gauge needles are used to inject the medication, with medication volumes not exceeding 2 mL. Common injection locations include the outer area of the upper arm, abdomen, thigh, upper back, and buttocks.[3]

Transdermal

The transdermal route of administration provides an effective method to administer medications that is noninvasive and has a relatively better safety profile as compared with intravenous administration. Many medications may be administered transdermally including nonsteroidal anti-inflammatory drugs (NSAIDs), opioids, local anesthetics, and even antidepressants.

The most obvious benefit of transdermal opioids is that it allows a total bypass of the GI tract when either there is a problem with absorption or, for the purposes of ENT surgeries, the GI tract may be unavailable. Transdermal release of opioids provides a steady concentration of the drug in the plasma, thus avoiding large fluctuations and providing a consistent level of analgesia. Other benefits include simplicity of administration, potential for long-term outpatient use, and improved quality of life.[4]

Rectal

The final route of administration we briefly discuss is the rectal route, which may also be considered when enteral administration is contraindicated. There are many different medications that have rectal formulations including laxatives, acetaminophen, NSAIDs, antiemetics, benzodiazepines, and opioids. The benefits of the rectal route of administration include allowing for delivery of medications that have poor stability or solubility that would be unable to tolerate the physiologic environment of the stomach and GI tract, low cost of rectal formulation of most medications, and ease of administration that does not require a health care provider. However, patient discomfort and/or refusal of rectal administration limits their practical use in the perioperative setting.[5]

ACETAMINOPHEN

Acetaminophen is a common, effective, and safe medication used as an over-the-counter pain reliever for daily life, but also plays an important role in multimodal analgesia in the perioperative setting. Unlike NSAIDs, another very common over-the-counter analgesic, acetaminophen does not interfere with platelet function or cause adverse reactions in patients with asthma or peptic ulcer disease. Although the mechanism of action is not entirely clear, it is thought to selectively inhibit cyclooxygenase in the central nervous system, although this inhibition is absent in the peripheral nervous system and stomach, accounting for its decreased incidence of ulcers and platelet interference. It has been proposed that the analgesic effects of acetaminophen come from agonism on the cannabinoid receptors, leading to increased levels of endogenous cannabinoids and results in analgesia and a sense of well-being.[5,6] Acetaminophen is available for various routes of administration including oral, intravenous, and rectal. The uptake of acetaminophen is the greatest via the intravenous route with very little absorption occurring via the GI tract. However, some studies suggest that there is not increased bioavailability with intravenous use compared with oral. One review article analyzed 6 randomized clinical trials and found that the bioavailability of 1000 mg of oral acetaminophen was 89% and concluded that there is no clear indication for intravenous acetaminophen over oral when a patient has a normally functioning GI tract. However, the intravenous formulation has a much faster onset of action and results in higher plasma concentrations of the drug, resulting in greater patient satisfaction and perceived pain relief as compared with oral administration. This review article found that intravenous acetaminophen decreased pain by 50% in 37% of patients and decreased opioid use by 30% at 4 hours and 16% at 6 hours.[7] A Cochrane review of 20 randomized, double-blind, placebo-controlled clinical trials found that the number needed to treat to achieve 50% pain relief after a single 1000-mg dose of acetaminophen as compared with placebo was 4.6 demonstrating acetaminophen's superiority to placebo and effectiveness as a stand-alone analgesic. Not only can acetaminophen be used alone, but when combined with other analgesics, such as opioids, a greater analgesic effect can be achieved. This same Cochrane Review showed that, in patients with moderate to severe acute postoperative pain, oral oxycodone at doses of more than 5 mg had greater efficacy and longer lasting analgesia when combined with acetaminophen.[8] Owing to its low side effect profile, efficacy, and ability to be given nonenterally, acetaminophen is a useful perioperative analgesic for ENT surgeries.[9]

NONSTEROIDAL ANTI-INFLAMMATORY DRUGS

NSAIDs are among the most common and effective nonopioid analgesic medications used not only over the counter, but also in the perioperative setting. There are many different types of nonselective NSAIDs including salicylates, proprionic acids, pyrazoles, acetic acids, oxicams, fenamates, and napthyl-alkanones, which all act by reversibly inhibiting cyclooxygenase 1 and 2, which is responsible for prostaglandin synthesis. Arachidonic acid is released from tissues as a result of damage, which is subsequently metabolized into prostaglandins that then lower the pain threshold and cause pain. The mechanism of action of NSAIDs is due to the inhibition of cyclooxygenase and, therefore, decreased prostaglandin synthesis.[9,10] NSAIDs also have a variety of routes of administration, including oral, intravenous, and transdermal, and have been used as local infiltration as the site of wounds or surgical incisions and even intranasally.[10] Intravenous ketorolac is the most common nonparenteral NSAID used postoperatively and intranasal ketorolac has recently been approved for use and has been shown to have effective analgesia in the postoperative setting.[11] The maximum dose of intravenous ketorolac is 30 mg every 6 hours for a maximum of 5 days. This dose should be decreased to 15 mg in patients age 65 or older. NSAIDs have been clearly shown to have superior analgesic effects as compared with acetaminophen in dental surgery with one review article demonstrating 8 studies that found NSAIDs were superior to acetaminophen in regards to pain scores postoperatively.[12] One systemic review found that NSAIDs, when given postoperatively, were effective in decreasing opioid requirements by 20% to 35% and also decreased the side effects of opioids, such as nausea, vomiting, and sedation.[11,13] Despite their effectiveness, NSAIDs do not come without risks. Chronic use of NSAIDs can commonly cause gastric ulcers and interfere with platelet inhibition, which is associated with a higher bleeding risk. However, short-term use of NSAIDs in the perioperative setting in terms of platelet inhibition and increased bleeding risk is less well-studied. Decreased prostaglandin synthesis may also be associated with impaired bone healing and acute renal injury. Cyclooxygenase-2 specific inhibitors, such as celecoxib, have a lower side effect profile, because the specificity of these drugs have little to no effect on platelet aggregation and the GI tract. They also offer similar analgesic profiles to nonspecific NSAIDs.[9–11] However, their role in the postoperative period, and especially for ENT surgeries, is limited because currently all available formulas in the United States are oral medications. Parecoxib has been approved in Europe and is available in the intravenous formulation; however, it has not been approved by the US Food and Drug Administration. NSAIDs are an effective analgesic class in the postoperative setting for ENT, especially dental surgeries.

OPIOIDS

ENT patients with significant acute postoperative pain or with chronic pain from an anatomic defect or malignancy would likely benefit from the use of opioid medications for analgesia. Opioid agonists such as hydrocodone, oxycodone, morphine, and many others act primarily at the mu-opioid receptor to provide analgesic effects. Although many opioids are administered orally, there are intravenous, intramuscular, intranasal, transdermal, and neuraxial formulations[14] available for patients who are physically unable to take the medications by mouth. In this discussion, we focus on intravenous and transdermal options, which are more commonly used and more pertinent to the otolaryngology patient population. As a word of caution, the recommendations provided do not account for specific patient comorbidities and may not be appropriate for patients with complex pain pathology, such as patients with a history of high-dose opioid use, opioid abuse disorder, or central pain disorders. In managing patients with a history of chronic pain, it is imperative to involve their outpatient chronic pain physicians and develop individualized pain management plans. Furthermore, in the inpatient setting, patients with high opioid requirements at baseline may benefit from consultations with the acute pain service, supportive care service, or similar services within the hospital that have experience managing patients with complicated pain.

In the postoperative setting, intravenous delivery of opioid medications is one of the most common methods of pain management. Especially in patients with difficulties with swallowing or with residual effects of anesthesia putting them at risk for aspiration, the intravenous route can provide analgesia reliably, quickly, and effectively. Intermittent boluses of opioid agonists such as morphine, hydromorphone, or fentanyl can be requested by the patient and delivered by the nursing staff. However, intermittent boluses typically require a significant dose of opioid per bolus as well as a greater demand on the nursing staff to both deliver the medication and to monitor for sedation and respiratory depression. This strategy is typically most appropriate in the postanesthesia care unit where close monitoring by the nursing staff is standard. Reliance on intermittent opioid boluses on the inpatient units, where there is typically a lack of continuous pulse oximetry and higher patient-to-nurse ratios, may lead to inadequate analgesia or greater adverse events.

For inpatient floor patients, a patient-controlled analgesia (PCA) device can provide immediate analgesia, at lower bolus doses, without requiring an increased nursing workload.[15,16] A PCA device for intravenous medications, most commonly opioids, involves the use of a microprocessor-controlled infusion pump[15] that delivers a preset amount of medication when activated by the patient. The medications used in PCAs are commonly pure mu-opioid agonist such as morphine, hydromorphone, and fentanyl, given their relatively rapid onset of action, high efficacy, and intermediate duration of action.[14]

The advantages of PCA use for postoperative pain management include patient autonomy, medication dosing as frequently as every 6 minutes and a consistent level of analgesia by avoiding peaks and troughs in medication plasma concentration.[15] By design, the PCA is intended to be activated by the patient, to decrease the risk of another individual overmedicating an already sedated patient. With increased sophistication of PCA devices, there is detailed tracking of opioid usage and may be real-time monitoring of end-tidal carbon dioxide as a proxy for adequate ventilation. The primary disadvantage of PCA usage is the lack of analgesic coverage while the patient is asleep, given the short to intermediate duration of action of the medications, which may result in uncontrolled pain once the patient awakens.[14]

PCA use is not appropriate for every patient, making it important to evaluate each individual for potential limitations. In particular, PCA use requires the patient to be cooperative with the ability to follow instructions, which can be difficult for young children, mentally delayed adults, patients with dementia or delirium, and those with a physical disability that would prevent manual activation of the PCA button. Even in able-bodied adults, an understanding of the duration of action of the medications and the lock-out interval is important for managing expectations and overall success of the pain management plan.

There are several important variables that determine how opioids are delivered by a PCA device. The most common parameters are demand dose, lock-out interval, and 1-hour maximum dose. Descriptions of these parameters are summarized in **Table 1**,

Table 1
Parameters, descriptions, and ranges related to PCA for various opioids

Parameter	Descriptions	Range
Initial loading dose	One-time dose at the time the PCA is started	Morphine: 1–3 mg Hydromorphone: 0.25–1 mg Fentanyl: 25–50 μg
Demand dose	Drug-specific amount delivered at the lock-out interval	Morphine: 0.5–2.5 mg Hydromorphone 0.1–0.5 mg Fentanyl: 5–25 μg
Lock-out interval	Minimum time between demand doses	5–20 min
1-Hour maximum dose	Maximum dose of medication that can be delivered within 1 h	Typically, total calculated by demand dose × doses per hour
Basal rate	Continuous infusion, delivered without patient activation. Consider for opioid tolerant patients	Depends on chronic opioid usage
Nursing bolus	Intermittent doses that can only be administered by nursing staff, to allow patient to "catch up"	Typical 2–3× demand dose, every 2–4 h

along with commonly used values to which they are set based on cited publications and various institutional protocols including Emory University and MD Anderson Cancer Center.[14,15,17] It is typically prudent to start at a lower dose before uptitrating the settings based on the patient's response. For example, a typical starting hydromorphone PCA order set includes a demand dose of 0.2 mg, every 6 minutes, with a 1-hour maximum dose of 2 mg. If the patient has a tolerance to opioids, they may require a higher regimen, with the goal of eventually weaning the PCA and transitioning to an oral regimen before patient discharge. In some instances, if their chronic opioid use is greater than 60 mg oral morphine equivalents, a continuous rate on the PCA or a separate long-acting medication can be added to the regimen to provide a basal analgesic effect. However, a continuous basal rate may detract from the safety of PCA. Without a continuous basal rate, if a patient becomes overly sedated, the patient stops pushing the demand button and stops receiving further opioid. With a continuous basal rate, a sedated patient would continue to receive opioid. Therefore, caution is recommended with continuous basal rate infusions.

One intravenous option for a long-acting opioid is methadone, a synthetic mu-receptor agonist, serotonin reuptake inhibitor, and N-methyl-D-aspartate (NMDA) receptor antagonist.[14,18] It has a variable half-life that is likely due to several factors, including lipophilicity and distribution, and results in a biphasic elimination pattern. Owing to an alpha elimination of 8 to 12 hours, methadone can provide analgesia for 6 to 8 hours after administration, and the beta elimination period of 30 to 60 hours allows for prevention of opioid withdrawal for greater than 24 hours.[14,18] As a result, methadone for analgesia should be dosed every 8 hours, whereas methadone for maintenance therapy for opioid or heroin addiction is dosed daily. For patients on chronic oral methadone therapy, conversion to intravenous has traditionally been a 2:1 ratio, although some providers have found a 1:0.7 ratio[19] to be more appropriate. However, with these patients it is highly recommended that the primary service obtain assistance from the acute pain service regarding an appropriate regimen so as to minimize respiratory depression and monitoring for QTc changes on the electrocardiogram. Even for patients naïve to methadone, several double-blinded randomized controlled trials have found intraoperative methadone use to be associated with reduced postoperative opioid requirements, decreased pain scores, and patient perception of pain management in cardiac surgeries[20] and spinal fusion.[21] This finding suggests that methadone can be a viable medication in the management of postoperative pain, possibly in other specialties including otolaryngology, although more research is needed to determine appropriate dosing, rate of respiratory depression, and whether there is a decrease in chronic postsurgical pain.[22]

One alternative to the use of a long-acting opioid such as methadone is to use an opioid that can be continuously delivered via a transdermal patch. Of the options on the market currently, two of the most commonly used are buprenorphine patches and fentanyl patches. Buprenorphine is a partial agonist at the mu opioid receptor, with a ceiling effect on respiratory depression but not on its analgesic properties.[23] At higher doses, buprenorphine has traditionally been used for treatment of and maintenance therapy for opioid use disorder. Recent research including a metanalysis of randomized controlled trials has shown that buprenorphine can provide noninferior analgesia for acute pain compared with traditional opioids.[24] In the transdermal formulation, branded as Butrans,[25] buprenorphine is a nonenteral option for postsurgical patients. Available doses for buprenorphine transdermal patches are 7.5 µg, 10 µg, 15 µg, and 20 µg/h patches, to be worn for 7 days before replacing.[25] However, even at the highest dose, the analgesic effect is limited and may not be appropriate for patients requiring more than 80 mg of oral morphine equivalents per day.[25]

Fentanyl is a high potency mu opioid agonist[26] that can be found in a transdermal patch and has been used for management of acute and chronic pain. Fentanyl patches have doses ranging from 12 µg/h up to 100 µg/h, which is equivalent to 30 to 240 mg of oral morphine equivalents per days, approximately, according to the Medicare opioid conversion table.[27] As a result, fentanyl patches can provide significantly higher opioid effects as compared with buprenorphine patches. Owing to its pharmacokinetics, the analgesic effect may be delayed by up to 12 hours after the initiation of the patch and the patch should be changed every 72 hours.[4] Owing to the delayed onset, fentanyl patches may be difficult to titrate in response to fluctuating acute postoperative surgical pain, but can provide the basal opioid level for opioid-tolerant patients.[4] It is important to be aware that skin temperature impacts the rate of absorption, meaning that febrile patients or those using external heating apparatuses may have increased levels of fentanyl.[4] Fentanyl patches also contain significantly higher amounts of drug product than what is delivered to the patient, so patches should never be tampered with or cut and used patches should be disposed of responsibly. Fentanyl can also be found in intranasal, buccal, and sublingual formations, although these avenues are used less frequently.

KETAMINE

The use of ketamine in multimodal analgesia in the postoperative setting has been rapidly gaining popularity owing to its efficacy and low side effect profile. Ketamine was first developed in 1970 and functions as an NMDA receptor antagonist, which blocks nociceptive and inflammatory pain transmission.[28] During tissue injury, glutamate is released from the dorsal horn of the spinal cord and upregulates the release of proinflammatory cytokines via binding of the NMDA receptor which leads to acute pain and ultimately central sensitization, opioid-induced hyperalgesia, and opioid tolerance. By acting as an NMDA receptor antagonist, ketamine has a role not only

Table 2
Mechanism of action and common dosages of several nonopioid medications and nonintravenous opioid formulations

Medication	Analgesic Mechanism of Action	Common Dosages
Acetaminophen	Selectively inhibits cyclooxygenase in CNS Agonism of cannabinoid receptors	IV: 1000 mg every 8 h PR: 650 mg every 4–6 h
NSAIDs	Nonselective: reversibly inhibit cyclooxygenase 1 and 2 Selective: selectively inhibit cyclooxygenase	Ketorolac 15–30 mg IM or IV every 6 h No cyclooxygenase-2 inhibitor is available for IM or IV administration
Fentanyl	Selective mu-receptor agonist	Transdermal: 12–50 μg/h reapplied every 72 h
Buprenorphine	Partial mu-receptor agonist	Transdermal: 5–20 μg/h, reapplied every 7 d
Ketamine	NMDA receptor antagonist	IV infusion: 0.1–1.2 mg/kg/h

Abbreviations: CNS, central nervous system; IM, intramuscular; IV, intravenous; PR, per rectum.

in the prevention of pain in the acute setting, but also in chronic pain conditions as well.[9] There have been multiple studies evaluating the effectiveness of ketamine for analgesia in the perioperative setting. A 2015 review article evaluating 39 clinical trials found that low-dose ketamine infusions with a rate of less than 1.2 mg/kg/h decreased opioid consumption by as much as 40% and decreased pain scores.[28] In a review article from 2011 that evaluated 70 randomized, double-blind, and placebo-controlled studies and involved 4701 patients, it was found that ketamine had an opioid-sparing effect that was most profound in more painful surgeries and surgeries that involved the upper abdomen and thorax. Disappointingly, this study found no significant opioid-sparing effect for tonsillectomies or head and neck surgeries.[29] However, a 2014 meta-analysis by Cho and colleagues[30] that examined children undergoing tonsillectomy found that preoperative local or systemic administration of ketamine before tonsillectomy had a statistically significant decrease in postoperative pain, decreased postoperative analgesic requirements, and increased time to first analgesic requirement without adverse side effects, including nausea, vomiting, sedation, or psychomimetic manifestations. Ketamine not only has a role in pain management in the opioid-naïve patient, but is also an excellent choice for opioid-dependent patients for whom standard postoperative pain regimens are ineffective. A study conducted by Loftus and colleagues[31] observing 101 opioid-dependent patients undergoing spinal surgery found that patients who received a bolus of ketamine followed by a low-dose infusion of 0.1 μg/kg/min had a nearly 40% decrease in morphine consumption over a 48-hour period and also reported 26% lower pain scores 6-week after surgery. Although the use of ketamine in the perioperative setting may have limited effectiveness for ENT surgeries in the opioid-naïve adult, it has been shown to be beneficial in children receiving ENT surgeries, specifically tonsillectomies, by reducing opioid consumption and has been shown to have a role in reducing opioid requirements in opioid-tolerant adults.

SUMMARY

ENT surgeries provide unique challenges to ensuring adequate postoperative pain control owing to the location and nature of surgeries that may require patients to be

NPO for prolonged periods of time, and that make enteral medication administration difficult or impossible. The are many alternative routes of medication administration that bypass the GI tract and are effective in the perioperative setting, such as intravenous, transdermal, subcutaneous, and rectal administration. Opioids remain an effective analgesic in the perioperative setting, but a multimodal approach to analgesia is paramount for providing safe and effective pain control. For chronic pain, guidelines from the Centers for Disease Control and Prevention recommend that, if opioid therapy is initiated, the clinician should prescribe an immediate release opioid instead of extended release opioid.[32] **Table 2** summarizes the mechanism of action and common dosages of various nonopioid medications as well as several transdermal opioid formulations. Application of a combination of opioid delivery via intravenous boluses, PCA, or transdermal patches along with the addition of adjuncts such as acetaminophen, NSAIDs, and/or ketamine can lead to improved analgesia, decreased opioids consumption, and increased patient satisfaction after ENT surgery.

DISCLOSURE

The authors have nothing to disclose.

REFERENCES

1. Capdevila X, Barthelet Y, Biboulet P, et al. Effects of perioperative analgesic technique on the surgical outcome and duration of rehabilitation after major knee surgery. Anesthesiology 1999;91(1):8–15.

2. Jin JF, Zhu LL, Chen M, et al. The optimal choice of medication administration route regarding intravenous, intramuscular, and subcutaneous injection. Patient Prefer Adherence 2015;9:923–42.

3. Annersten M, Willman A. Performing subcutaneous injections: a literature review. Worldviews Evid Based Nurs 2005;2:122–30.

4. Leppert W, Malec-Milewska M, Zajaczkowska R, et al. Transdermal and topical drug administration in the treatment of pain. Molecules 2018;23(3):681.

5. Hua S. Physiological and pharmaceutical considerations for rectal drug formulations. Front Pharmacol 2019;10:1196.

6. Ghanem CI, Pérez MJ, Manautou JE, et al. Acetaminophen from liver to brain: new insights into drug pharmacological action and toxicity. Pharmacol Res 2016;109:119–31.

7. Jibril F, Sharaby S, Mohamed A, et al. Intravenous versus oral acetaminophen for pain: systematic review of current evidence to support clinical decision-making. Can J Hosp Pharm 2015;68(3):238–47.

8. Gaskell H, Derry S, Moore RA, et al. Single dose oral oxycodone and oxycodone plus paracetamol (acetaminophen) for acute postoperative pain in adults. Cochrane Database Syst Rev 2009;(3):CD002763.

9. Helander EM, Menard BL, Harmon CM, et al. Multimodal analgesia, current concepts, and acute pain considerations. Curr Pain Headache Rep 2017;21:3. Available at: https://doi-org.proxy.library.emory.edu/10.1007/s11916-017-0607-y.

10. Reuben SS. Update on the role of nonsteroidal anti-inflammatory drugs and cox-ibs in the management of acute pain. Curr Opin Anaesthesiol 2007;20(5):440–50.

11. Pogatzki-Zahn E, Chandrasena C, Schug SA. Nonopioid analgesics for postoperative pain management. Curr Opin Anaesthesiol 2014;27(5):513–9.

12. Hyllested M, Jones S, Pedersen J, et al. Comparative effect of paracetamol, NSAIDs or their combination in postoperative pain management: a qualitative review. Br J Anaesth 2002;88(2):199–214.
13. Maund E, Mcdaid C, Rice S, et al. Paracetamol and selective and non-selective non-steroidal anti-inflammatory drugs for the reduction in morphine-related side-effects after major surgery: a systematic review. Br J Anaesth 2011; 106(3):292–7.
14. Benzon H. Postoperative pain and other acute pain syndromes. Practical management of pain. 5th edition. Philadelphia: Elsevier Mosby; 2014. p. 272–3.
15. Grass J. Patient-controlled analgesia. Anesth Analg 2005;101(5S):S44–61.
16. Hudcova J, McNicol E, Quah C, et al. Patient controlled opioid analgesia versus conventional opioid analgesia for postoperative pain. Cochrane Database Syst Rev 2006. https://doi.org/10.1002/14651858.CD003348.pub2.
17. Post-Operative Pain Management. In: The University of Texas MD Anderson Cancer Center. 2018. Available at: https://www.mdanderson.org/documents/for-physicians/algorithms/clinical-management/clin-management-post-op-pain-web-algorithm.pdf. Accessed December 15, 2019.
18. Methadone Hydrochloride Injection, FDA fact sheet. Available at: https://www.accessdata.fda.gov/drugsatfda_docs/label/2016/021624s006lbl.pdf. Accessed December 1, 2019.
19. Gonzalez-Barboteo J, Porta-Sales J, Sanchez D, et al. Conversion from parenteral to oral methadone. J Pain Palliat Care Pharmacother 2008;22(3):200–5.
20. Murphy GS, Szokol JW, Avram MJ, et al. Intraoperative methadone for the prevention of postoperative pain: a randomized, double-blinded clinical trial in cardiac surgical patients. Anesthesiology 2015;122(5):1112–22.
21. Murphy GS, Szokol JW, Avram MJ, et al. Clinical effectiveness and safety of intraoperative methadone in patients undergoing posterior spinal fusion surgery: a randomized, double-blinded, controlled trial. Anesthesiology 2017;126(5): 822–33.
22. Murphy G, Szokol J. Use of methadone in the perioperative period. Anesthesia Patient Safety Foundation Newletter 2018;32(3): Circulation 122,210.
23. Fishman M, Kim P. Buprenorphine for chronic pain: a systemic review. Curr Pain Headache Rep 2018;22(12):83.
24. White LD, Hodge A, Vlok R, et al. Efficacy and adverse effects of buprenorphine in acute pain management: systematic review and meta-analysis of randomised controlled trials. Br J Anaesth 2018;120(4):668–78.
25. Butrans, product website. Clinical Data, Dosing, and Important Safety Information and Indication. Available at: https://butrans.com/. Accessed December 1, 2019.
26. Drewes A, Jensen R, Nielsen L, et al. Differences between opioids: pharmacological, experimental, clinical, and economical perspectives. Br J Clin Pharmacol 2013;75(1):60–78.
27. Opioid Oral Morphine Milligram Equivalent (MME) Conversion Factors. Medicare. 2017. Available at: https://www.cms.gov/Medicare/Prescription-Drug-Coverage/PrescriptionDrugCovContra/Downloads/Opioid-Morphine-EQ-Conversion-Factors-April-2017.pdf. Accessed December 5, 2019.
28. Jouguelet-Lacoste J, La Colla L, Schilling D, et al. The use of intravenous infusion or single dose of low-dose ketamine for postoperative analgesia: a review of the current literature. Pain Med 2015;16(2):383–403.
29. Laskowski K, Stirling A, Mckay WP, et al. A systematic review of intravenous ketamine for postoperative analgesia. Can J Anaesth 2011;58:911–23.

30. Cho HK, Kim KW, Jeong YM, et al. Efficacy of ketamine in improving pain after tonsillectomy in children: meta-analysis. PLoS One 2014;9(6):e101259.
31. Loftus RW, Yeager MP, Clark JA, et al. Intraoperative ketamine reduces perioperative opiate consumption in opiate-dependent patients with chronic back pain undergoing back surgery. Anesthesiology 2010;1. https://doi.org/10.1097/aln.0b013e3181e90914.
32. CDC guideline for prescribing opioids for chronic pain. Available at: https://www.cdc.gov/drugoverdose/pdf/guidelines_at-a-glance-a.pdf. Accessed December 5, 2019.

Chronic Pain Management in Head and Neck Oncology

Michael A. Blasco, MD[a], Joehassin Cordero, MD[b], Yusuf Dundar, MD[b],*

KEYWORDS

- Pain • Chronic pain • Head and neck cancer • Integrative medicine
- Pain management

KEY POINTS

- Chronic pain is common in patients with head and neck cancer and is experienced during all phases of treatment, including survivorship. Patients with advanced cancers and with comorbid depression/anxiety are at increased risk of pain.
- Patients experience pain from a variety of causes, including tissue destruction, bone invasion, nerve compression, and alteration of central pain processing.
- Optimal pain control is achieved with a combination of nonopioid and opioid medications. World Health Organization guidelines support the use of nonsteroidal antiinflammatory drugs and oral opioids as the basis of maintenance pain control in chronic cancer pain.
- Adjuvant therapies, including antidepressants, anticonvulsants, interventional neurolysis, and acupuncture, may be offered to patients as part of a multimodal approach to pain control.

INTRODUCTION

Pain is epidemic in the head and neck cancer population.[1] Patients with head and neck cancer experience pain from a variety of sources, related to both the cancer itself as well as interventions used to treat the cancer. Pain may last for years after completing initial therapy, becoming an on-going challenge well after a patient is declared cured. Chronic pain, which is traditionally recognized as pain that persists beyond normal healing time,[2] is a common and frustrating problem for patients and providers, because pain may persist despite a lack of obvious inciting factors. Providers working with patients with head and neck cancer should be able to:

1. Identify risk factors for chronic pain

[a] Department of Otolaryngology–Head and Neck Surgery, Princess Margaret Cancer Centre/University Health Network, University of Toronto, 610 University Avenue, Toronto, Ontario M5G 2M9, Canada; [b] Department of Otolaryngology–Head and Neck Surgery, Texas Tech University Health Sciences Center, 3601 4th Street, Stop 8315, Lubbock, TX 79430-8315, USA
* Corresponding author.
E-mail address: Yusuf.Dundar@ttuhsc.edu

Otolaryngol Clin N Am 53 (2020) 865–875
https://doi.org/10.1016/j.otc.2020.05.015
0030-6665/20/© 2020 Elsevier Inc. All rights reserved.

oto.theclinics.com

2. Seek out treatable causes of chronic pain
3. Provide thoughtful, multimodal therapy in the treatment of chronic pain

EPIDEMIOLOGY

A large meta-analysis of 3300 patients with cancer reported high levels of pain during all phases of oncologic treatment: 59% in patients undergoing treatment, 33% in patients that had completed treatment, and 64% in patients with advanced or metastatic disease.[3] Of all types analyzed, patients with head and neck cancer reported the highest prevalence of pain at 70%. A prospective study of patients with head and neck cancer showed pain as a presenting symptom in 48%, with a quarter of all patients having chronic pain at 12 and 24 months after conclusion of therapy.[4] Chronic pain is frequently accompanied by physical impairments that affect the ability to treat pain, including dysphagia and trismus.[5]

TYPES OF PAIN

Cancer pain may be classified according to its mechanism (**Table 1**), and may broadly be categorized as either (1) nociceptive pain or (2) neuropathic pain.[6]

Nociceptive pain is defined as pain that arises from activation of peripheral nociceptors (nerve endings) caused by damage to nonneural tissue. Nociceptive pain arises in patients with head and neck cancer from a variety of causes:

- Tumor destruction of local tissues, particularly bone
- Diagnostic interventions, including needle or surgical biopsy
- Surgical tissue injury
- Acute effects of radiotherapy and chemotherapy, including mucositis and dermatitis
- Osteoradionecrosis of mandible, maxilla, or skull base

Neuropathic pain is defined as pain caused by a lesion of the somatosensory nervous system. Neuropathic pain in patients with head and neck cancer may be caused by tumor compression or invasion of structures of either the peripheral or central nervous system. Traditionally, pain arising despite no evidence of tissue damage or evidence of a lesion of the somatosensory nervous system was deemed neuropathic pain; however, the term nociplastic pain was recently adopted to help more fully characterize the neurobiology of pain.[6] Nociplastic pain may arise from alterations to peripheral and central nervous pain processing after long-standing exposure to nociceptive or neuropathic pain.[7–9]

RISK FACTORS

Discrete risk factors have been identified for increased pain in patients with head and neck cancer. Providers should be able to identify patients at risk for pain, particularly those with modifiable and treatable risk factors.

Tumor-Related Risk Factors

- Site: several studies describe an association with worse pain in oral cavity cancers compared with laryngeal or pharyngeal tumors.[4,10] This worse pain may be caused by the dense concentration of nerve endings in the oral cavity as well as the higher incidence of bone invasion in oral cancers.

Table 1 Cancer pain classified by neural mechanism			
Type		**Mechanism**	**Examples**
Nociceptive	Somatic	Stimulation of pain receptors on sensory nerve endings	Mucosal tumors, bone invasion
	Visceral		Lung metastasis
Neuropathic	Nerve compression	Stimulation of nervi nervorum	Mass effect on cranial nerves or spinal rootlets
	Peripheral nerve injury	Lowered firing threshold of sensory nerves	Cranial nerve invasion by tumor
	Central nerve injury	Alteration of pain processing	Intracranial invasion by skull base tumor
	Sympathetic injury	Dysfunction of autonomic nervous system	First-bite syndrome after parapharyngeal surgery

- Stage: pain tends to be worse in patients with advanced tumor sizes and T stages,[11–13] as well as for patients with TNM (tumor, node, metastasis) stage III and IV cancers.[14,15]

Treatment-Related Risk Factors

In general, patients receiving multimodal oncologic therapy (surgery with adjuvant radiotherapy, chemoradiotherapy) tend toward worse pain outcomes than those who receive surgery or radiation alone.[16–19] Outcomes comparing radiation versus surgery are less clear. Patients with oropharyngeal cancer treated with nonsurgical therapy have worse pain than patients treated with primary surgical therapy,[20] whereas total laryngectomy patients seem to have worse pain than patients treated with a laryngeal preservation approach.[13,21,22]

Patient-Related Risk Factors

Increased pain is associated with multiple sociodemographic factors. Younger patients tend to report worse pain than older patients.[12,23,24] Several studies have described an association between gender and pain, with women reporting worse pain scores than men,[12,25] although functional outcomes may be worse in male patients.[15] In addition, patients who are unemployed,[26] divorced,[27] and with low incomes[28] showed worse pain scores.

Psychological comorbidities are important risk factors for pain in patients with head and neck cancer. Both anxiety and depression are significantly associated with pain.[27,29] One study analyzed personality as a predictor of quality of life in patients with head and neck cancer.[30] Patients with head and neck cancer showing dispositional optimism as evaluated by the Life Orientation Test described less pain and better global quality of life compared with pessimists.

TREATMENT GUIDELINES

The World Health Organization (WHO) published updated guidelines in January 2019 for the pharmacologic management of cancer pain in adults and adolescents.[31] The WHO identifies 7 guiding principles in the management of cancer pain. These principles provide a framework for providers in their approach to developing optimum pain treatment plans (**Table 2**).

Table 2
World Health Organization recommendations for analgesic dosing

7. Cancer pain management should be integrated as part of cancer care

Recommendation	Explanation
By mouth	Oral administration is preferred whenever feasible because of high effectiveness and accessibility as well as low cost. Dysphagia and gastrostomy tube dependence may require use of alternate formulations
By the clock	Analgesics should be given at appropriate intervals, with fixed intervals for continuous pain relief. Dosage should be increased until the patient is comfortable, and the next dose is given before the previous dose's effect has worn off
For the individual	Individualized pain treatment is prescribed in the context of careful assessment of the patient, identification of the source of the pain (eg, nociceptive vs neuropathic), and to a degree that the patient finds acceptable to maintain a quality of life. The previous WHO guidelines included a pain management ladder, which escalated pharmacotherapy from nonopioid medications to weak opioids and then strong opioids. The current guidelines acknowledge individualized pain strategies rather than a generalized pain management plan
With attention to detail	Patients should be aware of adverse effects of treatments they are prescribed. The treatment plan should be written out in full for patients and their families, including medication names, reasons for use, dosage, and dosing intervals

1. The goal of optimal management of pain is to reduce pain to levels that allow an acceptable quality of life

Providers and patients should approach pain control with realistic expectations, because the complete elimination of pain in all patients is unfeasible. Therefore, the goal of pain management is to reduce pain to a degree that results in an acceptable quality of life for the patient.

2. Global assessment of the person should guide treatment, recognizing that individuals experience and express pain differently

Assessment and reassessment at regular intervals is encouraged to identify patients with pain, ensure treatment is appropriate and safe, and monitor side effects. The WHO provides multiple pain assessment tools to add in the evaluation of patients.

3. Safety of patients, carers, health care providers, communities, and societies must be assured

Providers are encouraged to practice opioid stewardship to ensure patient safety and minimize the effects of addiction and diversion on society. Attention should be paid to patients' psychological history, patterns of opioid consumption, and history of substance use and abuse.

4. A pain management plan includes pharmacologic treatments and may include psychosocial and spiritual care

The experience of pain is molded by the patient's social, cultural, and spiritual background in addition to the tumor biology. Psychosocial care, including spiritual and culturally appropriate counseling, is an essential part of holistic pain management.

5. Analgesics, including opioids, must be accessible: both available and affordable

The WHO identifies regulatory, legal, and economic policies as barriers to adequate pain relief, citing poor access and availability in low-income and middle-income nations.

6. Administration of analgesic medicine should be by mouth, by the clock, for the individual, and with attention to detail

Pain management should be integrated into the treatment plan throughout the patient's oncologic care, from diagnosis through treatment and beyond.

The WHO approach to cancer pain management has been validated in several large studies,[32,33] with less than 15% of patients reporting inadequate cancer pain relief when treated using the WHO guidelines. However, nonpharmacologic approaches to pain are not incorporated into the WHO guidelines. These strategies have become important tools in the management of head and neck cancer pain, as discussed later.

TREATMENT STRATEGIES
Initiation of Pain Relief

Treatment of pain in the head and neck is initiated after clinical assessment of the patient as well as evaluation of pain severity. Nonopioid analgesics, such as nonsteroidal antiinflammatory drugs (NSAIDs) and acetaminophen, should be started in all patients if no contraindications are present. Nonopioid analgesics may be appropriate as monotherapy in mild pain, but should be combined with opioids for patients in moderate to severe pain in order to achieve rapid and effective pain control.

Previous WHO guidelines recommended initiation of a weak opioid (eg, codeine) before starting a strong opioid, such as morphine or oxycodone (**Table 3**). One randomized trial comparing codeine with morphine in moderate cancer pain reported significantly reduced pain in the morphine group, with similar adverse effect profile and tolerability.[34] Furthermore, genetic variations in codeine metabolism, present in about 10% of the North American population, may result in either ineffective pain control or rapid intoxication after drug administration.[35,36] As a result, the WHO makes no specific recommendations about initiation of a weak opioid rather than a strong opioid in patients with moderate or severe cancer pain.

Combination analgesic formulations are commonly prescribed in the United States, usually hydrocodone or oxycodone combined with acetaminophen. Although convenient, consideration should be made toward prescribing these medications independently, to allow titration of the opioid dose up to an effective level while limiting the hepatotoxic or nephrotoxic effects of high-dose acetaminophen or NSAIDs.

Maintenance of Pain Relief

Round-the-clock pain control is achieved with appropriating dosing of[1] maintenance pain medicines, usually acetaminophen/NSAIDs with or without opioids, and[2] through management of breakthrough pain with rapid-acting analgesics. See **Table 4** for typical starting doses.

1. Maintenance pain control: the choice of analgesic medications for maintenance pain control has been intensely studied. Overall, high-quality data show that a combination of strong opioid and an NSAID provides the most reliable maintenance pain relief.[37–47] No study has shown a difference based on choice of opioid with regard to speed of pain relief, durable pain reduction, functional outcomes, or adverse advents. The choice of opioid should be tailored to the patient's response

Table 3
Medications for cancer pain management

Medicine Group	Medicine Class	Example Medicine
Nonopioids	Acetaminophen	Acetaminophen tablets, liquid, suppository
	NSAIDs	Ibuprofen tablets and liquids
		Naproxen tablets
		Ketorolac tablets and IV
		Celecoxib tablets
Opioids	Weak opioids	Codeine tablets and liquids
		Hydrocodone[a]
	Strong opioids	Morphine and hydromorphone tablets, liquid, IV
		Oxycodone tablets, liquid
		Fentanyl transdermal patch, IV
Adjuvants	Steroids	Dexamethasone, prednisone, methylprednisolone tablets
	Antidepressants	Amitriptyline tablets
		Venlafaxine tablets
	Anticonvulsants	Gabapentin tablets

Abbreviation: IV, intravenous.

[a] Hydrocodone is available in the United States only in combined formulations with acetaminophen or ibuprofen (see text).

Adapted from World Health Organization. Noncommunicable diseases and their risk factors. Guidelines for the pharmacological and radiotherapeutic management of cancer pain in adults and adolesecents 2019, Retrieved from https://www.who.int/ncds/management/palliative-care/cancer-pain-guidelines/en/.

to the analgesic, tolerability of side effects, and ability to adhere to the dosage schedule.

2. Breakthrough pain control: patients should have access to a rapid-acting opioid, such as immediate-release morphine or hydromorphone, in order to manage pain flares that occur in the setting of round-the-clock maintenance analgesia.

Adjunctive Medications

A variety of nonanalgesic medications have been used as adjuvant treatment in head and neck cancer pain. Their uses and limitations are reviewed here.

1. Steroids: steroids are occasionally prescribed to treat bone pain or neuropathic pain related to nerve compression. However, steroid use should be limited to as short a duration as possible because of toxicities including hyperglycemia, mood changes and delirium, and gastrointestinal bleeding.
2. Antidepressants: tricyclic antidepressants (TCAs, eg, amitriptyline) and selective serotonin-norepinephrine reuptake inhibitors (SNRIs, eg, venlafaxine) have shown good clinical efficacy in treating neuropathic pain.[48,49] In addition, TCAs and SNRIs are useful in the treatment of depression, which is epidemic in the head and neck cancer population.[50]
3. Anticonvulsants: gabapentin has shown good efficacy in patients with head and neck cancer as an adjuvant analgesic treating neuropathic pain both in the perioperative period[51] as well as during radiation therapy.[52] However, industry-sponsored trials of gabapentin have shown discrepancies in reporting of methods, analyses, and outcomes.[53,54] This has called into question the drug's efficacy despite widespread use in the treatment of neuropathic pain.

Table 4
Typical starting dosages of pain medicines

Medicine	Typical Starting Dosage	Notes
Acetaminophen	500–1000 mg orally every 6 h	Maximum dose 4 g daily
Ibuprofen	400–800 mg orally every 8 h	Take with food to reduce gastric side effects. Avoid in patients with bleeding risk Maximum dose 2400 mg
Morphine	5 mg orally every 4 h	No maximum dose
Fentanyl	25-μg transdermal patch every 72 h	No maximum dose
Amitriptyline	10–25 mg orally at bedtime	Anticholinergic side effects Maximum dose 100 mg daily

Adapted from World Health Organization. Noncommunicable diseases and their risk factors. Guidelines for the pharmacological and radiotherapeutic management of cancer pain in adults and adolesecents 2019, Retrieved from https://www.who.int/ncds/management/palliative-care/cancer-pain-guidelines/en/.

NONPHARMACOLOGIC INTERVENTIONS IN HEAD AND NECK CANCER PAIN
Interventional Techniques

When patients have persistent pain despite the appropriate use of multimodal systemic analgesics, interventional pain therapies may be considered. Neurolysis, deliberate injury of a nerve in order to interrupt transmission of pain signals, is an effective tool in the treatment of chronic head and neck pain. Local anesthetic blocks of sensory nerves may be used to select patients who would respond to more definitive neurolysis. If the patient's pain is alleviated by a local block, neurolysis should be considered and the patient offered referral to an interventional pain specialist. Examples of nerves amenable to neurolysis in the head and neck include the trigeminal ganglion and its branches, sphenopalatine ganglion, occipital nerve, superior laryngeal nerve, and glossopharyngeal nerve.

Integrative Therapies

Integrative medicine, also known as complementary and alternative medicine, is commonly used by patients with head and neck cancer, with at least a third to half reporting its use.[55–57] Integrative medicine includes natural products such as herbs, vitamins, and probiotics; mind-body techniques such as yoga, tai chi, and meditation; chiropractic manipulation; homeopathy; and acupuncture. Although the data for integrative medicine in the prevention or treatment of cancer are poor, there is extensive evidence supporting integrative medicine for symptom management.[58]

Acupuncture has perhaps the most robust body of literature supporting its use in head and neck oncology. Patients with chronic pain after neck dissection showed significant reductions in pain and dysfunction compared with patients randomized to usual care with analgesics and physical therapy.[59] Auricular acupuncture reduced pain intensity scores compared with placebo in patients with pain that was inadequately controlled with oral analgesics.[60] In addition, multiple trials have shown reduction of xerostomia in patients with head and neck cancer treated with acupuncture.[59,61,62]

SUMMARY

Pain is epidemic in patients with head and neck cancer. Providers involved in the care of patients with head and neck cancer should be able to describe the common pain syndromes experienced by these patients, identify patients at risk of pain, and provide multimodal treatment of chronic pain. Treatment of chronic pain encompasses analgesic medications; adjuvant pharmacotherapy, including antidepressants and anticonvulsants; interventional techniques; as well as integrative medicine.

DISCLOSURE

The authors have no financial conflicts of interest or funding sources for this article.

REFERENCES

1. Macfarlane TV, Wirth T, Ranasinghe S, et al. Head and neck cancer pain: systematic review of prevalence and associated factors. J Oral Maxillofac Res 2012; 3(1):e1.
2. Bonica JJ. The management of pain. Philadelphia: Lea & Febiger; 1953.
3. Van den beuken-van everdingen MH, De rijke JM, Kessels AG, et al. Prevalence of pain in patients with cancer: a systematic review of the past 40 years. Ann Oncol 2007;18(9):1437–49.
4. Chaplin JM, Morton RP. A prospective, longitudinal study of pain in head and neck cancer patients. Head Neck 1999;21(6):531–7.
5. Chua KS, Reddy SK, Lee MC, et al. Pain and loss of function in head and neck cancer survivors. J Pain Symptom Manage 1999;18(3):193–202.
6. International Association for the Study of Pain. IASP terminology. Available at: https://www.iasp-pain.org/Education/Content.aspx?ItemNumber=1698. Accessed November 29, 2019.
7. Coderre TJ, Katz J, Vaccarino AL, et al. Contribution of central neuroplasticity to pathological pain: review of clinical and experimental evidence. Pain 1993;52(3): 259–85.
8. Coderre TJ, Melzack R. Central neural mediators of secondary hyperalgesia following heat injury in rats: neuropeptides and excitatory amino acids. Neurosci Lett 1991;131(1):71–4.
9. Coderre TJ, Vaccarino AL, Melzack R. Central nervous system plasticity in the tonic pain response to subcutaneous formalin injection. Brain Res 1990;535(1): 155–8.
10. Borggreven PA, Verdonck-de leeuw IM, Muller MJ, et al. Quality of life and functional status in patients with cancer of the oral cavity and oropharynx: pretreatment values of a prospective study. Eur Arch Otorhinolaryngol 2007;264(6): 651–7.
11. Borggreven PA, Aaronson NK, Verdonck-de leeuw IM, et al. Quality of life after surgical treatment for oral and oropharyngeal cancer: a prospective longitudinal assessment of patients reconstructed by a microvascular flap. Oral Oncol 2007; 43(10):1034–42.
12. Infante-cossio P, Torres-carranza E, Cayuela A, et al. Quality of life in patients with oral and oropharyngeal cancer. Int J Oral Maxillofac Surg 2009;38(3):250–5.
13. Singer S, Wollbrück D, Wulke C, et al. Validation of the EORTC QLQ-C30 and EORTC QLQ-H&N35 in patients with laryngeal cancer after surgery. Head Neck 2009;31(1):64–76.
14. Schliephake H, Jamil MU. Prospective evaluation of quality of life after oncologic surgery for oral cancer. Int J Oral Maxillofac Surg 2002;31(4):427–33.
15. Connelly ST, Schmidt BL. Evaluation of pain in patients with oral squamous cell carcinoma. J Pain 2004;5(9):505–10.

16. Hamid OA, El fiky LM, Medani MM, et al. Laryngeal cancer in Egypt: quality of life measurement with different treatment modalities. Head Neck 2011;33(8):1162–9.

17. Korfage A, Schoen PJ, Raghoebar GM, et al. Five-year follow-up of oral functioning and quality of life in patients with oral cancer with implant-retained mandibular overdentures. Head Neck 2011;33(6):831–9.

18. Lotempio MM, Wang KH, Sadeghi A, et al. Comparison of quality of life outcomes in laryngeal cancer patients following chemoradiation vs. total laryngectomy. Otolaryngol Head Neck Surg 2005;132(6):948–53.

19. Nalbadian M, Nikolaidis V, Nikolaou A, et al. Psychometric properties of the EORTC head and neck-specific quality of life questionnaire in disease-free Greek patients with cancer of pharynx and larynx. Qual Life Res 2010;19(5):761–8.

20. Tschudi D, Stoeckli S, Schmid S. Quality of life after different treatment modalities for carcinoma of the oropharynx. Laryngoscope 2003;113(11):1949–54.

21. Müller R, Paneff J, Köllner V, et al. Quality of life of patients with laryngeal carcinoma: a post-treatment study. Eur Arch Otorhinolaryngol 2001;258(6):276–80.

22. Weinstein GS, El-sawy MM, Ruiz C, et al. Laryngeal preservation with supracricoid partial laryngectomy results in improved quality of life when compared with total laryngectomy. Laryngoscope 2001;111(2):191–9.

23. Sato J, Yamazaki Y, Satoh A, et al. Pain is associated with an endophytic cancer growth pattern in patients with oral squamous cell carcinoma before treatment. Odontology 2010;98(1):60–4.

24. Derks W, De leeuw RJ, Hordijk GJ, et al. Quality of life in elderly patients with head and neck cancer one year after diagnosis. Head Neck 2004;26(12): 1045–52.

25. Hammerlid E, Bjordal K, Ahlner-elmqvist M, et al. A prospective study of quality of life in head and neck cancer patients. Part I: at diagnosis. Laryngoscope 2001; 111(4 Pt 1):669–80.

26. Allison PJ. Alcohol consumption is associated with improved health-related quality of life in head and neck cancer patients. Oral Oncol 2002;38(1):81–6.

27. Chan JY, Lua LL, Starmer HH, et al. The relationship between depressive symptoms and initial quality of life and function in head and neck cancer. Laryngoscope 2011;121(6):1212–8.

28. Huang TL, Tsai WL, Chien CY, et al. Quality of life for head and neck cancer patients treated by combined modality therapy: the therapeutic benefit of technological advances in radiotherapy. Qual Life Res 2010;19(9):1243–54.

29. Zwahlen RA, Dannemann C, Grätz KW, et al. Quality of life and psychiatric morbidity in patients successfully treated for oral cavity squamous cell cancer and their wives. J Oral Maxillofac Surg 2008;66(6):1125–32.

30. Allison PJ, Guichard C, Gilain L. A prospective investigation of dispositional optimism as a predictor of health-related quality of life in head and neck cancer patients. Qual Life Res 2000;9(8):951–60.

31. World Health Organization. Guidelines for the pharmacological and radiotherapeutic management of cancer pain in adults and adolescents. 2019. Available at: https://www.who.int/ncds/management/palliative-care/cancer-pain-guidelines/en/. Accessed December 16, 2019.

32. Zech DF, Grond S, Lynch J, et al. Validation of World Health Organization guidelines for cancer pain relief: a 10-year prospective study. Pain 1995;63(1):65–76.

33. Schug SA, Zech D, Dörr U. Cancer pain management according to WHO analgesic guidelines. J Pain Symptom Manage 1990;5(1):27–32.

34. Bandieri E, Romero M, Ripamonti CI, et al. Randomized trial of low-dose morphine versus weak opioids in moderate cancer pain. J Clin Oncol 2016; 34(5):436–42.

35. Desmeules J, Gascon MP, Dayer P, et al. Impact of environmental and genetic factors on codeine analgesia. Eur J Clin Pharmacol 1991;41(1):23–6.

36. Gasche Y, Daali Y, Fathi M, et al. Codeine intoxication associated with ultrarapid CYP2D6 metabolism. N Engl J Med 2004;351(27):2827–31.

37. Kress HG, Koch ED, Kosturski H, et al. Direct conversion from tramadol to tapentadol prolonged release for moderate to severe, chronic malignant tumour-related pain. Eur J Pain 2016;20(9):1513–8.

38. Marinangeli F, Ciccozzi A, Aloisio L, et al. Improved cancer pain treatment using combined fentanyl-TTS and tramadol. Pain Pract 2007;7(4):307–12.

39. Wilder-smith CH, Schimke J, Osterwalder B, et al. Oral tramadol, a mu-opioid agonist and monoamine reuptake-blocker, and morphine for strong cancer-related pain. Ann Oncol 1994;5(2):141–6.

40. Staquet M, Gantt C, Machin D. Effect of a nitrogen analog of tetrahydrocannabinol on cancer pain. Clin Pharmacol Ther 1978;23(4):397–401.

41. Staquet M, Luyckx A, Van cauwenberge H. A double-blind comparison of alclofenac, pentazocine, and codeine with placebo control in pathologic pain. J Clin Pharmacol New Drugs 1971;11(6):450–5.

42. Minotti V, De angelis V, Righetti E, et al. Double-blind evaluation of short-term analgesic efficacy of orally administered diclofenac, diclofenac plus codeine, and diclofenac plus imipramine in chronic cancer pain. Pain 1998;74(2–3):133–7.

43. Poulain P, Denier W, Douma J, et al. Efficacy and safety of transdermal buprenorphine: a randomized, placebo-controlled trial in 289 patients with severe cancer pain. J Pain Symptom Manage 2008;36(2):117–25.

44. Ferrer-brechner T, Ganz P. Combination therapy with ibuprofen and methadone for chronic cancer pain. Am J Med 1984;77(1A):78–83.

45. Sittl R, Griessinger N, Likar R. Analgesic efficacy and tolerability of transdermal buprenorphine in patients with inadequately controlled chronic pain related to cancer and other disorders: a multicenter, randomized, double-blind, placebo-controlled trial. Clin Ther 2003;25(1):150–68.

46. Rodríguez M, Barutell C, Rull M, et al. Efficacy and tolerance of oral dipyrone versus oral morphine for cancer pain. Eur J Cancer 1994;30A(5):584–7.

47. Xiao Y, Liu J, Huang XE, et al. Clinical study on fluvoxamine combined with oxycodone prolonged-release tablets in treating patients with moderate to severe cancer pain. Asian Pac J Cancer Prev 2014;15(23):10445–9.

48. Mishra S, Bhatnagar S, Goyal GN, et al. A comparative efficacy of amitriptyline, gabapentin, and pregabalin in neuropathic cancer pain: a prospective randomized double-blind placebo-controlled study. Am J Hosp Palliat Care 2012;29(3): 177–82.

49. Fallon MT. Neuropathic pain in cancer. Br J Anaesth 2013;111(1):105–11.

50. Osazuwa-peters N, Simpson MC, Zhao L, et al. Suicide risk among cancer survivors: head and neck versus other cancers. Cancer 2018;124(20):4072–9.

51. Lee TS, Wang LL, Yi DI, et al. Opioid sparing multimodal analgesia treats pain after head and neck microvascular reconstruction. Laryngoscope 2020;130(7): 1686–91.

52. Hermann GM, Iovoli AJ, Platek AJ, et al. A single-institution, randomized, pilot study evaluating the efficacy of gabapentin and methadone for patients undergoing chemoradiation for head and neck squamous cell cancer. Cancer 2020; 126(7):1480–91.

53. Vedula SS, Bero L, Scherer RW, et al. Outcome reporting in industry-sponsored trials of gabapentin for off-label use. N Engl J Med 2009;361(20):1963–71.
54. Vedula SS, Li T, Dickersin K. Differences in reporting of analyses in internal company documents versus published trial reports: comparisons in industry-sponsored trials in off-label uses of gabapentin. PLoS Med 2013;10(1):e1001378.
55. Warrick PD, Irish JC, Morningstar M, et al. Use of alternative medicine among patients with head and neck cancer. Arch Otolaryngol Head Neck Surg 1999; 125(5):573–9.
56. Asher BF, Seidman M, Snyderman C. Complementary and alternative medicine in otolaryngology. Laryngoscope 2001;111(8):1383–9.
57. Molassiotis A, Ozden G, Platin N, et al. Complementary and alternative medicine use in patients with head and neck cancers in Europe. Eur J Cancer Care (Engl) 2006;15(1):19–24.
58. Matovina C, Birkeland AC, Zick S, et al. Integrative medicine in head and neck cancer. Otolaryngol Head Neck Surg 2017;156(2):228–37.
59. Pfister DG, Cassileth BR, Deng GE, et al. Acupuncture for pain and dysfunction after neck dissection: results of a randomized controlled trial. J Clin Oncol 2010; 28(15):2565–70.
60. Alimi D, Rubino C, Pichard-léandri E, et al. Analgesic effect of auricular acupuncture for cancer pain: a randomized, blinded, controlled trial. J Clin Oncol 2003; 21(22):4120–6.
61. Garcia MK, Meng Z, Rosenthal DI, et al. Effect of true and sham acupuncture on radiation-induced xerostomia among patients with head and neck cancer: a randomized clinical trial. JAMA Netw Open 2019;2(12):e1916910.
62. Simcock R, Fallowfield L, Monson K, et al. ARIX: a randomised trial of acupuncture v oral care sessions in patients with chronic xerostomia following treatment of head and neck cancer. Ann Oncol 2013;24(3):776–83.

54.

55.

56.

57.

58.

Controlled Substance Agreements and Other Best Opioid Prescription Practices

Melissa Straub, MD, MPH, Anna A. Pashkova, MD*

KEYWORDS

- Controlled substance agreements • Opioid prescribing best practices
- Chronic opioid prescription

KEY POINTS

- Prescription of controlled substances for chronic pain is complex, and given the known detrimental side effects, requires careful management between patient and provider.
- Part of responsible prescription of controlled substances for chronic pain can include a controlled substance agreement, which serves as an educational tool and an agreement between patient and provider.
- Best practices for chronic opioid prescription include ongoing monitoring for correct use, including routine drug screening, evaluating ongoing need for narcotic medications, and regularly reviewing the prescription monitoring program.

INTRODUCTION

Acute and chronic pain are common symptoms among patients presenting to surgical providers. At the initial consultation, patients may be opioid naïve or they may be on chronic analgesic therapy.[1] It is important for the surgical provider to evaluate both the current and potential postoperative pain needs of each patient to develop a personalized therapeutic plan for the perioperative future. For patients requiring chronic opioids, controlled substance agreements constitute a nonlegally binding agreement between the physician and provider outlining treatment goals and guidelines. Best prescription practices and expectations are outlined in the controlled substance agreement, including informed consent, regular checks of prescription drug monitoring program, regular toxicology screening, adhering to 1 provider/1 pharmacy, and regular reassessment of risk/benefit analysis of the treatment.

Department of Anesthesiology, Columbia University Medical Center, 622 West 168th Street, PH 5-505, New York, NY 10032, USA
* Corresponding author.
E-mail address: ap3762@cumc.columbia.edu

Otolaryngol Clin N Am 53 (2020) 877–883
https://doi.org/10.1016/j.otc.2020.05.017
0030-6665/20/© 2020 Elsevier Inc. All rights reserved.

CONTROLLED SUBSTANCE AGREEMENTS AND OTHER BEST OPIOID PRESCRIBING PRACTICES

Controlled substances, including opioids and benzodiazepines, are common medications that are used in the perioperative period. It is not uncommon for surgical procedures to represent the first time that patients may be exposed to opioids or other controlled substances. Yet, these substances can pose significant risk to patients. In 2016, drug overdose resulted in the death of an estimated 63,600 people in the United States, which was an increase of 21% from 2015, with more than 60% involving opioids.[2] Experts estimate that one-half of these overdoses were related to prescription opioids.[2] Given that 1 in 16 patients may become chronic users of opioids after surgical procedures, it is imperative that providers follow best practices when managing their pain.[2]

The US Department of Health and Human Services estimates that the cost of both acute and chronic pain to the United States is between $560 billion and $635 billion annually. Because many patients present to a variety of physician providers for management of their pain, management can prove difficult. Controlled substance use, in particular opioids, and their potential adverse consequences have increased since the 1990s. This escalation has been termed the "opioid epidemic" and drug-related deaths have tripled from 1999 to 2015.[3] Although these alarming statistics include prescribed sources, they also include alternative, nonprescription sources. In October 2017, a public health emergency was declared and in 2018 the "Initiative to Stop Opioid Abuse and Reduce Drug Supply and Demand" was released.

Despite these striking statistics, many controlled substances remain important components of acute, perioperative, and chronic pain management. However, providers may feel increasingly uncomfortable with prescribing these medications to patients. To this end, the rate of opioid prescriptions has been decreasing and greater numbers of providers are refusing to provide prescriptions for these medications.[1] Therefore, with their high potential for misuse, it is important for providers to understand current guidelines for both prescribing and monitoring appropriate use of these medications.

The initial approach to patients who may benefit from use of a controlled substance involves a careful evaluation of their underlying condition, with establishment of a clear diagnosis, involving obtaining a relevant workup and potentially offering surgical or other definitive intervention, should it be deemed appropriate. A comprehensive treatment plan should be established with clear, measurable outcomes that can be tracked over time, involving important clinical metrics, such as PEG score, improvements in quality of life, the ability to perform activities of daily living, or functional status (**Table 1**).[3] A multimodal and multidisciplinary treatment plan should be established, which may include medications, interventional pain management techniques, and physical or occupational therapy.[1] Providers should perform risk assessment while devising a personalized treatment plan for patients. This assessment should help to identify risk factors from relevant patient or family history and current biopsychosocial factors that may impact their ability to comply with different aspects of treatment plans.[1]

Once a provider has determined that a controlled substance is a necessary component of a patient's chronic treatment plan, they should enter into a mutual treatment agreement with the patient with clearly outlined goals and guidelines for their care (**Box 1**). This step is important for both providers and patients to understand responsible use of these medications and provide a framework for discussion before treatment initiation as well as should any potential discrepancies arise. This previously

Table 1
PEG score: used to assess pain and functioning
During the past week,
1. What number best describes your *Pain*?
0 = no pain   10 = worst pain imaginable
2. What number best describes how much your pain interfered with your *Enjoyment* of life?
0 = no interference   10 = complete interference
3. What number describes how much pain interfered with your *General activity*?
0 = no interference   10 = complete interference

The PEG score may be tracked to gauge benefit from chronic opioid use. To calculate PEG score, average scores from questions 1 through 3.

From Checklist for prescribing opioids for chronic pain. CDC. Available at: https://www.cdc.gov/drugoverdose/pdf/pdo_checklist-a.pdf.

has been described as a narcotic contract; however, this term carries significant stigma and does not encompass all potential agents for misuse, dependence, or addiction. Additionally, the use of the term contract can suggest legal connotations, so this language is discouraged. Therefore, many in the pain treatment community advocate for the term controlled substance agreement.

One of the most important tenants of a controlled substance agreement is the belief in shared decision making between the patient and the provider. A candid discussion should occur with the patient where information is provided regarding the risks, benefits, and alternatives to controlled substance use. The patient and provider should have a frank discussion regarding expectations of disease progression and functional goals of treatment. This patient-centric discussion should aim to incorporate the patient's values and preferences regarding their care in the setting of physician-guided treatment recommendations. During this discussion, it is important to assess each

Box 1
Common components of controlled substance agreements
Goals of treatment (improved functional status, benefits outweigh risks, reevaluation)
Risks of opioid treatment
Safe medication storage
No early refills (file police report if stolen)
Safe medication disposal
Regular toxicology screens/pill counts
No refills on nights/weekends
No illicit substances
No diversion
One prescribing provider only
One pharmacy for medications only

Data from G., Keough Forte, K., & Johnson McGee, S. (2016). Breaking the pain contract: A better controlled-substance agreement for patients on chronic opioid therapy. Cleve Clin J Med, 83(11), 827-35.

patient's health literacy and ensure that all essential medical information is communicated in a clear, understandable format. The provider should attempt to identify and educate the patient regarding any potential gaps in understanding.

It is important that the language that is used both during the discussion and with the formal controlled substance agreement highlights the partnership between the patient and the physician. Providers should avoid using language that promotes mistrust or is accusatory in nature. This style of communication may undermine the trust-building component of the agreement that is essential to a successful treatment plan and successful treatment of patients' pain. Instead, a focus on patient safety and shared decision making with an understanding of mutual respect can facilitate these goals can help establish a therapeutic alliance between patient and physician.

The goals of treatment should be outlined in the controlled substance agreement. It should be clear that the benefits versus the risks of opioids and other analgesics will continue to be reevaluated at regular time intervals, and the decision to wean off opioids may occur if the risks outweigh the benefits.

The controlled substance agreement can also serve as an important educational tool for the patient regarding not only appropriate use of the prescribed pharmacologic agent, but also other potential agents that can interact with the controlled substance. The agreement should clarify guidelines from the provider regarding the avoidance of other substances, such as alcohol and illicit drugs, while undergoing this type of therapy. The dangerous adverse effects, including respiratory depression and death, should be highlighted from concomitant use of the substances and agreement should be established between patient and provider regarding their use.

Plans for follow-up should be established so that patients and providers can have an ongoing dialogue and discussion regarding the treatment plan. Decisions can be made at these points regarding whether modification of the plan is necessary. Patients should be notified of the importance of keeping regular appointments with their provider while they are participating in a controlled substance agreement and that this is a requirement of continued prescription therapy.

Within the controlled substance agreement, best practices for these substances should be outlined and adhered to at subsequent patient visits as well as outlining practice policies (**Box 2**). One key element of this involves obtaining informed consent, including education regarding the potential risks and benefits of opioids. It is essential that patients understand the risks of overdose and death with the use of certain controlled substances. Clear guidelines should be given if overdose is suspected.

Box 2
Best practices for chronic opioid prescribing

Discuss risks/benefits of opioids

Complete a controlled substance agreement

Perform regular urine toxicology screening

Prescribe refills at office visits

Check prescription drug monitoring program

Assess PEG or other measurement of functional status

Consider naloxone prescription for patients on 50mg oral morphine equivalents or higher daily

Data from Dowell, D., Haegerich, T. M., & Chou, R. (2016). CDC guideline for prescribing opioids for chronic pain—United States, 2016. Jama, 315(15), 1624-1645.

The provider should consider prescribing naloxone to be used in case of accidental overdose to patients at higher risk. This includes patients with a history of overdose, history of substance use disorder, those concurrently taking benzodiazepines, and those on 50mg oral morphine equivalents daily or higher. The patient and those living in the household should be educated regarding naloxone use.[4]

There are several objectives of the physician–patient controlled substance agreement, among which is improved compliance with appropriate use of these medications by patients. A meta-analysis of various practice settings prescribing controlled substances showed modest improvement in patient compliance after the institution of controlled substance agreement.[5] A study looking at pain adherence in patients who had controlled substance agreement in a pain practice showed that this metric improved by 50% in patients.[6] After the introduction of controlled substance agreement in the treatment of noncancer chronic pain, patients were shown to have fewer primary care visits, fewer hospitalizations, and fewer specialty care visits.[7]

Physicians should review with the patient what their preferred pharmacy is and an agreement should be made to only fill controlled substance prescriptions at this location and only at the appropriately prescribed intervals with no early refills. Expectations should be described, including how refill requests are managed after hours and on weekends. An agreement should be established regarding management if medication is lost, stolen, or misplaced, with an understanding that a police report must be filed. Physicians should routinely review the prescription drug monitoring program to ensure that patients are compliant. As a part of the controlled substance agreement, patients should understand that their prescribing physician will be routinely reviewing this information. In accordance with this, both the patient and the physician should agree that the physician involved in the controlled substance agreement should be the only provider prescribing controlled substances and the patient should not attempt to obtain these medications from outside sources.

Additional measures may be used, including pill counts, where patients should be instructed to bring in their medications and providers can count the remaining pills. This measure can help to ensure that patients are taking the pills throughout the prescription interval at an appropriate rate as prescribed. It is important for patients to understand that they should not be taking the controlled substance more frequently than prescribed. Patients should be instructed that they should bring their medications in their original packaging for this counting to occur.

Patients should also be counseled regarding the appropriate disposal of controlled substances, should they have excess. Patients should be educated regarding the inappropriateness and illegal nature of giving or selling their medications to other individuals. They should be counseled on keeping their medications in a secure location, where others do not have access. Part of the controlled substance agreement should include routine urine screening for both the presence of the prescribed agent as well as the absence of other nonprescribed agents.

The controlled substance agreement should outline whom the physician is able to communicate with regarding the patient's use of certain pharmacologic agents. Many of these agreements inform patients that the physician will be able to communicate with the patient's primary care provider and other consultants. These details should be clearly agreed upon before treatment initiation.

Both the prescribing physician and the patient should be provided with a copy of the agreed-upon controlled substance agreement. This step can provide the patient with a reference in case questions arise, as well as promote standard office practices. This document may aid in avoiding both conflict and confusion between patients and providers. This step can help the patient to understand standard practices and destigmatize regular toxicology screenings and other protocols. Guidelines may outline appropriate contact with office staff members and require the avoidance of combative, coercive, or abusive behavior toward these individuals.

It is important for physicians prescribing controlled substances to be transparent in their controlled substance agreement policies and apply them universally to the patients who they treat using the aforementioned medications. Studies have shown that physicians' ability to predict which patients will misuse controlled substances is only slightly better than chance alone.[8]

An additional benefit of obtaining a controlled substance agreement is that it can provide documentation that informed consent was obtained. Patients should understand both the potential benefits of pain relief and the known adverse consequences associated with controlled substance use. These agreements should outline issues such as respiratory depression, tolerance, dependence, addiction, and constipation. Females of child-bearing age should understand the risk of the controlled substance in case of pregnancy. Patients should also understand that controlled substances may provide incomplete relief of their pain and that their treatment expectations should be established. Patients should be counseled about avoiding abrupt discontinuation of these agents. Discussion should ensue regarding the symptoms and risks of withdrawal with certain agents. The controlled substance agreement may be a potential opportunity to give instructions regarding the potential dangers of driving or operating heavy machinery while using controlled substances. The controlled substance agreement can also set the expectation that the controlled substance would be discontinued if the controlled substance agreement is violated.

As a part of their ongoing care, patients and providers should routinely evaluate the continued need of controlled substances as a part of their care plan. Alternative therapies should always be sought, and providers and patients should discuss the potential for tapering off the controlled substance at the earliest possible point in time.

The controlled substance agreement is another potential avenue to outline the multimodal nature of a treatment plan for the patient. As part of the therapeutic alliance, the providers may request or require that the patient is compliant with other aspects of pain treatment. This process can include a variety of other modalities, including physical therapy, psychotherapy, or behavioral counseling.[9]

SUMMARY

The controlled substance agreement is a nonlegal agreement between the provider and the patient that serves as a valuable tool for setting expectations and guidelines for chronic opioid therapy. It may be used to outline best opioid prescription practices and destigmatize practice policies, such as regular monitoring of prescription drug monitoring program and regular toxicology screenings. It can also outline treatment guidelines, such as regular reassessment of treatment benefits versus risks. It may set expectations for discontinuation of therapy if deemed appropriate. Because many surgical patients present with acute or chronic pain, the surgeon must be versed in best opioid prescription guidelines for the safe management of these medications.

REFERENCES

1. U.S. Department of Health and Human Services. Pain management best practices inter-agency task force report: updates, gaps, inconsistencies, and recommendations. Retrieved from U. S. Department of Health and Human Services website.

2019. Available at: https://www.hhs.gov/ash/advisory-committees/pain/reports/index.html. Accessed December 10. 2019.

2. Overton HN, Hanna MN, Bruhn WE, et al. Opioid-prescribing guidelines for common surgical procedures: an expert panel consensus. J Am Coll Surg 2018; 227(4):411–8.

3. Checklist for prescribing opioids for chronic pain. CDC. Available at: https://www.cdc.gov/drugoverdose/pdf/pdo_checklist-a.pdf. Accessed December 10. 2019.

4. Dowell D, Haegerich TM, Chou R. CDC guideline for prescribing opioids for chronic pain—United States, 2016. JAMA 2016;315(15):1624–45.

5. Starrels JL, Becker WC, Alford DP, et al. Systematic review: treatment agreements and urine drug testing to reduce opioid misuse in patients with chronic pain. Ann Intern Med 2010;152(11):712–20.

6. Manchikanti L, Manchukonda R, Damron KS, et al. Does adherence monitoring reduce controlled substance abuse in chronic pain patients? Pain Physician 2006;9(1):57–60.

7. Philpot LM, Ramar P, Elrashidi MY, et al. A before and after analysis of health care utilization by patients enrolled in opioid controlled substance agreements for chronic noncancer pain. Mayo Clin Proc 2018;93(No. 10):1431–9.

8. Bronstein K, Passik S, Munitz L, et al. Can clinicians accurately predict which patients are misusing their medications? J Pain 2011;12(4):P3.

9. Collen M. Analysis of controlled substance agreements from private practice physicians. J Pain Palliat Care Pharmacother 2009;23(4):357–64.

Pain Psychology for Surgeons and Otolaryngologists

Nomita Sonty, MPhil, PhD

KEYWORDS

- Pain management • Pain beliefs • Resilience • Catastrophization
- Preprocedure psychological screening • Psychological therapy

KEY POINTS

- Pain experience is the result of an interplay between psychological, social, environmental, and biological factors.
- Pain beliefs and pain expression influence and are influenced by learning history, perception of pain, and threat appraisal.
- Catastrophization, which consists of rumination, magnification of symptoms, and feelings of helplessness, is a predictor of poor prognosis.
- Readiness for change and patient expectations influence response to treatment.
- Psychological techniques can be incorporated by surgeons and otolaryngologists to manage procedure-related anxiety.

INTRODUCTION

More than 115 million emergency room visits each year are for management of acute pain, a condition characterized by an inciting event, occurring suddenly, and with a duration of less than 3 months to 6 months. In the years 2006 to 2010, an estimated 28 million inpatient surgical procedures and 48 million ambulatory surgeries, respectively, were reported in the United States[1,2]; 50% of patients undergoing surgery on the oral, pharyngeal, and laryngeal region as well as on the neck and salivary glands had a visual analog scale score higher than 40 mm on day 1 on a scale of 0 mm to 100 mm. A multivariate analysis of these data revealed that preoperative pain, pain catastrophizing, and the anatomic site of operation were independent predictors of postoperative pain.[3] Despite this knowledge and recent medical advances, acute pain often is undertreated and contributes to increases in health care costs and lengths of stay in the hospitals. Moreover, poorly controlled postoperative pain leads

Department of Anesthesiology, PH-5, College of Physicians and Surgeons, Columbia University, 622 West 168th Street, New York, NY 10032, USA
E-mail address: ns331@cumc.columbia.edu

Otolaryngol Clin N Am 53 (2020) 885–895
https://doi.org/10.1016/j.otc.2020.05.018
0030-6665/20/© 2020 Elsevier Inc. All rights reserved.

to increased anxiety and is seen as a contributor to the development of chronic pain. In a comprehensive report, the Institute of Medicine[4] noted that approximately 100 million Americans suffer from chronic pain. Furthermore, the US Department of Health and Human Services[5] identified educational gaps in pain management for medical practitioners and highlighted the pivotal role of psychological aspects of pain and its management in medical training. Finally, aside from the physiologic benefit of better pain control, "there is a moral imperative to do our best to avert patients' needless suffering from pain."[6]

It is now understood that pain is more nociception. Historically, however, physiologic pain was considered a distinct entity separate from any psychological contributions. Furthermore, if assessed as psychological it was assumed that the pain was "all in the patient's head." This often carried with it a stigma and a disparaging interpretation that the pain was not real, a figment of the patient's imagination, and was being perpetuated for secondary gain. This provider attribution resulted in a conflictual relationship between patient and provider, minimized the patient's pain complaints, and often led to undertreatment of pain. As early as 1954, John Bonica[7] commented in his book, *The Management of Pain*, that "...there has emerged a sketch plan of the pain apparatus with its receptors, conducting fibers.... (but) medicine has overlooked the fact that the activity of this apparatus is subject to a constantly changing influence of the mind." Pain was now being recognized as complex because patients had (1) pain in the absence of pathology, (2) pathology in the absence of pain, (3) individual differences in responses to identical treatments, and (4) a poor response to surgical procedures and medications that were known to consistently eliminate pain.[8]

The understanding that pain is a multifaceted construct resulted in the conceptualization of the biopsychosocial model, one that recognizes that the experience of pain is the result of complex interactions among biological, psychological, and social factors.[9] The current definition of chronic pain is that it is an "unpleasant sensory and emotional experience with actual or potential tissue damage or described in terms of such damage."[10] Therefore, pain is subjective and it reflects a perception of the sensation, appraisal of threat, and interpretation of sensory input and has social ramifications. In short, the recognition that the experience of pain was more than nociception created a platform upon which to examine "the constantly changing influences of the mind."[7]

This article is based on a summary of selected literature and clinical experience in pain psychology. It highlights relevant psychological factors that influence acute and chronic pain with the aim of preparing the practitioner to understand patient presentations and broaden interpretation of behaviors, which otherwise might be seen as challenging. Also included are factors that can influence an optimal surgical outcome and psychological approaches to pain management.

PSYCHOLOGICAL FACTORS THAT INFLUENCE PAIN RESPONSE AND TREATMENT OUTCOME
Learning

One of the first few psychological factors to be explored was the role of learning in maintaining pain.[11] The importance of reward or punishment, otherwise known as operant conditioning, was identified as being an important process in reinforcing pain and its associated behaviors. It also became evident that there was a difference between the experience of pain and exhibiting pain behaviors. Recognizing the role of pain behaviors in communicating pain experience led to a body of research attempting to objectively examine these behaviors. It also became evident that pain behaviors that may have started due to operant processes were not as dependent on the original circumstances as much as they were on the communicative function of these behaviors.[8] Over the years, numerous taxonomies to measure quantitative and qualitative dimensions of pain behaviors were developed. Follick and colleagues[12] confirmed that 4 behaviors—partial movement, limitation statements, sounds, and position shifts—identified 88.9% of their pain subjects. Keefe and Hill,[13] in an experimental study, found significant differences between pain patients and controls on 5 specific pain behaviors: guarding, bracing, rubbing the painful area, grimacing, and sighing. Pain behaviors often occur in an interpersonal domain and can be strengthened by the response of others in the environment when they react to these behaviors in a rewarding manner.[14]

A second form of learning is through classical conditioning, which refers to the repeated pairing of 2 stimuli, 1 of which is a neutral stimulus and results in a response being elicited by both stimuli. Classical conditioning, also known as respondent conditioning, may maintain and generalize pain behaviors through avoidance, behaviors that may have been initially learned through operant conditioning.[15] Therefore, avoidance of a painful stimuli perpetuates the cycle pain-avoidance-pain because the fearful stimuli never is confronted. Finally, learning and reinforcement occur not only through personal experience but also through observation and modeling influences that come from family and culture.

Affect

Affective distress in the form of depression, anger, and anxiety is a common comorbid condition associated with acute and chronic pain. There is a plethora of research documenting the relationship between depression, anxiety, and pain.[16] Research on affective factors has examined the interactive effects of preexisting mood disorders on pain, mood disorders that emerged after onset of pain, and those aggravated by the chronicity of pain. Anxiety disorders and chronic pain share common underlying cognitive and behavioral processes. Therefore, "selective attention directed toward threatening information, such as bodily sensation leads to greater arousal. Because of this attentional process, those with high anxiety sensitivity may be primed, such that even minor painful stimuli are amplified."[17] Surprisingly, there is limited information on chronic pain or acute pain after ear, nose, and throat surgery. The few studies available have identified that the type and location of surgery, delay in returning to work after 2 weeks following a routine otolaryngologic surgery, amount of preoperative pain, amount of preoperative anxiety, and catastrophization are predictors of poor outcome. Additionally, expectations of high levels of postoperative pain were mediated by catastrophization and also predictive of poor recovery.[18,19] For more detailed information on this topic, readers are referred to Salas and colleagues.[20]

Personality and Early Life Adversities

Over the years, there have been many attempts to find a specific personality type associated with pain but with little success. Engel[21] broadened the scope and presented a model showing the interaction between personality traits, dispositions, and biological factors in determining an individual's experience and response to pain. More recently, descriptive research using Cloninger's Temperament and Character Inventory has shown that individuals who are fearful, are pessimistic, are sensitive to criticism, have a high need for reassurance (high harm avoidant), and have difficulty with defining and setting realistic goals (lower self-directedness) reflect the personality features of chronic pain sufferers. These characteristics also were found in those suffering from anxiety and depressive disorders,[22] highlighting the closely interwoven relationships between personality, mood disorders, and pain. Early life adversities, including neglect, physical and sexual abuse, and rejection, were found to create opportunities for developing a conditioned response to certain stimuli, which, in turn, influenced reaction to pain in adulthood. These reactions were mediated by distress and poor sleep but also buffered by resilience, optimism, and control.[23] Research on resilient personality has shown that positive characteristics, such as optimism, acceptance, and purpose in life, decrease maladaptive coping.[24]

Social Support

The beneficial effects of social support on physiologic and psychological health are well documented[25] so also are the detrimental effects of isolation and unsatisfactory relationships. In a systematic review, Krahé and colleagues[26] concluded that modulation of pain based on interpersonal factors depended on (1) the degree to which social partners were active or perceived by the partners to possess a possibility of action, (2) the degree to which partners could perceive the intentions of their social partners, (3) preexisting relationship prior to pain onset, and (4) individual differences in relating to others.

Sociocultural Factors and Pain Disparities

Ethnicity influences pain by its cultural context. Mistrust of the health care system, fear of addiction, and limited access to resources, including health information, are factors that influence pain outcome. Culturally normative explanations and expectations determine whether pain is seen as a normal part of life or as a pathologic state.[27] Health inequities are an inherent part of socioeconomic disadvantage and ethnic minority status. Both these factors can result in high-impact chronic pain and poor access to and quality of pain care.[28]

Cognitions and Pain Beliefs

It is well documented that patients' beliefs about their pain, its controllability, and self-efficacy influence chronicity and treatment outcome. Negative outcomes in neuromodulation surgical procedures are associated with beliefs that the pain is purely physical, means loss of a productive life, and responds only to medical or surgical methods.[29]

More recently, there has been an emphasis on positive characteristics, such as social support, appropriate expectations, and effective coping skills, in buffering the adverse effects of chronic pain. When confronted with adversity, such as chronic pain, the individual initially resorts to a customary style of coping. When this style is not successful in the context of unexpected acute pain or unrelenting chronic pain, the person is forced to acquire more adaptive methods of coping. Active or passive coping is considered an individual's effort to manage real or perceived stress. Active coping strategies include engagement in activity in spite of pain whereas passive strategies result in withdrawal from activity.[30] Extant research reveals that passive or avoidant coping strategies are strongly associated with higher pain-related disability.

Chronic pain can contribute to rekindling preexisting maladaptive ways of thinking or creating new ones. These distorted beliefs about self or situation, otherwise known as cognitive errors, add to the complexity of the pain response by decreasing function and increasing distress. Burns[31] lists 10 cognitive errors often seen in maladaptive coping. Here are a few of those most commonly seen in patients with pain:

1. All-or-nothing thinking or categorical/black and white thinking: "As long as I have pain I will not be happy."

2. Over-generalization—coming to a general conclusion based on a single event: "All medicines aggravate my tinnitus.... I know because when I applied capsaicin cream for my neck pain my ears started to worsen."
3. Discounting the positive: "Yes today is a good day but it doesn't matter because I still have pain."
4. Magnification: "If I walk around the block today, I will not be able to walk again for a week."

Catastrophization is the misinterpretation of an event as a catastrophe. It is personalized and is selectively attended to by the person in pain.[32] Through a cycle of rumination, magnification, and helplessness, catastrophic thinking is maintained. Fear avoidance has been found to play a key role in catastrophization.[33] In addition, functional magnetic resonance imaging research supports these findings and demonstrates that catastrophization is significantly associated with the anticipation of pain (medial frontal cortex and cerebellum), attention to pain (dorsal contralateral anterior, dorsolateral prefrontal cortex, and claustrum), and emotional aspects of pain.[34]

Resilience

In the past few years, the concept of resilience has been getting a fair amount of attention because it is seen as a buffer between pain and disability. The 3 forms of resilience outcomes seen in a successful adaptation to chronic pain are (1) recovery or the extent to which the person regains equilibrium after adversity; (2) sustainability or the perseverance of desirable actions, goal pursuits, and social engagements that are sources of positive emotion and self-esteem; and (3) growth or the realization that one can grow from adverse experiences by becoming aware of one's capabilities.[35]

Readiness for Change

The concept, readiness for change, was developed for improving treatment adherence in smoking cessation and substance abuse and later applied by Jensen[36] to pain management. This model assumes that people pass through different stages of readiness, ranging from precontemplation to contemplation to preparation to action and to maintenance as they transition from maladaptive to adaptive behaviors. It also assumes that behavior change is a process and that people can be helped to move from 1 stage to the next. Motivational interviewing has been used successfully to enhance progression through these stages and adherence to treatment in different pain conditions.[37] Therefore, for a successful outcome, it is important to match a patient's stage of readiness to the intervention. When there is a mismatch between a patient's readiness and the treatment option offered, there likely is poorer treatment adherence and a poorer outcome.

ASSESSING BEHAVIORAL APPROPRIATENESS FOR SURGERY

Often, a thorough presurgical evaluation inclusive of psychological components is helpful in ensuring that a patient is psychiatrically stable, understands the procedure and process, has appropriate outcome expectations, and is treatment adherent. In addition to a clinical assessment, providers can use questionnaires or self-report measures to obtain systematic information regarding pain levels, psychiatric symptomatology, suicidality, and function. Risk factors for a poor outcome in patients undergoing neuromodulation procedures (ie procedures using neuromodulation to improve chronic pain) were identified as the following: (1) longer pain chronicity, (2) ongoing psychological distress, (3) current pain-related catastrophizing, (4) a history of untreated abuse or trauma, (5) current nicotine or substance abuse, (6) poor social support, and (7) significant cognitive deficits.[38]

A brief screening to assess risk prior to a procedure includes the following factors:

1. Pain: pain intensity frequently is assessed using a numeric rating scale of 0 to 10, where 0 = no pain and 10 = worst pain. Additionally, obtaining information on pain descriptors, pain duration, pain frequency and functional ability is helpful in understanding the pain in a more nuanced manner.
2. Psychiatric illness: patients with untreated psychiatric illnesses are seen as poor responders from a pain perspective for elective surgery, especially for the type of procedure that requires reliable feedback from a patient. If a patient is seeing a mental health provider, it often is helpful to obtain corollary information from the provider regarding a patient's psychiatric stability.
3. Substance abuse: Patients should be assessed for active or untreated substance abuse.
4. Capacity to make decisions: assess the patient's capacity to understand the technology, the procedure, and the risks versus benefits.
5. Treatment adherence: procedures requiring lifestyle changes, regular medication use, or compliance with any postoperative recommendations need patients to adhere to them for the best possible outcome. It is helpful to obtain historical information on the patient's response to previous treatments and adherence habits.
6. Expectations: for an optimal outcome, clarity regarding a patient's expectations is necessary. It gives the provider an opportunity to educate the patient if expectations are unrealistic. A mismatch between patient and provider expectation can affect a patient's overall response to treatment.
7. Functional goals: it is helpful to identify what type of improvement in function a patient hopes to regain after the procedure.
8. Response to unsatisfactory surgical outcome: determine how catastrophic a failed procedure or intervention will be for the patient.
9. Summarize and provide preparatory information for upcoming surgery: it is helpful to provide a patient with information regarding the upcoming procedure, not only from a consent perspective but also to enhance cognitive and emotional readiness for the procedure. The information can be of 2 forms: procedural information, which includes the mechanics of the procedure, and sensory information, which includes the pain and other sensations a patient might experience after the procedure. With respect to sensory information, it is helpful to inform the patient how long these acute sensory symptoms may last.[32] It is important to ask patients what they would like to know and recognize their personality type to determine how much information should be provided. For example, in order to manage their health-related anxiety, an obsessive personality–style patient may need detailed information, take notes during the appointment, and ask many questions. Other patients can become more anxious when detailed medical information is provided.

Upon completion of the screening, the practitioner may make the following recommendations for an elective procedure:

1. No psychological risks or vulnerabilities identified. Proceed with procedure.
2. Some risks in the form of unrealistic expectations identified. Provide psychoeducation and then proceed with procedure.
3. Moderate risk identified, such as untreated depression, anxiety, or substance abuse: refer to mental health provider for treatment. Re-evaluate in 3 months to 6 months.

PSYCHOTHERAPEUTIC APPROACHES TO PAIN MANAGEMENT

There is a long history of psychological therapies used as an integral part of comprehensive pain management. Although these strategies are used by mental health practitioners, a few of these approaches may simplified and incorporated into medical and surgical practices.

Therapies based on operant behavioral approaches use principles of learning and reinforcement in order to change behavior. In vivo exposure to painful or anxiety-provoking stimuli is one such technique. In this technique, patients are progressively exposed to a stimulus that they have been avoiding for fear that it will cause pain. This gradual engagement with the stimuli, which may at this time result in minimal to no pain, helps patients learn that their expectations about pain associated with this stimulus is unrealistic. For this technique to succeed, a graded hierarchy of pain-related anxiety-provoking activities may need to be created and patient taught a relaxation exercise. In addition, educating patients about their pain and the associated stimulus is helpful.

Tip: educate patients regarding the procedure and refer them to resources they may use for more information, including videos.

Cognitive behavior therapy (CBT) is considered the gold standard for psychological intervention of pain[39] and focuses on changing maladaptive beliefs, emotional responses, and behavior. CBT for chronic pain is based on 2 broad principles. The first is "feelings of pain and aspects of emotional, physical, and social functioning impacted by pain are both related *and* separable…problems with functioning related to pain can be addressed even if the pain is not targeted directly and remains unchanged. The second principle is that psychological factors can influence the experience of pain itself."[40] CBT is a short term-structured form of therapy and includes techniques, such as monitoring of thoughts, feelings, and behaviors related to pain and distress; cognitive restructuring; relaxation exercises; behavioral activation; assertiveness skills; and personalized daily activity and pain management schedules. Workbooks, such as *Managing Pain Before It Manages You* by Margaret Caudill,[41] can be helpful in providing psychoeducation for the chronic pain patient. Calm and Headspace are 2 apps that are popular among patients with pain, anxiety, and sleep issues. Health Journeys has produced several CDs, MP3s and a streaming app by Belleruth Naparstek to promote successful surgery, to help with anxiety and panic, and to ease pain.

Tip: understand a patient's thoughts and feeling regarding the procedure and reassure by educating and managing anxiety.

Mindfulness-based stress reduction often is an 8-week training program, developed by Jon Kabat-Zinn,[42] that emphasizes intensive mindfulness training through mindful daily meditation. Mindfulness is considered a nonjudgmental acceptance and awareness of the present, including physical sensations, emotions, thoughts, and impulses in order to reduce pain and suffering. This form of therapy helps individuals see pain as discrete events and not as a continuous pattern through their life. Meditation has been shown to decrease preprocedure anxiety and postprocedure recovery. There are many mindfulness meditation apps that can be used as adjuncts in treatment. Mindfulness Coach is a helpful app to promote this skill.

Tip: encourage patients to learn breathing and relaxation techniques to decrease preprocedure anxiety.

The acceptance commitment therapy (ACT) therapeutic approach falls broadly under CBT and includes methods of acceptance, mindfulness, activation, and behavior change.[41] A central aspect of ACT is psychological flexibility, which is the capacity of an individual to change behavior based on values. ACT supports active behavioral engagement in spite of pain and the willingness to tolerate pain in order to engage in a purposeful activity without emphasizing reduction of pain.[39]

Tip: encourage patients to continue to be actively engaged in valued activities in spite of the pain.

There are several models of group therapy that are offered for patients suffering with chronic pain and their goals can be 1 or all of the following: (1) psychoeducation, (2) providing social support, and (3) building a repertoire of coping skills, including relaxation exercises and mindfulness practice. In practices that do have a multidisciplinary team, it is not unusual to have a support group organized by a nurse or a nurse practitioner. At ColumbiaDoctors Pain Medicine, time-limited pain and spirituality groups were offered, co-led by a pain psychologist and a hospital chaplain to address pain, grief, and existential issues. In some cities, peer groups are available. Internet-based peer groups also are being offered.

Tip: encourage patients to participate in disease-specific or procedure-specific groups to find support and information from their peers.

Biofeedback often is used as an adjunct to other psychotherapies. It enables an individual to change physiologic activity by learning from the feedback provided from their bodily responses (muscle tension, surface skin temperature, heart rate, electroencephalogram, and galvanic skin response) on a monitor. With repeated practice, patients learn the association between their physiologic response and their thoughts and feelings and how to modify them. Biofeedback has been found effective in the management of headache disorders, in particular tension headaches.

Hypnosis is an adjunctive treatment in the management of chronic and acute pain and has been found efficacious in decreasing pain and distress compared with standard care.[43] Although medical procedures often are a source of acute pain and anxiety, patients can be taught to manage the anxiety with images that promote a deeply relaxed state. When in this state, they are provided the anxiety-provoking cues but are asked to continue to stay in the relaxed state. Posthypnotic cues are provided and suggestions for going through surgery in a relaxed manner are given. Readers are referred to a comprehensive article on clinical hypnosis in the treatment of pain by McKernan and colleagues[44] for a more detailed review.

TECHNOLOGY TO IMPROVE PSYCHOLOGICAL INTERVENTIONS

Technology to improve psychological interventions is a relatively new approach to providing psychological services and has the potential for significant growth. In a detailed discussion on the use of technology in pain management, Eccleston and colleagues[45] acknowledge the complexity of this approach and suggest that technologies can achieve 3 main therapeutic functions: improve access to psychological interventions, improve psychological interventions themselves, and directly alter pain experience. Smartphones, interactive apps, and virtual reality systems are a few examples of extending psychological interventions outside the clinical setting. Apps, such as Calm and Headspace, have become popular. The shift from traditional to technology-based therapeutics is an interdisciplinary challenge and Eccleston and colleagues[45] emphasize that the focus should not be on achieving similar results to face-to-face therapy but on using technology to improve treatment via innovation.

REFERRAL TO MENTAL HEALTH PRACTITIONERS

When patients present with active psychiatric symptoms, substance abuse, drug-seeking behavior, and nonadherence to treatment, they may benefit from a referral to a pain-trained mental health professional. Referral to a psychiatrist may be necessary for pharmacotherapy related to pain and psychiatric symptoms. Licensed, pain-trained clinical psychologists are skilled in various forms of individual, family, and group therapies. Some psychologists have additional training in CBT for insomnia for managing pain-associated sleep disorders.

REFERENCES

1. Hall MJ, Schwartzman A, Zhang J, et al. Ambulatory surgery data from hospitals and ambulatory surgery centers: United States, 2010. Natl Health Stat Report 2017;102:1–15.
2. Tighe P, Buckenmaier CC III, Boezaart AP, et al. Acute pain medicine in the United States: a status report. Pain Med 2015;16(9):1806–26.
3. Sommer M, Geurts JW, Stessel B, et al. Prevalence and predictors of postoperative pain after ear, nose, and throat surgery. Arch Otolaryngol Head Neck Surg 2009;135(2):124–30.
4. Institute of Medicine. Relieving pain in America: a blueprint for transforming prevention, care, education and research. Washington, DC: National Academies Press; 2011.
5. U.S. Department of Health and Human Services. Pain management best practices inter-agency task force final report – 2019. Updates, gaps, inconsistencies, and recommendations.
6. Brennan F, Carr DB, Cousins MJ. Pain management: A fundamental human right. Anesth Analg 2007;105(1):205–21.
7. Bonica JJ. The management of pain. Philadelphia: Lea & Febiger; 1954.
8. Turk DC, Flor H. Chronic pain: a biobehavioral perspective. In: Gatchel RJ, Turk DC, editors. Psychosocial factors in pain: critical perspectives. New York: The Guilford Press; 1999. p. 18–34.
9. Wandner LD, Prasad R, Ramezani A, et al. Core competencies for the emerging specialty of pain psychology. Am Psychol 2019;74(4):432–44.
10. IASP 1979 in PAIN, number 6, page 250.
11. Fordyce W. Behavioral science and chronic pain. Postgrad Med J 1984;60: 865–8.
12. Follick MJ, Ahern DK, Aberger EW. Development of an audiovisual taxonomy of pain behavior: Reliability and discriminant validity. Health Psychol 1985;4:555–68.
13. Keefe FJ, Hill RW. An objective approach to quantifying pain behavior and gait patterns in low back pain patients. Pain 1985;21(2):153–61.
14. Gil KM, Keefe FJ, Crisson JE. Social support and pain behavior. Pain 1987;29(2): 209–17.
15. Main CJ, Keefe FJ, Jensen MP, et al. Fordyce's behavioral methods for chronic pain and illness. Philadelphia: Wolters Kluwer; 2014.
16. de Heer EW, Gerrits MM, Beekman AT, et al. Published online 2014 Oct 15 The Association of Depression and Anxiety with Pain: A Study from NESDA. PLoS One 2014;9(10).
17. Turk DC, Monarch ES. Psychological approaches to pain management. In: Turk DC, Gatchel RJ, editors. Psychological approaches to pain management, a practitioner's handbook. 3rd edition. New York: Guilford Press; 2018. p. 3–24.

18. Granot M, Ferber SG. The roles of pain catastrophizing and anxiety in the prediction of postoperative pain intensity: a prospective study. Clin J Pain 2005;21(5): 439–45.

19. Pavlin DJ, Sullivan MJ, Freund PR, et al. Catastrophizing: a risk factor for postsurgical pain. Clin J Pain 2005;21(1):83–90.

20. Salas E, Kishino N, Dersh J, et al. Psychological disorders and chronic pain: are there cause and effect relationships. In: Turk DC, Gatchel RJ, editors. Psychological approaches to pain management, a practitioner's handbook. 3rd edition. New York: Guilford Press; 2018. p. 25–44.

21. Engel GL. The need for a new medical model: A challenge for biomedicine. Science 1977;196:4286.

22. Naylor B, Boag S, Gustin SM. New evidence for a pain personality? A critical review of the last 120 years of pain and personality. Scand J Pain 2017;17:58–67.

23. Mathur A, Graham-Engeland JE, Slavish DC, et al. Recalled early life adversity and pain: the role of mood, sleep, optimism, and control. J Behav Med 2018; 41(4):504–15.

24. Smith BW, Tooley EM, Montague EO, et al. The role of resilience and purpose in life in habituation to heat and cold pain. J Pain 2009;10(5):493–500.

25. Kikusui T, Winslow JT, Mori Y. Social buffering: relief from stress and anxiety. Philos Trans R Soc Lond B Biol Sci 2006;361(1476):2215–28.

26. Krahé C, Springer A, Weinman JA, et al. The social modulation of pain: others as predictive signals of salience - a systematic review. Front Hum Neurosci 2013; 7:386.

27. Peacock S, Patel S. Cultural influences on pain. Rev Pain 2008;1(2):6–9.

28. Janevic MR, McLaughlin SJ, Heapy AA, et al. Racial and socioeconomic disparities in disabling chronic pain: Findings from the health and retirement study. J Pain 2017;18(12):1459–67.

29. Doleys DM, Cianfrini L. Evaluating patients for neuromodulation procedures. In: Turk DC, Gatchel RJ, editors. Psychological approaches to pain management, a practitioner's handbook. 3rd edition. New York: Guilford Press; 2018.

30. Jensen MP, Turner JA, Romano JM, et al. Coping with chronic pain: a critical review of the literature. Pain 1991;47(3):249–83.

31. Burns DD. The feeling good handbook: using the new mood therapy in everyday life. New York: W Morrow; 1989.

32. Gorczyca R, Filip R, Walczak E. Psychological aspects of pain. Ann Agric Environ Med 2013;1(Special issue):23–7.

33. Crombez G, Eccleston C, Van Damme S, et al. Fear-avoidance model of chronic pain: the next generation. Clin J Pain 2012;28(6):475–83.

34. Gracely RH, Geisser ME, Giesecke T. Pain catastrophizing and neural responses to pain among persons with fibromyalgia. Brain 2004;127(Pt 4):835–43.

35. Sturgeon JA, Zautra AJ. Resilience: a new paradigm for adaptation to chronic pain. Curr Pain Headache Rep 2010;14(2):105–12.

36. Jensen MP. Enhancing motivation to change in pain treatment. In: Turk DC, Gatchel RJ, editors. Psychological approaches to pain management, a practitioner's handbook. 3rd edition. New York: Guilford Press; 2018. p. 71–95.

37. Ang D, Kesavalu R, Lydon JR, et al. Exercise-based motivational interviewing for female patients with fibromyalgia: a case series. Clin Rheumatol 2007;26(11): 1843–9.

38. Campbell CM, Jamison RN, Edwards RR. Psychological screening/phenotyping as predictors for spinal cord stimulation. Curr Pain Headache Rep 2013; 17(1):307.

39. Day MA, Thorn BE, Burns JW. The continuing evolution of biopsychosocial interventions for chronic pain. J Cogn Psychother 2012;26(2):114–29.
40. McCracken LM, Vowles KE. Acceptance and commitment therapy and mindfulness for chronic pain: model, process, and progress. Am Psychol 2014;69(2): 178–87.
41. Caudill M, Benson H. Managing Pain before it manages you. 3rd edition. New York: The Guilford Press; 2016.
42. Kabat-Zinn J. Full catastrophe living: using the wisdom of your body and mind to face stress, pain, and illness. New York: Delta Trade Paperbacks; 1991.
43. Kendrick C, Sliwinski J, Yu Y, et al. Hypnosis for acute procedural pain: a critical review. Int J Clin Exp Hypn 2016;64(1):75–115.
44. McKernan LC, Nash MR, Patterson DR. Clinical hypnosis in the treatment of acute and chronic pain. In: Turk DC, Gatchel RJ, editors. Psychological approaches to pain management, a practitioner's handbook. 3rd edition. New York: Guilford Press; 2018.
45. Eccleston C, Tabor A, Keogh E. Using advanced technologies to improve access to treatment, to improve treatment and to directly alter experience. In: Turk DC, Gatchel RJ, editors. Psychological approaches to pain management, a practitioner's handbook. 3rd edition. New York: Guilford Press; 2018.

Sinus Headache
Differential Diagnosis and an Evidence-Based Approach

Raymond Kim, MBChB, PhD, Zara M. Patel, MD*

KEYWORDS

- Headache • Sinus headache • Facial pain
- International Classification of Headache Disorders • Sinusitis • Rhinosinusitis
- Chronic rhinosinusitis

KEY POINTS

- Rhinologic symptoms and headaches are common, and some patients will have both even though they may not be related.
- International Headache Society classification has replaced the term "headache secondary to disorders of sinuses" with "headache secondary to disorders of the nose or paranasal sinuses," and this category only includes headache associated with sinusitis.
- There is international consensus to include facial pressure/pain as one of the symptoms associated with sinusitis, but also opposing evidence that eliminating this may increase the specificity of clinical diagnosis of chronic rhinosinusitis.
- Recognition of the broad differential diagnoses and a multidisciplinary approach are crucial in optimal management of headache disorders.

INTRODUCTION

The World Health Organization (WHO) ranks headache as 1 of the 10 most disabling conditions globally, and 1 of the 5 most disabling conditions in female individuals. An international collaboration of nongovernment organizations and WHO has identified 46% of the adult population with an active headache disorder, with 3% of the population having chronic daily headache. Of these patients, more than 10% were identified to be suffering from migraines, and approximately 40% tension-type headache, in which the total societal burden of the latter is thought to be even higher than migraines because of the high prevalence.[1] Furthermore, pain has been found to be the strongest predictor of depression after controlling for other variables, and vice versa, which contributes to the significant decline in quality of life.[2]

Department of Otolaryngology–Head and Neck Surgery, Stanford University School of Medicine, 801 Welch Road, Stanford, CA 94305, USA
* Corresponding author.
E-mail address: zmpatel@stanford.edu

Otolaryngol Clin N Am 53 (2020) 897–904
https://doi.org/10.1016/j.otc.2020.05.019
0030-6665/20/© 2020 Elsevier Inc. All rights reserved.

The International Classification of Headache Disorders, 3rd edition (ICHD-3) is an evidence-based approach to the differential diagnoses, and the subsequent classifications of headache disorders (**Table 1**).[3] Although the vast majority of headache disorders are able to be, and should be managed in the primary care setting, often there has not been adequate training in the diagnosis and treatment of headaches.[4] Neurologists, neurosurgeons, dental/oromaxillofacial specialists, pain specialists, and otolaryngologists are some of the specialists who often receive referrals from primary care physicians for the diagnosis and management of headaches. Patients are often able to describe the location of the pain, but the identification of the origin of the pain is often identifiable only after careful workup and evaluation by the treating physician.

Sinus Headache

The term "sinus headache" has been superseded by the diagnosis "headache attributed to disorder of the nose or paranasal sinuses" in ICHD-3 because the former has been applied both to primary headache disorders and to headache supposedly attributed to various conditions involving nasal or sinus structures.[3] Unfortunately, this distinction has yet to filter through to patients and even many treating physicians.

The new definition excludes primary headache disorders and is defined as headache caused by a disorder of the nose and/or paranasal sinuses and associated with other symptoms and/or clinical signs of the disorder. The subclassifications are headache attributed to acute rhinosinusitis and headache attributed to chronic or recurring rhinosinusitis (**Tables 2** and **3**).[3] The diagnostic criteria of these subcategories are highly evidence based and valuable in defining "sinus headache" to patients and referring physicians.

Rhinosinusitis

Rhinosinusitis is the only sinonasal condition that the ICHD-3 has included in association with "headache attributed to disorder of the nose or paranasal sinuses." The International Consensus on Allergy and Rhinology publication[5] defines acute rhinosinusitis (ARS) as sinonasal inflammation lasting less than 4 weeks associated with the sudden onset of symptoms, which must include nasal blockage/

Table 1		
The International Classification of Headache Disorders		
Primary Headaches	**Secondary Headaches**	**Other**
1. Migraine	1. Trauma or injury to the head and/or neck	1. Painful lesions of the cranial nerves and other facial pain
2. Tension-type headache	2. Cranial and/or cervical vascular disorder	2. Other headache disorders
3. Trigeminal autonomic cephalgias	3. Substance or its withdrawal	
4. Other primary headache disorders	4. Infection	
	5. Disorder of homeostasis	
	6. Disorder of the cranium, neck, eyes, ears, nose, sinuses, teeth, mouth, or other facial or cervical structure	
	7. Psychiatric disorder	

From Stovner LJ, Hagen K, Jensen R, et al. The Global Burden of Headache: A Documentation of Headache Prevalence and Disability Worldwide. *Cephalalgia.* 2016;27(3):193-210.

Table 2
Diagnostic criteria of headache attributed to disorder of the nose or paranasal sinuses: acute rhinosinusitis

A. Any headache fulfilling criterion C
B. Clinical, nasal, endoscopic and/or imaging evidence of acute rhinosinusitis
C. Evidence of causation demonstrated by at least 2 of the following:
  1. Headache has developed in temporal relation to the onset of rhinosinusitis
  2. Either or both of the following:
    a. Headache has significantly worsened in parallel with worsening of the rhinosinusitis
    b. Headache has significantly improved or resolved in parallel with improvement in or resolution of the rhinosinusitis
  3. Headache is exacerbated by pressure applied over the paranasal sinuses
  4. In the case of a unilateral rhinosinusitis, headache is localized and ipsilateral to it
D. Not better accounted for by another International Classification of Headache Disorders, 3rd edition diagnosis.

Note:
  Migraine and *Tension-type headache* can be mistaken for *Headache attributed to acute rhinosinusitis* because of similarity in location of the headache, and in case of migraine, because of the commonly accompanying nasal autonomic symptoms. The presence or absence of purulent nasal discharge and/or other features diagnostic of acute rhinosinusitis help to differentiate these conditions.
Comments:
  Pain due to pathology in the nasal mucosa or related structures is usually perceived as frontal or facial, but may be referred more posteriorly. Simply finding pathological changes on imaging of acute rhinosinusitis, correlating with the patient's pain description, is not enough to secure the diagnosis. Treatment response to local anesthesia is compelling evidence, but may also not be pathognomonic. An episode of migraine may be triggered or exacerbated by nasal or sinus pathology.

From Headache Classification Committee of the International Headache Society (IHS) The International Classification of Headache Disorders, 3rd edition. Cephalalgia. 2018;38(1):1-211.

obstruction/congestion or nasal discharge (anterior/posterior) and facial pain/pressure or reduction/loss of smell. A diagnosis of chronic rhinosinusitis is made when the symptoms of nasal obstruction/congestion/blockage, nasal drainage (mucopurulent) that may drain anteriorly or posteriorly, facial pain/pressure/fullness, and decreased or loss of sense of smell persist over 12 weeks. Recurrent ARS has been defined as 4 episodes per year of ARS with distinct symptom-free intervals between episodes. Patients may also experience acute exacerbations of chronic rhinosinusitis when a previous diagnosis of chronic rhinosinusitis exists, and a sudden worsening of symptoms occurs, with a return to baseline symptoms following treatment. This consensus document also supports facial pressure/headache as one of the symptoms of all the aforementioned types of sinusitis. This is supported by the American Academy of Otolaryngology Head and Neck Surgery clinical practice guideline, which includes facial pain-pressure-fullness as one of the cardinal symptoms of rhinosinusitis.[6]

However, there is also evidence demonstrating that rhinosinusitis does not necessarily lead to facial pain or headache, where more than 80% of patients with visible purulence endoscopically had no facial pain,[7] and a significant proportion of patients with facial pain and sinusitis had persistent symptoms postoperatively.[7–9] Aggregate evidence suggests that headache and facial pain are symptoms experienced by some patients with rhinosinusitis, but not universally, and the contradicting evidence may be a reflection of the complexity of correctly diagnosing and classifying a headache

Table 3
Diagnostic criteria of headache attributed to disorder of the nose or paranasal sinuses: chronic or recurring rhinosinusitis

A. Any headache fulfilling criterion C
B. Clinical, nasal endoscopic and/or imaging evidence of current or past infection or other inflammatory process within the paranasal sinuses
C. Evidence of causation demonstrated by at least 2 of the following:
   1. Headache has developed in temporal relation to the onset of chronic rhinosinusitis
   2. Headache waxes and wanes in parallel with the degree of sinus congestion and other symptoms of chronic rhinosinusitis
   3. Headache is exacerbated by pressure applied over the paranasal sinuses
   4. In the case of a unilateral rhinosinusitis, headache is localized and ipsilateral to it
D. Not better accounted for by another International Classification of Headache Disorders, 3rd edition diagnosis.

Comment:
It has been questioned whether chronic sinus pathology can produce persistent headache. Recent studies seem to support such causation. However, pathological changes seen on imaging or endoscopy correlating with the patient's pain description are not on their own enough to secure this diagnosis.

From Headache Classification Committee of the International Headache Society (IHS) The International Classification of Headache Disorders, 3rd edition. Cephalalgia. 2018;38(1):1-211.

disorder. Furthermore, potential origins of pain from the nose and paranasal sinuses is not limited to rhinosinusitis, and certainly goes beyond inflammatory processes. However, these are classified under separate headings in ICHD-3 (eg, secondary to cranial and/or cervical vascular disorder, painful lesions of the cranial nerves and other facial pain). Therefore it is still pertinent for the otolaryngologist to have a systematic approach to the diagnosis and management of patients with headache disorders beyond simply considering whether there is presence of sinus inflammation.

Pain Pathway Overview

Headache and facial pain are thought to be secondary to central sensitization of the trigeminal nucleus by myofascial, vascular, or supraspinal input.[10] This sensitization is thought to increase pain from established disease, or provoke pain in the absence of disease. Pain also has a marked emotional and psychological overlay, but the presence of these does not exclude an underlying organic pathology.

The skin of the face and scalp has sensory fibers mainly in the ophthalmic and maxillary divisions of the trigeminal nerve, with minor contribution from the facial nerve, in which the greater superficial petrosal branch supplies the periauricular region. The mucosa of the sinus ostia, turbinates, and the nasal septum also gain supply from the first and second division of the trigeminal nerve.

The frontal sinus innervation is via the dural and cutaneous branches of the ophthalmic nerve. Anterior ethmoid air cells gain innervation via the anterior ethmoid nerve, and supraorbital nerves, both branches of the ophthalmic nerve. The posterior ethmoid and sphenoid air cells are by both the maxillary nerve, via the orbital and lateral posterior superior nasal branches of the pterygopalatine ganglion, and the posterior ethmoid nerve, a branch of the ophthalmic nerve. The maxillary sinus is supplied by the infraorbital, superior alveolar branches, and greater palatine branches of the maxillary nerve.

Otalgia often overlaps with headache disorders as well,[11,12] which is not surprising, given the sensory innervation of the ear is derived from trigeminal, facial, glossopharyngeal, vagus, and cervical plexus nerve branches, all with overlapping regions of innervation.

Anatomic Approach

The ICHD-3 covers secondary headache or facial pain according to anatomic subsites,[3] and provides an excellent framework:

- Headache attributed to disorder of cranial bone
- Headache attributed to disorder of the neck
  - Cervicogenic headache
  - Headache attributed to retropharyngeal tendonitis
  - Headache attributed to craniocervical dystonia
- Headache attributed to disorder of the eyes
  - Headache attributed to acute angle-closure glaucoma
  - Headache attributed to refractive error
  - Headache attributed to ocular inflammatory disorder
  - Trochlear headache
- Headache attributed to disorder of the ears
- Headache attributed to disorder of the nose or paranasal sinuses
  - Headache attributed to ARS
  - Headache attributed to chronic or recurring rhinosinusitis
- Headache attributed to disorder of the teeth
- Headache attributed to temporomandibular disorder
- Headache attributed to inflammation of the stylohyoid ligament
- Headache or facial pain attributed to other disorder of cranium, neck, eyes, ears, nose, sinuses, teeth, mouth, or other facial or cervical structure

Another way of approaching the origin of headache in the paranasal sinus region anatomically, beyond rhinosinusitis already discussed, would be to consider the tissue types of the craniocervical region. A vascular cause may present as migraine, cluster headache, paroxysmal hemicrania, or temporal arteritis. Several neuralgias have also been described, including trigeminal, glossopharyngeal, post-herpetic neuralgias, and SUNCT (short-lasting unilateral neuralgiform headache and conjunctival injection and tearing). Contact point headache from nasal septal spur[13,14] would be an example of neuralgia, as would be Eagle syndrome. An odontogenic/masticatory headache could include dentin or enamel periodontium defects causing dental pain, temporomandibular joint dysfunction, and myofascial pain.

Management

The same systematic approach taken by otolaryngologists in treating any patient applies to the management of patients with "sinus headache," beginning with obtaining a comprehensive history. This should go beyond a sinonasal history, and cover the full head and neck region, including eyes and oromaxillofacial region, as evidenced by the aforementioned differential diagnoses. Also critical is obtaining history regarding primary headache disorders, particularly when 70% of the adult population report having had episodic tension-type headaches,[9] and the percentages of the adult population with an active headache disorder are 46% for headache overall, 11% for migraine,

42% for tension-type headache, and 3% for chronic daily headache.[1] Migraines can present in numerous ways, with multiple commonly overlapping symptoms associated with true sinus issues, like nasal congestion and rhinorrhea, and triggered by weather changes, allergies, and environmental irritants, making the distinction difficult for those without computed tomography (CT) and endoscopy at their disposal.[15,16] It is important for otolaryngologists to be aware that migraines can often be without aura, and may be bilateral.

A nasal endoscopy alone should not be deemed sufficient when managing patients with "sinus headache," and a comprehensive head and neck examination, including neurologic examination is required. Further targeted examination (eg, temporomandibular joint) may be necessary based on the patient history. A CT scan of the paranasal sinuses may follow depending on the history and nasal endoscopy findings, and any sinus disease should of course be treated appropriately. Other than acute and chronic rhinosinusitis, as classified by the ICHD-3 as conditions leading to headache from nose and paranasal sinuses, recurrent acute sinusitis, various anatomic variations, including middle turbinate concha bullosa, mucosal contact points,[17,18] and barotrauma,[19] are conditions that may lead to medical and/or surgical interventions by otolaryngologists. If one of these interventions is considered, especially surgery, an in-depth discussion about etiologies of headache and how surgery may or may not relieve this symptom if the sinuses turn out not to be the primary cause in the end, is wise.

For non-sinogenic causes of headache on history, examination, and imaging, input from other specialties is often required, as well as ongoing communication with the referring primary care physician. Given the high prevalence of migraines, empiric treatment with triptans may have a role,[20-22] along with a referral to a neurologist, so the patient can carry information to the neurologist about whether or not they responded and time to true diagnosis and treatment is not wasted. Although a neurology referral is often indicated, otolaryngologists should have a working understanding of the more common headache syndromes and their treatment options, so they can get patients started on something with likely benefit while waiting for the specialist appointment. Examples include triptans for migraines, high-flow oxygen for cluster headaches, massage and physical therapy for tension headaches, and indomethacin for hemicrania continua or paroxysmal hemicrania continua.[20]

SUMMARY

Nasal symptoms, such as nasal obstruction and rhinorrhea, are extremely prevalent, and may or may not be associated with underlying primary headache disorders. Headache is one of the most common disorders of the nervous system.[15] The International Consensus Statement on Allergy and Rhinology, the American Academy of Otolaryngology Head & Neck Surgery, and the International Headache Society all support facial pain/pressure to be associated with rhinosinusitis. However, the differential diagnoses of headache disorders are plentiful and any one of those mentioned previously may coexist with nasal symptoms. In fact, eliminating facial pain and headache from the clinical diagnostic criteria for chronic rhinosinusitis was found to have a significantly improved specificity for diagnosis of sinusitis as confirmed via CT or nasal endoscopy.[16] Otolaryngologists are one of the multiple groups of physicians who assess and manage patients with headache disorders, and it is critical to have a systematic framework when approaching patients, and to practice a multidisciplinary approach to the assessment and management of sinus headache.

REFERENCES

1. Stovner LJ, Hagen K, Jensen R, et al. The global burden of headache: a documentation of headache prevalence and disability worldwide. Cephalalgia 2016; 27(3):193–210.
2. Lerman SF, Rudich Z, Brill S, et al. Longitudinal associations between depression, anxiety, pain, and pain-related disability in chronic pain patients. Psychosom Med 2015;77(3):333–41.
3. Headache Classification Committee of the International Headache Society (IHS) The International Classification of Headache Disorders, 3rd edition. Cephalalgia 2018;38(1):1–211.
4. Steiner TJ, Jensen R, Katsarava Z, et al. Aids to management of headache disorders in primary care (2nd edition) : on behalf of the European Headache Federation and Lifting The Burden: the Global Campaign against Headache. J Headache Pain 2019;20(1):57–62.
5. Orlandi RR, Kingdom TT, Hwang PH, et al. International Consensus Statement on Allergy and Rhinology: rhinosinusitis. Int Forum Allergy Rhinol 2016;6(Suppl 1): S22–209.
6. Rosenfeld RM, Piccirillo JF, Chandrasekhar SS, et al. Clinical practice guideline (update): adult sinusitis. Otolaryngol Head Neck Surg 2015;152(2 Suppl):S1–39.
7. West B, Jones NS. Endoscopy-negative, computed tomography-negative facial pain in a nasal clinic. Laryngoscope 2001;111(4 Pt 1):581–6.
8. Tarabichi M. Characteristics of sinus-related pain. Otolaryngol Head Neck Surg 2000;122(6):842–7.
9. De Corso E, Kar M, Cantone E, et al. Facial pain: sinus or not? Acta Otorhinolaryngol Ital 2018;38(6):485–96.
10. Olesen AE, Andresen T, Staahl C, et al. Human experimental pain models for assessing the therapeutic efficacy of analgesic drugs. Simonsen U. Pharmacol Rev 2012;64(3):722–79.
11. Maciel LFO, Landim FS, Vasconcelos BC. Otological findings and other symptoms related to temporomandibular disorders in young people. Br J Oral Maxillofac Surg 2018;56(8):739–43.
12. Stepan L, Shaw C-KL, Oue S. Temporomandibular disorder in otolaryngology: systematic review. J Laryngol Otol 2017;131(S1):S50–6.
13. Altin F, Haci C, Alimoglu Y, et al. Is septoplasty effective rhinogenic headache in patients with isolated contact point between inferior turbinate and septal spur? Am J Otolaryngol 2019;40(3):364–7.
14. Wang J, Yin J-S, Peng H. Investigation of diagnosis and surgical treatment of mucosal contact point headache. Ear Nose Throat J 2016;95(6):E39–44.
15. Saylor D, Steiner TJ. The global burden of headache. Semin Neurol 2018;38(2): 182–90.
16. Hirsch SD, Reiter ER, DiNardo LJ, et al. Elimination of pain improves specificity of clinical diagnostic criteria for adult chronic rhinosinusitis. Laryngoscope 2017; 127:1011–6.
17. Sollini G, Mazzola F, Iandelli A, et al. Sino-nasal anatomical variations in rhinogenic headache pathogenesis. J Craniofac Surg 2019;30(5):1503–5.
18. Herzallah IR, Hamed MA, Salem SM, et al. Mucosal contact points and paranasal sinus pneumatization: does radiology predict headache causality? Laryngoscope 2015;125(9):2021–6.
19. Jamil RT, Reilly A, Cooper JS. Sinus squeeze (barosinusitis, aerosinusitis). Treasure Island (FL): StatPearls Publishing; 2020.

20. Patel ZM, Kennedy DW, Setzen M, et al. "Sinus headache": rhinogenic headache or migraine? An evidence-based guide to diagnosis and treatment. Int Forum Allergy Rhinol 2013;3(3):221–30.
21. Lal D, Rounds A, Dodick DW. Comprehensive management of patients presenting to the otolaryngologist for sinus pressure, pain, or headache. Laryngoscope 2015;125(2):303–10.
22. Hu S, Helman S, Filip P, et al. The role of the otolaryngologist in the evaluation and management of headaches. Am J Otolaryngol 2019;40(1):115–20.

Quality Improvement in Pain Medicine

Jordyn P. Lucas, MD, John D. Cramer, MD*

KEYWORDS

- Opioid crisis • Overprescription • Multimodal analgesia • HCHAPs
- Joint commission

KEY POINTS

- The opioid crisis was created in part by bringing to light the lack of recognition of pain and encouragement of heavily addressing pain.
- Efforts have been made to address policies that have contributed to the overprescription of opioids.
- Multimodal analgesic plans and creating prescriber guidelines has an impact on the amount of opioids prescribed and consumed among patients.

INTRODUCTION

The United States is in the midst of an opioid epidemic and grappling with how to address pain and safely steward these potentially dangerous medications. Pain management is a challenging issue among doctors and patients. The challenges of addressing pain stem from a multitude of factors including the subjectivity associated with pain and the dependence paired with opioid use and abuse. It is difficult for practitioners to objectify pain, which in turn leaves some patients overtreated and others suffering.

NATIONAL EFFORTS TO ASSESS PAIN

Over the last 30 years, there have been several cultural shifts in the approach to pain and use of opioids. In the early 1990s, a pivotal report released by the president of the American Pain Society brought to light the shortcomings of pain management and highlighted the issue of undertreatment of analgesic-responsive acute pain and chronic cancer pain.[1] The issue was thought to be embedded in the failure of patients in reporting their pain to health care providers, the inability of nurses to be able to adjust the dose of pain medication, and the reluctance of physicians to use opioids.[2]

Department of Otolaryngology–Head and Neck Surgery, Wayne State University School of Medicine, 4201 St Antoine Street, UHC 5E, Detroit, MI 48201, USA
* Corresponding author.
E-mail address: jdcramer@med.wayne.edu

Otolaryngol Clin N Am 53 (2020) 905–913
https://doi.org/10.1016/j.otc.2020.05.020
0030-6665/20/© 2020 Elsevier Inc. All rights reserved.

oto.theclinics.com

Also emphasized in this report was the therapeutic use of opiate analgesics and the "rare result of addiction." This coincided with relaxation in regulations for opioid prescribing, and marketing by pharmaceutical companies. As a result, opioid prescribing in the United States soared.[1] Currently, the country contains approximately 5% of the world's population and consumes more than 99% of the world's hydrocodone with similar rates among other opioid preparations.[3]

National policies have reflected these cultural attitudes. Policies designed by the Centers for Medicare and Medicaid Services (CMS), the Joint Commission on Accreditation of Healthcare Organizations (Joint Commission), and others that improve the quality of treatment of pain may have also inadvertently contributed to the rising use of opioids. It is important for otolaryngologists to understand how these policies have changed over time to understand how incentives to address pain have evolved.

First in 2000, Dr O'Leary, president of the Joint Commission, announced new standards of care for pain, mandating that health care organizations assess pain at each encounter with the patient, incorporating pain as the "fifth vital sign" into widespread use.[4] Responsibility was placed on health care organizations to incorporate a systematic assessment of pain and to use quantitative measures of pain, such as 10-point scale.[4] Institutions that wished to be in compliance with the Joint Commission became responsible for the assessment and management of pain in all patients. Skeptics of these new standards argued that requiring patients to be screened for the presence of pain and making it a "patient's right" issue fostered overreliance on opioids.[5]

Next, in 2006 the Hospital Consumer Assessment of Healthcare Providers and Systems (HCAHPS) survey was introduced as a method for measuring patients' experiences at US hospitals that accentuated the importance of pain control for patients. This publicly reported survey consists of 29 questions completed by patients within 48 hours to 6 weeks after discharge regarding their hospital stay. The topics questioned include multiple components of hospital care, including pain control (**Box 1**).[6] These questions initially focused on assessing how often pain was well controlled and whether or not the hospital staff did everything possible to control pain. Because of the correlation of the timing of filling potential opioid prescriptions on discharge and completion of the HCAHPS survey, it has been hypothesized that this survey could inadvertently incentivize clinicians to overprescribe opioids on discharge to ensure sufficient ratings and reimbursement.

The significance of the HCAHPS measures was further elevated in 2010 when the Patient Protection and Affordable Care Act included HCAHPS among the measures to be used to calculate value-based incentive payments in the Hospital Value-Based Purchasing program. CMS uses this program to incentivize hospitals to improve the quality of care. As data on the opioid epidemic became more apparent there has been recognition that these policies need to be adapted.

Box 1
HCAHPS questions related to pain

During this hospital stay, did you need medicine for pain?

During this hospital stay, how often was your pain well controlled?

During this hospital stay, how often did the hospital staff do everything they could to help you with your pain?

UNINTENDED COSTS OF SATISFACTION: THE OPIOID EPIDEMIC

These policies, which encourage aggressive treatment of pain, combined with opioid manufacturers heavily pushing opioids as a safe and effective treatment and a cultural shift in attitudes about pain contributed to the rise in opioid abuse and overdose. As a result of the combined effects opioid consumption tripled in the United States between 2000 and 2012.[3] Even as efforts to aggressively treat pain were ramping up, reports from institutions across the nation began to recognize adverse drug reactions associated with increased opioid usage. In 2005, a large prospective study found that the incidence of opioid-related oversedation and respiratory depression events more than doubled following implantation of a numerical pain treatment protocol.[7] Gradually, evidence of problems from overuse of opioids emerged and by 2012 it became clear that there was a rising epidemic of opioid abuse and overdose.[8] Sadly, since 2000 more than 300,000 Americans have died as a result of opioid overdose.[9]

NATIONAL EFFORTS TO RESPOND TO THE OPIOID EPIDEMIC

Although neither the Joint Commission's Pain Management Standards nor the HCAHPS survey explicitly promote opioid use, the focus on aggressive pain management may have contributed to increases in prescribing. In response to the opioid epidemic, these organizations have made changes to address the embedded issues.

By 2004, the Joint Commission removed the phrase "pain as the fifth vital sign" from the Accreditation Standards Manual and by 2009 the requirement that pain be assessed in all patients was also removed. In 2011, a statement was added encouraging the use of pharmacologic and nonpharmacologic strategies for pain control, and examples of nonpharmacologic strategies to be tried.[2] On January 1, 2018 the Joint Commission revised the pain assessment and management standards to encourage safe opioid use and pain control. These new requirements call for educational resources for licensed independent practitioners; referrals to pain management specialists in cases of complex pain management needs; an online prescription drug monitoring program accessible to practitioners and pharmacists; the development of realistic expectations and goals that are understood by the patient for the degree, duration, and reduction of pain; and regular monitoring of opioid use and prescription by the organization.

Similarly, the HCAHPS survey questions discussing pain control in the hospital have undergone an evolution. Beginning in 2018, CMS announced that it would remove pain management questions from its determination of hospital payments. Pain management questions are now refined to focus on the health care organizations' communication with patients about pain during the hospital stay instead of focusing on how well pain was controlled. **Box 2** displays the new HCAHPS pain questions.

Box 2
Revised HCAHPS questions

During this hospital stay, did you have pain?

During this hospital stay, how often did hospital staff talk with you about how much pain you had?

During this hospital stay, how often did hospital staff talk with you about how to treat your pain?

It is important for surgeons to understand that the quality metrics assessing pain have changed such that incentives to potentially overtreat pain have been removed. Furthermore, although providers may have felt pressured to aggressively treat pain to improve satisfaction scores, recent data indicate that this belief may be unfounded. A hospital level cohort study of 31,481 patients that underwent surgery at 47 different hospitals across Michigan looking at postoperative opioid prescribing and HCAHPS pain measures, found there to be no correlation between postoperative opioid prescribing and HCAHPS scores.[10]

USING A QUALITY IMPROVEMENT FRAMEWORK TO ADDRESS OPIOID PRESCRIBING

Postoperative pain control is highly variable and ripe for quality improvement. One of the grandfathers of the modern quality improvement, Dr W. Edwards Deming, is quoted, "Uncontrolled variation is the enemy of quality."[11] Standardizing postoperative opioid prescribing and using multimodal nonopioid analgesia are two strategies that can address this variation and minimize excess opioids. Excess opioid prescribing places patients at risk of developing opioid dependency and communities at risk because of diversion.

Wide variation exists in prescribing for postoperative pain control.[12] A prospective study of patients undergoing thyroidectomy, parathyroidectomy, parotidectomy, sialendoscopy, and transoral robotic surgery identified that more than 50% of postoperative opioids went unused.[13] As expected there was wide variation in opioid consumption from a mean of 30 morphine milligram equivalent (MME; equivalent to four tablets of 5 mg oxycodone) for parathyroidectomy to 221 MME for transoral robotic surgery (equivalent to 30 tablets of 5 mg oxycodone). Numerous other studies have similarly found wide variation. Many otolaryngology departments have used a quality improvement framework to investigate this variation and improve pain management while minimizing opioid prescribing.

INCORPORATION OF MULTIMODAL ANALGESIA

Postoperative pain control and opioid consumption depend on the complete perioperative pain control strategy used. Preoperative education, medications given before incision, and postoperative medications all impact patients' perceived pain after surgery and it is necessary to consider the entire perioperative pain control strategy used. Postoperatively, the number of opioid tablets prescribed may anchor patients' expectations for pain and influence opioid consumption. Overall, patients consume five additional pills for every 10 pills overprescribed.[14] Another source of variation in postoperative opioid consumption depends on concomitant analgesia modalities. Combinations of multiple scheduled nonopioid pain medications have been increasingly used by many surgeons to replace and/or decrease postoperative opioids. Given the risks of subsequent opioid addiction developing from short-term opioids for acute pain, multimodal nonopioid therapy should be favored for mild to moderately painful surgeries.

Although the risk of bleeding from nonsteroidal anti-inflammatory drugs (NSAIDs) is low,[15] many surgeons concerned about the potential risk of bleeding have been hesitant to use NSAIDs postoperatively. However, NSAIDs are a diverse family of medications with different potential risks of bleeding depending on the proportion of cyclooxygenase (COX)-1 inhibition. Celecoxib is a selective COX-2 inhibitor that has been associated with fewer negative systemic effects, such as gastric ulceration and bleeding.[16] Celecoxib has recently been incorporated in nonopioid pain management regimens,[17] whereas other surgeons encourage use of nonselective NSAIDs, such as ibuprofen.[18]

SUCCESSFUL CASE STUDIES IN OTOLARYNGOLOGY

Recently, several examples of multimodal nonopioid analgesia for mild to moderately painful otolaryngologic surgeries have demonstrated success. Many of these examples have used a quality improvement framework including components of a Plan-Do-Study-Act cycle addressing excess opioid prescribing. These examples illustrate the potential of quality improvement methodology to iteratively improve care for patients. The University of Nebraska conducted a series of studies that illustrate some of the potential benefits of incorporation of evidence-based best practices and iterative quality improvement.

In an initial pilot evaluation of prospectively collected data on adults who underwent outpatient thyroid, parathyroid, and parotid surgery they investigated the use of a multimodal analgesia strategy incorporating acetaminophen, ibuprofen, and gabapentin.[19] This study included 64 patients and found that 61% of patients were able to avoid postoperative opioid use on discharge. These authors rapidly expanded on this pilot study and published a follow-up of 588 patients soon afterward illustrating how an initial pilot study can rapidly expand. They identified that adherence with the multimodal pathway increased to 88% over time, whereas the need for postoperative opioid prescriptions reduced to 1.9%.[20] Furthermore, incorporating NSAIDs was safe and did not lead to an increase risk of bleeding.[20] Among 1702 patients undergoing thyroid and parathyroid surgery from a different institution, investigators found that prescriptions for opioids were reduced after initiation of preoperative patient education and the use of nonopioid medications.[12]

To understand how to apply some of these data to other procedures in otolaryngology it is necessary to understand the variation that exists in postoperative pain and opioid requirements. In one of the landmark studies that provides a framework for this question, investigators prospectively studied postoperative pain and opioid consumption in 70,764 patients undergoing 179 different operations.[21] Among these a total of nine otolaryngology operations were included. Eight of nine otolaryngologic operations were rated among the least painful with maximum pain scores of 2.3 to 4.4/10 points. These surgeries including septoplasty, thyroidectomy, facial fracture reduction, rhinoplasty, endoscopic sinus surgery, middle ear surgery, salivary gland surgery, and lymph node biopsy.[21] Tonsillectomy was the only otolaryngologic surgery identified as a high-pain surgery. These data indicate that most otolaryngologic surgery produces mild to moderate pain and that multimodal analgesia pathways, such as those used in the thyroid/parathyroid surgery examples, can be applied.

In highly painful operations, such as, tonsillectomy, other oral cavity/oropharyngeal surgery, and major head and neck oncologic surgery, opioids may be required in addition to other multimodal strategies. A retrospective cohort study of patients undergoing free tissue transfer for head and neck reconstruction analyzed a group of 28 patients receiving multimodal analgesia and 37 patients undergoing a standard opioid-based analgesia.[22] Patients receiving multimodal analgesia received preoperative patient counseling; preoperative oral acetaminophen and gabapentin; intraoperative acetaminophen; and postoperative acetaminophen, gabapentin, celecoxib, and ketorolac. Further analgesia involved intravenous fentanyl pushes for breakthrough pain. The number of morphine equivalent doses for the multimodal analgesia cohort was 10.0 compared with 89.6 in the control cohort. Postoperative bleeding was similar between the two groups. The median number of MME doses prescribed at discharge was 0 for the multimodal analgesia cohort and 300 for the control cohort. This example shows the importance of a thorough treatment course beginning preoperatively and involving counseling and nonmedicinal measures.

Another example in highly painful head and neck cancer surgery undergoing free tissue transfer examined a simpler multimodal pathway incorporating COX-2 inhibitors. In this retrospective matched-cohort study of 147 patients, the effect of 200 mg of celecoxib scheduled twice daily through the feeding tube for a minimum of 5 days starting on postoperative Day 1 was investigated.[17] Oral opioids were offered to both patient cohorts in a scheduled manner and as needed and PRN intravenous opioids for severe pain that could be up-titrated depending on pain levels. Treatment with celecoxib was associated with significantly decreased mean use of intravenous and total opioids. Celecoxib patients used a mean of 1.5 mg of intravenous MME per day versus 5.3 mg of IV MME per day in the control group. Looking at cohorts that underwent the most common ablative procedure (composite oral resection), oral MME, intravenous MME, and total MME were all statistically significantly decreased in the celecoxib group compared with the noncelecoxib group. There were no statistically significant differences in the incidence of complications between the two groups. Of note, there was no difference in cardiovascular complications between the two groups.

Incorporation of Plan-Do-Study-Act agendas aimed at decreasing opioid prescriptions and subsequent consumption in the perioperative period require overcoming several barriers to become successful quality improvement initiatives. **Box 3** displays examples of potential barriers to quality improvement in perioperative pain control.

GUIDELINES TO STANDARDIZE CARE

The final challenge is standardizing and disseminating evidence-based recommendations for postoperative pain control. Simply lowering the default reset prescription quantity for opioid prescriptions has changed practice. Investigators at Yale lowered the amount of pills autopopulated in the electronic medical record (EMR) when prescribing discharge analgesia from 30 to 12. They looked at preintervention and postintervention prescriptions and found an overall decrease in opioids prescribed from 30 to 20, with no statistical significant increase in refill rates.[23] Furthermore, decreasing the amount of pills prescribed decreased consumption of opioids.

Another high-impact example used a quality improvement framework across multiple hospital systems in the Michigan Surgical Quality Collaborative. Investigators

---

Box 3
Potential barriers to quality improvement in perioperative pain control

Clinicians comfort using NSAIDs (nonselective or selective inhibitors) in the perioperative setting

Time to educate patients about multimodal analgesia

Need to develop systems to assess pain and refill medications for the minority of patients with high pain and/or opioid requirements after surgery

Cost of some multimodal analgesia strategies, such as liposomal bupivacaine

Patient perceptions that opioids are necessary

Patients hesitancy to dispose of unused opioids

Lack of collaboration among anesthesia, nurses, and surgeons in creating multimodal analgesic plans beginning preoperatively

---

Box 4
Strategies for quality improvement in perioperative pain control

Incorporate multimodal analgesia for all patients unless contraindicated
  Consider preventive analgesia with preoperative acetaminophen/NSAIDs/gabapentin
  Use of long-acting local and/or regional anesthesia whenever possible
  Scheduled acetaminophen
  Scheduled NSAIDs (nonselective COX-1 and -2 inhibitors or selective COX-2 inhibitors)
  Limit opioid prescribing if necessary
  Limit the usage of preset postoperative order sets, which include PRN opioids

Protocolize analgesia and opioid prescribing (update EMR default settings)

Develop patient educational resources to standardize multimodal analgesia

Educate patients about the risks of opioids including abuse and fatal overdose

Educate patients about disposal of unused opioids

Educate patients on the average number of opioids used by the general population after undergoing specific procedure

Partner with other health care stakeholders (anesthesia, nurses, residents, pharmacists) to encourage implementation

Ongoing monitoring of use of multimodal analgesia, opioid usage, patient pain, and satisfaction with pathway

---

designed guidelines for pain control and opioid prescribing for various general/vascular and gynecologic procedures and examined their impact in this statewide quality-improvement collaborative. Investigators found that after guideline implementation, prescription of postoperative opioids decreased in size from 26 ± 2 pills in the preguideline period to 18 ± 3 pills after the guidelines were released.[24] Opioid consumption also decreased, with no changes in satisfaction or pain scores.

In response to evidence that postoperative opioid prescribing guidelines decrease opioid prescribing without compromising patient satisfaction,[18,25] the American Academy of Otolaryngology – Head and Neck Surgery has sponsored a single specialty guideline directed at opioid and analgesic prescribing for acute postoperative pain in otolaryngology. These guidelines are targeted at common otolaryngology procedures; however, it is hoped that they will provide a framework that could be applied to less common procedures. Instituting prescribing recommendations for one procedure may result in decreased prescribing for other related procedures from spillover.[24] **Box 4** synthesizes several quality improvement strategies in perioperative pain control that could be used including multimodal analgesia, lowering default quantities on the EMR, and postoperative opioid prescribing guidelines.

SUMMARY

Efforts to make pain control a quality metric to compare hospitals may have incentivized overuse of opioids in the past. Fortunately, in response to the opioid epidemic, these incentives have been refined to remove any enticement to prescribe opioids. Although previous efforts to improve patient satisfaction by improving pain control may have had unintended consequences, the quality improvement framework also provides techniques to respond to this crisis. Several surgical specialties, including otolaryngology, have demonstrated that quality improvement efforts using prescriber guidelines and multimodal analgesia can address postoperative pain, maintain patient satisfaction, and minimize the use of opioids.

DISCLOSURE

None.

REFERENCES

1. Max MB. Improving outcomes of analgesic treatment: is education enough? Ann Intern Med 1990;113(11):885–9.
2. Baker DW. The Joint Commission's pain standards: origins and evolution. Oakbrook Terrace (IL): The Joint Commission; 2017.
3. Manchikanti L, Kaye AM, Knezevic NN, et al. Responsible, safe, and effective prescription of opioids for chronic non-cancer pain: American Society of Interventional Pain Physicians (ASIPP) Guidelines. Pain Physician 2017;20(2S):S3–92.
4. Phillips DM. JCAHO pain management standards are unveiled. JAMA 2000; 284(4):428.
5. Hansen G. Assessment and management of pain. JAMA 2000;284(18):2317–8.
6. Centers for Medicare & Medicaid Services. HCAHPS fact sheet. 2009. Available at: http://www.hcahpsonline.org/files/HCAHPS%20Fact%20Sheet,%20revised1,%203-31-09.pdf. Accessed November 20, 2017.
7. Vila H, Smith RA, Augustyniak MJ, et al. The efficacy and safety of pain management before and after implementation of hospital-wide pain management standards: is patient safety compromised by treatment based solely on numerical pain ratings? Anesth Analg 2005;101(2):474–80, table of contents.
8. Alexander GC, Kruszewski SP, Webster DW. Rethinking opioid prescribing to protect patient safety and public health. JAMA 2012;308(18):1865–6.
9. CDC New Significant Changes in Drug Overdose Deaths [Press Release] March 18, 2018.
10. Lee JS, Hu HM, Brummett CM, et al. Postoperative opioid prescribing and the pain scores on Hospital Consumer Assessment of Healthcare Providers and Systems Survey. JAMA 2017;317(19):2013–5.
11. Deming WE, William E. The essential Deming: leadership principles from the father of quality. New York: McGraw-Hill; 2013.
12. Shindo M, Lim J, Leon E, et al. Opioid prescribing practice and needs in thyroid and parathyroid surgery. JAMA Otolaryngol Neck Surg 2018;144(12):1098.
13. Dang S, Duffy A, Li JC, et al. Postoperative opioid-prescribing practices in otolaryngology: a multiphasic study. Laryngoscope 2019;130(3):659–65.
14. Clarke H, Soneji N, Ko DT, et al. Rates and risk factors for prolonged opioid use after major surgery: population based cohort study. BMJ 2014;348:g1251.
15. Riggin L, Ramakrishna J, Sommer DD, et al. A 2013 updated systematic review & meta-analysis of 36 randomized controlled trials; no apparent effects of non steroidal anti-inflammatory agents on the risk of bleeding after tonsillectomy. Clin Otolaryngol 2013;38(2):115–29.
16. Nissen SE, Yeomans ND, Solomon DH, et al. Cardiovascular safety of celecoxib, naproxen, or ibuprofen for arthritis. N Engl J Med 2016;375(26):2519–29.
17. Straube S, Derry S, McQuay HJ, et al. Effect of preoperative COX-II-selective NSAIDs (coxibs) on postoperative outcomes: a systematic review of randomized studies. Acta Anaesthesiol Scand 2005;49(5):601–13.
18. Vu JV, Howard RA, Gunaseelan V, et al. Statewide implementation of postoperative opioid prescribing guidelines. N Engl J Med 2019;381(7):680–2.
19. Oltman J, Militsakh O, D'Agostino M, et al. Multimodal analgesia in outpatient head and neck surgery. JAMA Otolaryngol Neck Surg 2017;143(12):1207.

20. Militsakh O, Lydiatt W, Lydiatt D, et al. Development of multimodal analgesia pathways in outpatient thyroid and parathyroid surgery and association with post-operative opioid prescription patterns. JAMA Otolaryngol Head Neck Surg 2018; 144(11):1023–9.
21. Gerbershagen HJ, Aduckathil S, van Wijck AJM, et al. Pain intensity on the first day after surgery. Anesthesiology 2013;118(4):934–44.
22. Eggerstedt M, Stenson KM, Ramirez EA, et al. Association of perioperative opioid-sparing multimodal analgesia with narcotic use and pain control after head and neck free flap reconstruction. JAMA Facial Plast Surg 2019;21(5):446.
23. Chiu AS, Jean RA, Hoag JR, et al. Association of lowering default pill counts in electronic medical record systems with postoperative opioid prescribing. JAMA Surg 2018;153(11):1012.
24. Howard R, Fry B, Gunaseelan V, et al. Association of opioid prescribing with opioid consumption after surgery in Michigan. JAMA Surg 2019;154(1):e184234.
25. Hannoun C. Les Annales de l'Institut Pasteur, 100 ans après. Ann Inst Pasteur Virol 1988;139:5–8.

Special Article Series: Intentionally Shaping the Future of Otolaryngology

Editor

JENNIFER A. VILLWOCK

OTOLARYNGOLOGIC CLINICS OF NORTH AMERICA

www.oto.theclinics.com

Consulting Editor
SUJANA S. CHANDRASEKHAR

October 2020 • Volume 53 • Number 5

Foreword

Diversity: A Necessity in the Otolaryngology Workforce

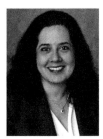

Sujana S. Chandrasekhar, MD, FACS, FAAOHNS
Consulting Editor

This Special Article Series, Intentionally Shaping the Future of Otolaryngology, is designed for otolaryngologists and health care leaders to reflect upon where we are and where we would like to be. It is clear that sitting back and waiting for change to happen is not adequate.

Dr Jennifer Villwock has thoughtfully curated this series, which offers 2 articles per issue of *Otolaryngologic Clinics of North America*, starting with the August 2020 issue. The 2 articles in the current issue directly approach workforce issues in Otolaryngology–Head and Neck Surgery. Dr Cass' article tells us where we are; Drs Villwock and Francis' article tells us why we need to be deliberate about expanding our physicians so that they represent more accurately the patients for whom we give care.

This does not mean that a physician of one background or circumstance cannot correctly care for a patient from another. We each care for people who both look like us and do not look like us, who come from similar and different socioeconomic and cultural backgrounds, and whose overall life experience varies, or does not, from ours. Deliberate actions that enhance diversity in our workforce enhance each of us and the care that all of our patients receive.

Diversity relates to race, ethnicity, socioeconomic status, sex, gender identity, sexual orientation, and disability. As the Mission Statement of the Ohio State Wexner Medical Center reads: "We celebrate and learn from our diversity. We see diversity as the uniqueness each of us brings to achieving our shared mission and goals. We recognize and value different perspectives, characteristics, experiences and attributes of each individual in creating an environment where we thrive on and benefit from our differences."[1]

Being deliberate about diversity from education to service to leadership is vitally important. The articles that follow articulate this clearly. I hope you enjoy reading

Otolaryngol Clin N Am 53 (2020) xxiii–xxiv
https://doi.org/10.1016/j.otc.2020.07.003
0030-6665/20/© 2020 Published by Elsevier Inc.

them as much as I did, and I hope you share this important information with your medical community.

Sujana S. Chandrasekhar, MD, FACS, FAAOHNS
Consulting Editor, Otolaryngologic Clinics of North America

Past President, American Academy of Otolaryngology–Head and Neck Surgery

Secretary-Treasurer, American Otological Society

Partner, ENT & Allergy Associates LLP
18 East 48th Street, 2nd Floor, New York, NY 10017, USA

Clinical Professor, Department of Otolaryngology–Head and Neck Surgery
Zucker School of Medicine at Hofstra-Northwell, Hempstead, NY, USA

Clinical Associate Professor, Department of Otolaryngology–Head and Neck Surgery
Icahn School of Medicine at Mount Sinai, New York, NY, USA

E-mail address:
ssc@nyotology.com

REFERENCE

1. Available at: https://medicine.osu.edu/diversity/mission. Accessed July 13, 2020.

Preface

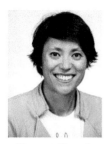

Jennifer A. Villwock, MD
Editor

These articles on leadership, diversity, and inclusion are being written, reviewed, and published in undoubtedly turbulent times. We are forging forward despite the uncertainties inherent in a global pandemic while simultaneously confronting hard realities about our society and embedded systemic issues. For example, the stark racial disparities, and disproportionate burden borne by minority populations, in COVID-19 outcomes are headline news. Conversations about how health is not biologically predetermined, but a complex interplay of factors, including housing conditions, chronic stress, employment status, racial discrimination, access to healthy food, inequities in our health care systems, and other sociodemographic factors can no longer be avoided.[1,2] Those of us in medicine are considered essential workers. Educating ourselves on these issues, amplifying the voices of our colleagues and communities for whom this is their lived experience, and learning how, despite our good intentions, we contribute to these issues is an equally critical part of our essential work.

As Maya Angelou said, "Do the best you can until you know better. Then when you know better, do better." We sincerely hope that the articles in this special issue provide the data and context to better understand where we are, where we hope to go, and how to do better.

Drs Cass and Smith provide a synthesis of the recent literature regarding the otolaryngology workforce and how this has evolved over the course of the past few decades in their timely article, "Current State of the Otolaryngology Workforce." They also describe projections of the future, such as anticipated physician shortfalls, increasing numbers of midlevel providers, continued room for improvement with respect to workforce diversity, and the need to better engage underserved communities.

In "What is Diversity and Why Does it Matter," Dr Francis and I discuss how health outcomes are impacted by diversity, challenges inherent in trying to define diversity,

Otolaryngol Clin N Am 53 (2020) xxv–xxvi
https://doi.org/10.1016/j.otc.2020.07.004
0030-6665/20/© 2020 Published by Elsevier Inc.

how we all benefit when our teams are diverse, and the responsibility we all share in addressing disparities in diversity and inclusion.

Jennifer A. Villwock, MD
Department of Otolaryngology
Head and Neck Surgery
Kansas University
University of Kansas Medical Center
3901 Rainbow Boulevard, MS 3010
Kansas City, KS 66160, USA

E-mail address:
jvillwock@kumc.edu

REFERENCES

1. Webb Hooper M, Nápoles AM, Pérez-Stable EJ. COVID-19 and racial/ethnic disparities. JAMA 2020. https://doi.org/10.1001/jama.2020.8598.
2. Chowkwanyun M, Reed AL Jr. Racial health disparities and Covid-19–caution and context. N Engl J Med 2020. https://doi.org/10.1056/NEJMp2012910.

The Current State of the Otolaryngology Workforce

Lauren M. Cass, MD, MPH*, Joshua B. Smith, MD

KEYWORDS

- Otolaryngology • Workforce • Diversity • Public health

KEY POINTS

- A shortage of otolaryngologists is predicted, caused by aging of both the population and the workforce.
- Action to increase the adequacy of the supply of otolaryngologists is critical, as is the need to emphasize delivery of care suited to the unique otolaryngic needs of the elderly.
- The number of fellowship training positions continues to increase.
- The otolaryngology workforce does not reflect the demographic makeup of the United States population, and efforts to diversify the specialty are needed.

INTRODUCTION

Owing in large part to the growing and aging of the United States population, the supply of otolaryngologists, and physicians in general, is expected to fall short of demand in the coming decades.[1–4] In addition, workforce composition and diversity are also critically important to delivering high-value care. Evaluation of the current workforce is a challenging, but vital, undertaking. This article reviews what is known about salient factors affecting the otolaryngology workforce, anticipated areas of concerns, and where there are gaps in knowledge.

OTOLARYNGOLOGY WORKFORCE SUPPLY
Calculating the Workforce

In its simplest form, physician workforce supply is calculated by the summation of current physicians with future graduates minus those exiting the workforce, and it is usually reported as a normalized measure of physicians per 100,000 population or patients per 1 physician. An adequate supply of otolaryngologists in the United States has been loosely estimated in the range of 2.3 to 3.5 full-time equivalents per 100,000,

Department of Otolaryngology Head and Neck Surgery, The University of Kansas Medical Center, 3901 Rainbow Boulevard, MS 3010, Kansas City, KS 66106, USA
* Corresponding author.
E-mail address: Lcass@kumc.edu
Twitter: @JBSmithMD (J.B.S.)

Otolaryngol Clin N Am 53 (2020) 915–926
https://doi.org/10.1016/j.otc.2020.05.016
0030-6665/20/© 2020 Elsevier Inc. All rights reserved.

an estimate that grew from work performed in the 1990s based largely on models extrapolated from health maintenance organizations.[5,6] Although this definition of adequacy omits important factors such as the distribution, diversity, and capability of the workforce, these crude ratios are nonetheless useful for comparison purposes.

Historical and Current Workforce Estimates

Over the last 25 years, published estimates of current otolaryngologist-to-population ratios were adequate, but estimates varied based on data source[2,3,7-9] (**Table 1**). Estimates from otolaryngology-specific sources tend to be higher than those from other sources.[8]

Predictions of Shortages in the Workforce

Despite adequate current workforce estimates, there seems to be consensus that there is an anticipated shortage of otolaryngologists.[2,3,10,11]

The most recent and comprehensive model of the shortage and potential mitigations strategies was put forth by Kim and colleagues.[11] Three supply scenarios were modeled, taking into account population growth, demand created by increased insurance coverage with the passage of the Affordable Care Act, and the increase in gross domestic product as it relates to increases in health care spending. Assuming static otolaryngology supply ratios, they predicted various estimates of workforce need. They then modeled different workforce changes to estimate whether these would meet the needs. Manipulation of productivity, residency growth, augmentation by nurse practitioners (NPs) and physician's assistants (PAs), reducing the length of residency, and delaying retirement were all studied. Without changes in residency positions or increases in retirement age, a deficit of 2500 otolaryngologists is expected by 2025. Extending the retirement age to 75 years alleviates some of the shortage; most other measures did not make up for predicted shortfalls. These models are limited by assumptions that are largely not derived from otolaryngology-specific

Table 1
Published estimates of the otolaryngology workforce

	Data Source	Data Year	Otolaryngologists per 100,000 Population
Pillsbury et al,[7] 2000	AMA Masterfile	1997	3.36
Cannon et al,[2] 2004	Area Resource file, AMA Physicians professional data	2000 2001 2002	3.16 3.16 3.21
Williams et al,[3] 2009	ABMS certificates	2005	3.16
Hughes et al,[8] 2016	AMA self-reported specialties, ABMS, AAO-HNS, ABOto, ACS	2009–2014	3.7
AAMC Physician Specialty Reports,[9] 2018	AMA Masterfile	2017	2.92

Abbreviations: AAMC, Association of American Medical Colleges; AAO-HNS, American Academy of Otolaryngology–Head and Neck Surgery; ABMS, American Board of Medical Specialties; ABOto, American Board of Otolaryngology; ACS, American College of Surgeons; AMA, American Medical Association.
Data from Refs.[1-3,7,8]

data. In addition to the manipulations of the workforce suggested by Kim and colleagues,[11] other ways to affect the supply of the workforce may include redistributing the workforce and improving the efficiency of the current workforce with innovative practices.

Although the need-specific workforce demand may not be precisely defined by any model, it is undeniable that the demand for otolaryngic care will continue to grow as the baby boomer generation ages and the aging otolaryngology workforce plans to retire.

Residency Training

Graduating residents form the bulk of new workforce members and most heavily influence the long-term workforce supply. Over the past 14 years (2006–2020) the number of residency positions listed through the National Residency Match Program (NRMP) has grown from 264 to 350 categorical positions. Historically, otolaryngology has enjoyed a steady and competitive supply of applicants to fill these positions. However, after peak interest between 2013 and 2015, applications decreased precipitously. In 2017, an unprecedented 4.6% of positions went unfilled. In 2018, there were fewer US MD (Doctor of Medicine) senior applicants than positions, and 3.8% of positions did not fill. The 2020 match experienced a surge with 505 applicants vying for 350 positions.[12] Although the reasons for these dramatic swings in applicants is not well understood, there is renewed focus on, and commitment to, the recruitment of future otolaryngologists with emphasis on mentorship, early exposure of the specialty to medical students, and reconsidering traditional metrics that do not correlate with resident success.[13]

The long-term supply of the otolaryngology workforce is most influenced by recruiting new otolaryngologists, and the ability to readily titrate residency positions is vital to scaling the workforce. Between 2013 and 2017, the number of new residency positions only grew by 1.1% per year. Reports of larger increases between 2017 and 2020 (from 315 to 350 positions) are mostly caused by the merging of preexisting osteopathic residency programs into the NRMP match.[12] The federal government funds most graduate medical education, but funding has remained essentially stagnant since the passage of the Balanced Budget Act of 1997. There have been recent pushes to expand medical school enrollment to address projected physician shortfalls. However, these have not been accompanied by proportional increases in residency positions.[8]

Alternative methods to circumvent the residency bottleneck have been proposed, such as decreasing the duration of residency from 5 years to 4 years and reallocating the resultant year's worth of positions to expand the number of entering residents. However, this would still not completely correct projected shortfalls, and the impact on quality and competence of graduating otolaryngologists is unknown.[11]

Fellowship Training

Fellowship training affects the workforce in several important ways. It extends the training period before otolaryngologists fully enter the workforce, potentially limits the range of services fellowship-trained otolaryngologists choose to provide, and can influence practice location and scope. Many residents plan to pursue fellowship training after residency. A 2010 cross-sectional survey of otolaryngology residents found that between 40% and 60% of senior residents were interested in pursuing fellowship training; 30% to 40% of senior residents were interested in academic careers.[14] Although new otolaryngologists are interested, there may not be openings in academia. Although academic department chairs had an average of 6 new hires between 2009 and 2014, mainly because of expanding departments, most intended to hire fewer new staff in the next 5 years, and many emphasize hiring generalists rather than specialists.[15]

Meanwhile, the number of fellowship positions has been steadily growing. According to their respective subspecialty Web sites, the current total number of pediatric, laryngology, rhinology, head and neck, and neurotology fellowship positions offered is approximately 140 to 150 per year. This number does not include facial plastic and reconstructive surgery fellowships, which are sponsored both by otolaryngology and plastic surgery. Although all of these positions may not fill each year, this number represents nearly half of the graduating residency class.

A recent study by Lin and colleagues[16] noted an increase in US fellowship-trained head and neck surgeons of 1.62 per year over the last 20 years. Of these graduates, greater than 70% practice with academic affiliation and 98% practice in urban locations. Neurotology has fewer fellowship positions (23 per year) and a length of 2 years, which slows the rate of growth of new neurotologists into the workforce. However, workforce analysis of neurotologists by Vrabec[17] in 2013 concluded that the supply of neurotologists was probably already adequate and raised concerns about the surgeons' competition for case volume needed to stay proficient. In pediatric otolaryngology, fellows entered academic practice most of the time (54.7%).[18] Rhinology fellowships have grown the most dramatically, from 3 in 1996 to 29 positions in 2017.[19] The Rhinology Training Council was established in 2016 by the American Rhinologic Society (ARS) to advise the ARS Board of Directors on key criteria to ensure both trainee success and good patient outcomes.[20] In 2020, 35 training programs were listed on the Web site with several training multiple fellows per year.[21] A survey of rhinology faculty found that around 60% of faculty thought that too many fellows were being trained for the number needed for academic and private practice positions, as well as for societal need.[22]

Foreign-Trained Otolaryngologists

Foreign-trained otolaryngologists make up 7.5% of the otolaryngology workforce, which is a small, but significant, percentage.[23] Foreign-trained physicians are required to overcome numerous obstacles for the opportunity to practice in the United States and this can act as a bottleneck to expansion of the workforce. They must work through the requirements of the Educational Commission for Foreign Medical Graduates for certification, which include passing US Medical Licensing Examinations step1, both step 2 examinations, and completing a US residency. According to the NRMP, between 2007 and 2020, 53 non-US international medical graduates were accepted into otolaryngology residency positions, filling 1.3% of the total offered positions over that duration. US international medical graduates were accepted to 20 (0.5%) positions over the same time period. Although information about the practice patterns of foreign-trained otolaryngologists is not known, foreign-trained physicians in general are more likely to practice in areas with greater poverty, less education, and greater percentage of minorities.[23]

Nurse Practitioners and Physician Assistants

To cope with increased societal demands and a workforce slow to expand, increased reliance on advanced practice providers (APPs), such as NPs and PAs, may be needed. Although the total number of PAs is growing with more choosing surgical subspecialties (27% in 2013), there are few PAs within otolaryngology.[24,25] According to the National Certification Commission of Physicians Assistants, only about 1% (921) of certified PAs in 2018 practiced within otolaryngology.[26] This number results in a 10:1

ratio of otolaryngologists to otolaryngology PAs. Otolaryngology PAs are predominantly white (86.2%), female (75.5%), young (median age, 37 years), and work in office-based private practice settings (62.9%).[26] Although 12% of PAs practice in rural settings, only 5% of rural PAs work in the surgical subspecialties.[24] Less is known about NPs in otolaryngology, but the Society for Otorhinolaryngology and Head-Neck Nurses (SOHN) reports a membership of 1100 nurses.

The potential benefits of collaborative care between physicians and APPs are numerous and include increased patient access to otolaryngic care, improved physician efficiency, and improvement in quality of care. These collaborations can exist along a spectrum of collaborative arrangement from scribe to near-independent practitioner.[27,28] However, the upfront investment in training an APP for a particular practice can be significant. Scope of practice for both PAs and NPs is determined at the state level. NPs are more likely to practice independently in the 23 states in which this is allowed and regulated by the state nursing board.[29] However, even independently practicing APPs tend to perform less intensive services, potentially reducing the benefits of adding more APPs to the workforce.[11] In addition, despite the potential benefit of PAs and NPs to extend the workforce, even under the most aggressive growth conditions, increases in both NPs and PAs failed to remedy projected overall physician workforce shortages.[30]

Workforce Diversity

Otolaryngology does not reflect the diversity of the US population. For example, women are 17.1% of practicing otolaryngologists even though they comprise most of the American population. At present, women occupy 36.3% of residency positions compared with only 8.1% in 2000.[2,9] Despite their increased representation in otolaryngology, women remain underrepresented in positions of leadership at the institutional and society levels.[31–34]

Minority populations in the United States are rapidly increasing, with projections showing non-Hispanic white people will no longer be the majority as early as 2045. Among other surgical specialties, otolaryngology continues to lag behind in representation of minorities and women.[9,35,36] **(Table 2)**. Schwartz and colleagues[37] reported that annual growth rates among African American and Native American residents in otolaryngology were not statistically significant, stalling at around 2% per year. The growth rate for Hispanic Americans in otolaryngology was statistically significant, but occurring at only half the growth rate of the Hispanic American population in the United States.[37]

Improving the gender, racial, and ethnic diversity of the otolaryngology workforce is critical for providing culturally competent care to our nation's burgeoning minority communities.

Productivity

When considering workforce supply, it is assumed that each physician provides the same amount of work. However, this may not be true. Common productivity measures include full-time equivalents equal to 40 hours of work per week, or relative value units. Within otolaryngology, no robust data exist on differences in productivity measures among different sections of the workforce. However, among all US physicians, there are trends toward more part-time work now than in the past and this may vary by age and gender.[38] Younger physicians and physicians closer to retirement may be more likely to choose reduction in hours.[38] There also may be reasons to consider differences in the medical versus surgical otolaryngology workforce. In 1 large retirement

Table 2
Demographics of the otolaryngology workforce across 10 years (2007–2018) compared with all specialties and the United States population (2017)

| | 2007 | | 2017 | | |
	Otolaryngology	All Specialties	Otolaryngology	All Specialties	United States
Total	9220	764,783	9526	892,856	321 million
Female (%)	11.2	28.3	17.1	35.2	50.8
Female Residents/ Fellows (%)	27.5	44.6	36.2	45.6	—
Age>55 y (%)	41.5	37.6	47.0	44.1	27.6
Ethnicity (%)					
Asian	23.0	27.5	13.8	17.1	5.4
Black	3.0	6.3	2.4	5.0	12.7
AIAN/NHPI	0.4	0.8	0.2	1.3	1.0
White	69.0	59.8	66.5	56.2	73.0
Other/ Unknown	4.6	5.5	12.3	13.7	4.8
Hispanic	6.7	9.9	3.5	5.8	17.6

Some columns do not sum to 100% because of differences in race classification among sources.
Abbreviations: AIAN, American Indian and Alaska Native; NHPI, Native Hawaiian and Pacific Islander.
From Association of American Medical Colleges. Specialty Physician Data 2018; Association of American Medical Colleges. Diversity in Medicine: Facts and Figures 2018; American Community Survey Demographic and Housing Estimates, 5-year estimates, 2013-2017.

survey of otolaryngologists, half of respondents more than 60 years of age who were still practicing indicated that they no longer practiced in the operating room.[39]

Practice Type

The practice setting of otolaryngologists continues to change. Between 2001 and 2009, otolaryngologists moved toward group practice (37.8% to 53.4%) and away from solo practice (30.1% to 25.1%).[8] The 2017 American Academy of Otolaryngology–Head and Neck Surgery Foundation Socioeconomic Survey data suggest that around 57% of otolaryngologists are in private practice. Practice type can influence the accessibility of patients to otolaryngologists based on insurance status. Physician-scientists represent a meager proportion of otolaryngologists but are vital to the health and progress of the specialty. A report by Gail Neely and colleagues[40] found that only 127 otolaryngologists (1.2% of the workforce at the time of publication) had received funding or were currently funded by the National Institutes of Health. Key barriers to increasing the number of physician-scientists in the workforce are thought to include a lack of available research dollars, the poor integration of medical training and research training in current medical school and residency curricula, and difficulty in obtaining guidance and mentoring by early-career physician-scientists.[41]

Aging Workforce and Retirement

Mirroring the rest of the population, the otolaryngology workforce is getting older. Data from the Association of American Medical Colleges between 2007 and 2018 show that the average age of otolaryngologists is greater than the average age of physicians at large (see **Table 1**). In addition, in the last 10 years, the average age has increased in the specialty. In 2007, 41.5% of otolaryngologists were more than 55 years of age versus 47% in 2018. Older physicians more quickly exit the workforce via retirement and may further accelerate the workforce shortage.

Although the most impactful long-term influence on workforce is recruitment of new otolaryngologists, the most impactful short-term influence on workforce supply is physician retirement. Survey data suggest that the average age for retirement for otolaryngologists is around the early to mid-60s. A survey of 865 otolaryngologists was conducted in 1999 to determine their thoughts on retirement.[39] Thirteen percent of respondents planned to retire before 60 years old, 37% between 61 and 65 years, 23% between 66 and 70 years, 16% between 71% and 75%, and 11% planned to retire after 75 years old.[39] For those respondents who had already retired, 43% said the major motivator for retirement was the "hassle factor," which the investigators describe as influences of managed care, government intrusions, hospital administrative interference, and health maintenance organization influences.[39] Among reasons for retirement reported in the 2004 updated workforce report, practice hassles (59.3%) rank among the top with age (46.8%) and finances (60.7%).[2] Another survey was performed in 2002 among 138 retired otolaryngologists from the southern geographic region of the American Laryngological, Rhinological and Otological Society.[42] Among the 126 men and 12 women respondents, the average age for retirement was 63.4 years for men and 62 years for women. In workforce modeling performed by Kim and colleagues,[11] delaying retirement age to 75 years was able to meet physician shortages in some models. Judging by physician responses in these studies, this solution does not seem reasonable. However, specific information on the age of retirement of the current otolaryngology workforce is unknown.

DEMAND FOR OTOLARYNGIC CARE AND HEALTH DISPARITIES

Ensuring an adequate workforce relies on an understanding of the multifaceted need for otolaryngic care. Although it is easy to measure demand as surgeon per population size, this metric is too simple to assess the unique needs of specific populations among various geographic regions and with certain otolaryngic conditions.

Underserved Populations

Underserved populations extend beyond those physically distant from otolaryngologists. Underserved populations may face economic, cultural, linguistic, or systemic barriers to medical care. A 2017 report by Shay and colleagues[43] showed that black and Hispanic children are significantly less likely to be diagnosed with frequent ear infections, hay fever, streptococcal pharyngitis, and sinusitis compared with white children, likely owing to a disparity in health care access rather than in disease incidence. Perhaps the most robust disparities in otolaryngology have been documented with regard to head and neck cancer, where it has been shown that outcomes are affected by race and ethnicity, insurance status, and socioeconomic status.[44–46]

However, disparities are not absolved through increased access to care. Vulnerable populations are more likely to receive care that is incongruent with evidence-based practice guidelines and at low-volume centers.[47] For example, nonwhite patients and those covered by Medicaid were more likely to receive pituitary surgery at low-volume centers and were more likely to develop complications postoperatively.[48] African American patients are more likely to undergo thyroidectomy by low-volume surgeons and are less likely than white patients to undergo appropriate adjuvant radioactive iodine therapy for well-differentiated thyroid cancer.[49] The persistence of health care disparities among these vulnerable populations despite physical closeness to health care providers highlights the importance of addressing systemic sources of inequality within health care.

Geriatric Otolaryngology

According to US census data, the overall population is projected to grow 9.7% in the next 15 years.[50] Those less than 18 years old are expected to increase by 3.6%, but the population aged 65 years and older is projected to increase by 39% and those aged 85 years and older are projected to increase by 76%. Although the general increase in population affects the demand for otolaryngic care, the dramatic increase in geriatric patients gives rise to the need for a different type of care. Geriatric patients have unique needs; a host of complex medical comorbidities; different therapeutic responses; distinct treatment preferences; and other complicating cognitive, mobility, and social factors.[51] To anticipate the needs of otolaryngologists to successfully treat geriatric patients, the American Academy of Otolaryngology Head and Neck Surgery has made available educational documents on their Web site on topics unique to geriatric patients.[52] In addition, the American Society of Geriatric Otolaryngology was founded in 2007 "to promote the generation and dissemination of knowledge to benefit the geriatric patient with disorders of the ears, nose, throat, head and neck."[53]

Geographic Region

Otolaryngologists are not evenly distributed among regions of the United States and the disparity of distribution of physicians, surgeons, and otolaryngologists has been noted for decades.[1,3,7,54] In 2000, Pillsbury and colleagues[7] reported differences in supply among various regions, with estimates ranging from 2.71 per 100,000 in the southwest to 3.64 per 100,000 in the mid-Atlantic states. It continues to be true that most otolaryngologists practice in metropolitan areas. Vickery and colleagues[55] found that 61.8% of physicians worked in areas that comprised only 55.3% of the total US population and that two-thirds of US counties had no practicing otolaryngologist. Gadkaree and colleagues[54] evaluated the distribution of otolaryngologists at the county level and among hospital referral regions in 2020. Rural counties had fewer otolaryngologists per population and, on multivariable analysis, county-level otolaryngology density was positively associated with highest education quartile and highest income quartile. The concentration of otolaryngologists among high-income urban areas further exacerbates health care disparities.

Although there are known supply deficiencies among rural areas, data on population size, resource level, and insurance funding needed to sustain an otolaryngology practice are unknown. Telemedicine may alleviate some of the disparity in rural areas. Telemedicine has been practiced to reach remote locations in Alaska for many years but uptake in the continental United States does not seem to be common.[56] In Iowa, visiting consultant clinics have improved access of rural residents to otolaryngologists but this comes at a cost of high monthly driving on the part of the otolaryngologists.[57] Other creative solutions or financial incentives may be necessary to serve the otolaryngic needs of patients in rural areas.

Limitations

Several important considerations about workforce estimations and predictions are worth mentioning. Although a ratio of providers to population is easy to measure and compare, it falls short in assessing whether the workforce is adequately diverse, appropriately geographically distributed, or best equipped to care for the needs of those it is intended to serve. Second, modeling of workforce supply and demand is an inexact science and is necessarily fraught with errors in assumptions, inclusions, and omissions of known and unknown variables. Although some known variables are considered here, other unpredictable factors not discussed have the ability to change outputs considerably and include improvements in technology; changes to conditions that are within (or out of) the domain of otolaryngic care; large structural shifts in health care delivery, such as telehealth; and major changes to payment structures through policy change. Predictions of workforce supply and demand should be carefully considered within the context of these major limitations.

SUMMARY

Multiple studies and projections indicate a coming shortage of otolaryngologists, particularly in the setting of the large aging baby boomer segment of the population, which affects both need for health care services and the workforce itself. In addition, increasing equity in otolaryngology, including, but not limited to, diversity of the workforce, adequate supply of otolaryngologists versed in geriatric care, and improving access to otolaryngic care in undeserved groups, remains a critical need. Targeted efforts to address each of these issues are needed.

DISCLOSURE

The authors have nothing to disclose.

REFERENCES

1. Association of American Medical Colleges. 2019 update: the complexities of physician supply and demand: projections from 2017 to 2032. 2019. Available at: https://www.aamc.org/system/files/c/2/31-2019_update_-_the_complexities_of_physician_supply_and_demand_-_projections_from_2017-2032.pdf. Accessed April 29, 2020.
2. Cannon CR, Giaimo EM, Lee TL, et al. Special report: reassessment of the ORL-HNS workforce: perceptions and realities. Otolaryngol Head Neck Surg 2004; 131:1–15.
3. Williams TE, Satiani B, Thomas A, et al. The impending shortage and the estimated cost of training the future surgical workforce. Ann Surg 2009;250(4):590–6.
4. Bhattacharyya N. The increasing workload in head and neck surgery: an epidemiologic analysis. Laryngoscope 2011;121(1):111–5.
5. Anderson GF, Han KC, Miller RH, et al. A comparison of three methods for estimating the requirements for medical specialists: the case of otolaryngologists. Health Serv Res 1997;32(2):139–53.
6. Mulhausen R. Physician need. JAMA 1989;261(13):1930.
7. Pillsbury HC, Cannon CR, Sedory Holzer SE, et al. The workforce in otolaryngology-head and neck surgery: moving into the next millennium. Otolaryngol Head Neck Surg 2000;123(3):341–56.
8. Hughes CA, McMenamin P, Mehta V, et al. Otolaryngology workforce analysis. Laryngoscope 2016;126(December):S5–11.
9. Association of American Medical Colleges. 2018 physician specialty data report. 2018. Available at: Https://Www.Aamc.Org/Data-Reports/Workforce/Report/Physician-Specialty-Data-Report. Accessed April 29, 2020.
10. Cooper RA. There's a shortage of specialists. Is anyone listening? Acad Med 2002;77(8):761–6.

11. Kim JSC, Cooper RA, Kennedy DW. Otolaryngology-head and neck surgery physician work force issues: an analysis for future specialty planning. Otolaryngol Head Neck Surg 2012;146(2):196–202.

12. National Resident Matching Program. Results and Data 2020 Main Residency Match®. 2020. Available at: www.nrmp.org. Accessed May 7, 2020.

13. Chang CWD, Gray ST, Malekzadeh S, et al. Cultivating and recruiting future otolaryngology residents: shaping the tributary. Otolaryngol Head Neck Surg 2019;160(1):8–10.

14. Golub JS, Ossoff RH, Johns MM, et al. Fellowship and career path preferences in residents of otolaryngology-head and neck surgery. Laryngoscope 2011;121(4): 882–7.

15. Lin J, Kacker A, Trujillo O, et al. Status and trends of general otolaryngology in academia. Laryngoscope 2016;126(9):1995–8.

16. Lin Y, Patel D, Ramsey T, et al. Trends in head and neck fellowship graduates in the United States from 1997 to 2017. Head Neck 2020;42(5):1024–30.

17. Vrabec JT. Workforce analysis of neurotologists in the United States. Otol Neurotol 2013;34(4):755–61.

18. Espinel A, Poley M, Zalzal GH, et al. Trends in U.S. pediatric otolaryngology fellowship training. JAMA Otolaryngol Head Neck Surg 2015;141(10):919–22.

19. Heineman TE, Ramakrishnan V, Hwang PH, et al. Workforce analysis of practicing rhinologists in the united states. Laryngoscope 2020;130(5):1116–21.

20. Rhinology Training Council. Available at: https://www.american-rhinologic.org/ rhinology-training-council. Accessed May 7, 2020.

21. Fellowship Programs. Available at: https://www.american-rhinologic.org/ program-list. Accessed May 7, 2020.

22. Riley CA, Soneru CP, Husain Q, et al. Faculty attitudes toward rhinology fellowship training: a survey of rhinology fellowship programs. Am J Rhinol Allergy 2019;33(1):8–16.

23. American Immigration Council. Foreign-Trained Doctors Are Critical to Serving Many U.S. Communities. 2018. Available at: Https://Www.Americanimmigrationcouncil.Org/ Research/Foreign-Trained-Doctors-Are-Critical-Serving-Many-Us-Communities. Accessed April 29, 2020.

24. Cawley JF, Lane S, Smith N, et al. Physician assistants in rural communities. J Am Acad Physician Assist 2016;29(1):42–5.

25. Morgan P, Everett CM, Humeniuk KM, et al. Physician assistant specialty choice. J Am Acad Physician Assist 2016;29(7):46–52.

26. National Commission on Certification of Physician Assistants. 2018 statistical profile of certified physician assistants by specialty. 2018. Available at: https://prodcmsstoragesa. blob.core.windows.net/uploads/files/2018StatisticalProfileofCertifiedPAsbySpecialty1.pdf. Accessed May 5, 2020.

27. Reger C, Kennedy DW. Changing practice models in otolaryngology-head and neck surgery: the role for collaborative practice. Otolaryngol Head Neck Surg 2009;141:670–3.

28. Norris B, Harris T, Stringer S. Effective use of physician extenders in an outpatient otolaryngology setting. Laryngoscope 2011;121(11):2317–21.

29. State Practice Environment. Available at: https://www.aanp.org/advocacy/state/ state-practice-environment. Accessed May 5, 2020.

30. Sargen M, Hooker RS, Cooper RA. Gaps in the supply of physicians, advance practice nurses, and physician assistants. J Am Coll Surg 2011;212(6):991–9.

31. Glauser W. Rise of women in medicine not matched by leadership roles. CMAJ 2018;190(15):E479–80.

32. Litvack JR, Wick EH, Whipple ME. Trends in female leadership at high-profile otolaryngology journals, 1997-2017. Laryngoscope 2019;129(9):2031–5.

33. Eloy JA, Svider P, Chandrasekhar SS, et al. Gender disparities in scholarly productivity within academic otolaryngology departments. Otolaryngol Head Neck Surg 2013;148(2):215–22.

34. Blumenthal DM, Bergmark RW, Raol N, et al. Sex differences in faculty rank among academic surgeons in the United States in 2014. Ann Surg 2018; 268(2):193–200.

35. Ukatu CC, Welby Berra L, Wu Q, et al. The state of diversity based on race, ethnicity, and sex in otolaryngology in 2016. Laryngoscope 2019. https://doi.org/10.1002/lary.28447.

36. Association of American Medical Colleges. Diversity in medicine: facts and figures 2019. 2019. Available at: https://www.aamc.org/data-reports/workforce/report/diversity-medicine-facts-and-figures-2019. Accessed May 11, 2020.

37. Schwartz JS, Young M, Velly AM, et al. The evolution of racial, ethnic, and gender diversity in US otolaryngology residency programs. Otolaryngol Head Neck Surg 2013;149(1):71–6.

38. Staiger DO, Auerbach DI, Buerhaus PI. Trends in the work hours of physicians in the United States. JAMA 2010;303(8):747–53.

39. Ward NO, Pratt LW. Otolaryngologists older than 60 years: results of and reflections on survey responses from 865 colleagues regarding retirement. Arch Otolaryngol Head Neck Surg 1999;125(3):263–8.

40. Gail Neely J, Smith RJ, Graboyes EM, et al. Guide to academic research career development. Laryngoscope Investig Otolaryngol 2016;1(1):19–24.

41. Milewicz DM, Lorenz RG, Dermody TS, et al. Rescuing the physician-scientist workforce: the time for action is now. J Clin Invest 2015;125(10):3742–7.

42. Mcguirt WF, Mcguirt WF. Otolaryngology retirement profile in the southeastern United States. Laryngoscope 2002;112(2):213–5.

43. Shay S, Shapiro NL, Bhattacharyya N. Pediatric otolaryngologic conditions: racial and socioeconomic disparities in the United States. Laryngoscope 2017;127(3): 746–52.

44. Shin JY, Yoon JK, Shin AK, et al. The influence of insurance status on treatment and outcomes in oral cavity cancer: an analysis on 46,373 patients. Int J Oral Maxillofac Surg 2018;47(10):1250–7.

45. Thompson-Harvey A, Yetukuri M, Hansen AR, et al. Rising incidence of late-stage head and neck cancer in the United States. Cancer 2020;126(5):1090–101.

46. Pagedar NA, Davis AB, Sperry SM, et al. Population analysis of socioeconomic status and otolaryngologist distribution on head and neck cancer outcomes. Head Neck 2019;41(4):1046–52.

47. Smedley BD, Stith AY, Nelson AR. Unequal treatment: confronting racial and ethnic disparities in health care (with CD). Washington, DC: National Academies Press; 2003. https://doi.org/10.17226/12875.

48. Goljo E, Parasher AK, Iloreta AM, et al. Racial, ethnic, and socioeconomic disparities in pituitary surgery outcomes. Laryngoscope 2016;126(4):808–14.

49. Al-Qurayshi Z, Randolph GW, Srivastav S, et al. Outcomes in thyroid surgery are affected by racial, economic, and healthcare system demographics. Laryngoscope 2016;126(9):2194–9.

50. Census Bureau US. 2017 National Population Projections Datasets. Available at: Https://Www.Census.Gov/Data/Tables/2017/Demo/Popproj/2017-Summary-Tables.Html. Accessed April 29 2020.

51. Eibling D, Kost K. The emerging field of geriatric otolaryngology. Otolaryngol Clin North Am 2018;51(4):847–52.
52. Geriatric Care Otolaryngology Online. Available at: https://www.entnet.org/content/geriatric-care-otolaryngology-online. Accessed April 29, 2020.
53. American Society of Geriatric Otolaryngology. Available at: http://geriatricotolaryngology.org/. Accessed April 29, 2020.
54. Gadkaree SK, Mccarty JC, Siu J, et al. Variation in the geographic distribution of the otolaryngology workforce: a national geospatial analysis. Otolaryngol Head Neck Surg 2020;162(5):649–57.
55. Vickery TW, Weterings R, Cabrera-Muffly C. Geographic distribution of otolaryngologists in the United States. Ear Nose Throat J 2016;95(6):218–23.
56. Kokesh J, Ferguson AS, Patricoski C. The alaska experience using store-and-forward telemedicine for ENT care in alaska. Otolaryngol Clin North Am 2011;44(6):1359–74.
57. Gruca TS, Nam I, Tracy R. Reaching rural patients through otolaryngology visiting consultant clinics. Otolaryngol Head Neck Surg 2014;151(6):895–8.

Diversity and Inclusion— Why Does It Matter

Carrie L. Francis, MD*, Jennifer A. Villwock, MD

KEYWORDS

- Medical education • Diversity • Inclusion • Underrepresented in medicine

KEY POINTS

- The US population is becoming increasingly diverse. In otolaryngology, racial, ethnic, and socioeconomic disparities have been identified in adult and pediatric populations.
- Competent health care systems can improve the efficiency of staff, patient satisfaction, and outcomes of care like unnecessary testing or differences in referral patterns.
- Otolaryngology has historically lagged behind other specialties with respect to diversity, equity and inclusion and remains one of the least diverse specialties as it relates to gender, race, ethnicity and other identities.

The US population is becoming increasingly diverse. Such a nation requires a culturally competent and diverse physician workforce.[1] Minoritized communities have higher rates of disease and receive lower quality care than White people. Women of color have staggering infant mortality rates compared with their white counterparts. In otolaryngology, racial, ethnic, and socioeconomic disparities have been identified in adult and pediatric populations.[2–6] Cultural competence, diversity, equity and inclusion (DEI) alone may not be enough. Without a critical lens toward structural racism sociodemographic-based health disparities will become more pronounced.[7–9] Cultural competence values equality, acknowledges historical injustice and incorporates culture into communication, relationship buildling, and adaptation to meet unique needs.[7,10]. Structural competence values equity and focuses on the elements of health influenced by systems and policy.[8,9] Additionally, there is a growing recognition that structural competence is essential to the practice of high-quality medicine.[8,9]

Structurally competent health care systems can improve the efficiency of staff, patient satisfaction, and outcomes of care, like unnecessary testing or differences in referral or treatment patterns. The presence of cross-cultural issues, political and socioeconomic forces highlight the need to be aware of the diverse experiences of patients and how these have an impact on how care is rendered and received.[11] Concordance in racial or ethnic patient-physician relationships result in improved

Department of Otolaryngology, Head & Neck Surgery, University of Kansas Medical Center, 3901 Rainbow Boulevard, MS 3010, Kansas City, KS, USA
* Corresponding author.
E-mail address: cfrancis@kumc.edu

Otolaryngol Clin N Am 53 (2020) 927–934
https://doi.org/10.1016/j.otc.2020.05.021

perception of communication, increased patient satisfaction, and improved appropriate health care utilization.[12] Conversely, poorly handled cross-cultural issues can result in patient noncompliance, delays in obtaining consent, unnecessary tests, and lower quality of care.[13] The American College of Surgeons Code of Professional Conduct states that "a good surgeon is more than a technician," with the possession of an "altruistic commitment to each patient's unique biologic, psychological, social, cultural, and spiritual needs" a critical component of good surgical practice. The Medical Professionalism Project—initiated by the American Board of Internal Medicine Foundation, American College of Physicians Foundation, and European Federation of Internal Medicine—also includes a commitment to social justice among baseline characteristics of professionalism.[14]

Attaining diversity, equity and inclusivity (DEI) is not always instinctive. It requires careful thought so that potential biases can be addressed. A commonly heard challenge to DEI is that it is hard to define diversity in objective and easily quantifiable terms. Additionally, many aspects of diversity are closely tied to identities. Thus, prioritizing certain components of diversity can be inherently threatening if it is perceived that some aspects of identity are more worthy than others. It also challenges deeply ingrained beliefs in meritocracy. Just as no one wants their hard work and resultant achievements negated by the belief that successes are because they are the token other, no one wants to believe that their accomplishments are secondary to their privilege. Yet, studies have shown that rigid beliefs in meritocracy can exacerbate inequality—the paradox of meritocracy.[15,16] In environments that prioritize meritocracy, it is easy to prioritize the belief that one is impartial. This can lead to lack of monitoring or scrutinizing behavior—creating an environment where there is disadvantage among underrepresented groups and unfair advantage among traditionally dominant groups. This is complicated further by the fact that ideals, such as diversity and meritocracy, may be nested in broader institutional or cultural environments simultaneously characterized with bias.[17] Additionally, progress in DEI requires something that cannot be mandated: buy-in.[18] This can be difficult to achieve because it relates to the challenges, discussed previously, and more. Simply creating requirements or mandatory training will not suffice and can be counterproductive. Diversity projects devoid of practical benefits are unlikely to gain support.[19] Top-down leadership is a must. Enlist broadly, listen, be transparent and accountable, and empower with recognition and support. Those involved must understand the importance of DEI for the specialty as well as its direct link to the quality of health care otolaryngologists provide.[20]

It also is critical to keep in mind that outward appearance is not the sole component of diversity. Although minoritized groups certainly are underrepresented in medicine (URiM), so are individuals from rural backgrounds and disadvantaged backgrounds and first-in-family physicians. Otolaryngology historically has lagged behind other specialties with respect to DEI. Today, it remains one of the least diverse specialties, with women as well as racial and ethnic minorities significantly underrepresented.[12] Between 1975 and 2010, there was an increase in the number of female otolaryngology residents but minimal improvements in racially and ethnically underrepresented groups.[21] In the decade since, there have been no significant gains in gender representation, and Hispanics and African Americans continue to be the most underrepresented groups in the field.[12] In a 2020 study, women and nonwhite applicants prioritized program diversity and placed higher emphasis on racially and gender-congruent mentors compared with their white and male peers.[22] In this study, however, several subjects noted that few programs had substantial diversity, making diversity less of a consideration. Yet, would diversity be a larger consideration in applicant decision making if diverse and inclusive programs were commonplace?

Application to the field of otolaryngology is a highly competitive process that seems to intensify every year.[23] Well-intentioned desires to select the best residents likely have created a hidden curriculum, similar to that seen in medical school, where certain backgrounds, activities, and histories carry different values. For example, during the selection process, a history of success in peer-reviewed research publications is likely viewed differently from similar success in financially necessitated work outside of medicine.[24,25] It is no surprise that successful applicants to medical school are coming from increasingly affluent backgrounds.[26,27] It has been postulated that the test preparation industry has transitioned medical education from a professional aspiration, earned through effort and study, to one that can be purchased with financial investment in test and application support services.[28] Additionally, the leadership and service activities that commonly populate resumes may better reflect the privilege of the applicants rather than their potential.[1,25]

It has been suggested that rather than a *glass ceiling*, a more apt term is *glass labyrinth*. Ceiling implies a linear trajectory with an assumed obvious solution: smash through the ceiling. Similar to a labyrinth, issues common for underrepresented groups in medicine are complex and multidimensional, requiring a variety of strategies to succeed. Many women report undercurrents of bias, difficulties in navigating professional life as the "other," special challenges in managing highly gendered doctor-nurse relationships, and struggles with work-life issues.[29] Workarounds include carefully constructed elements of self to be more well received by others, reliance on nonconfrontational strategies, keeping social distance, displaying professional symbols to overtly reinforce credibility and belonging, and downplaying otherness in appearance and voice. Creation of these dual identities may not resonate with true sense of self and lead to feelings of loss of authenticity.[29] Groups traditionally URiM, especially African Americans, remain less likely to be promoted even after controlling for percentage of time in clinical duties, years as a faculty member, and measures of academic productivity. Many have described these inequities as a minority tax, a considerable barrier that makes advancement in rank and leadership, among other successes, difficult to achieve.[30–32] Additionally, minority faculty are more likely to report feelings of loneliness and isolation, leading to lower levels of career satisfaction and job retention.[33] This has long-term ramifications in terms of role modeling, mentorship, sponsorship, and ability of individuals from underrepresented groups to have an impact on institutional culture. Health systems and departments with longitudinal DEI initiatives that include the stated efforts, as well as parity in pay, have made an impact on recruitment and retention.[34]

Some people argue that the moral or ethical framework for DEI is unnecessary because the business case for DEI is supported by a preponderance of evidence of improved outcomes with increased diversity. In fields that require complex thought and problem-solving, diversity leads to greater complexity of thought, improved troubleshooting abilities, and innovations.[19] Diverse educational environments allow for opportunities to challenge stereotypes and cultural assumptions.[35] As Columbia Business School Professor Dr. Katherine Phillips notes, "diversity jolts us into cognitive action in ways the homogeneity simply does not."[36,37] Simply interacting with individuals who are different forces the entire group to prepare more comprehensively, anticipate alternative viewpoints, and expect that reaching consensus will take effort. For example, elegant social science experiments investigating the impact of group composition on problem solving consistently demonstrate the benefits of diversity. When each group member is given unique information critical to solving a murder mystery, the progress of homogenous groups is hindered by assumptions that everyone already holds the same information and shares the same perspective.[38] Additionally, simply adding social diversity makes people believe that differences in perspective might exist.[37] Simultaneously expanding and refining thought processes and taking into account diverse experiences and perspectives are critical to appropriately addressing many of the complex problems facing medicine and otolaryngology today, such as the opioid epidemic, issues of adherence to treatment recommendations, and enhanced, shared, decision-making processes between clinicians and patients. Yet, decades after the business case for DEI was made, great strides in diversity, equity, or inclusivity have not been made. There is a business case for DEI but let it not be forgotten that the lack of DEI is a moral wrong that should be addressed and eliminated. Many ethical models have been used to support the elimination of health disparity; these frameworks can be applied easily to the physician workforce. The lack of a diverse workforce can perpetuate disparity and have an impact on the health outcomes of minority groups but also decreases the health of society as a whole.[20,39]

When will we know that "enough" is being done to support and achieve DEI? Ruth Bader Ginsberg famously responded to the question of when there will be enough women on the supreme court with, "When there are nine."[40,41] The "Global Gender Gap Report 2020" by the World Economic Forum suggests that the global gender gap can be closed in just under 100 years. In North America, it is expected in 150 years.[42] Other scholars have found that racial discrimination in hiring practices has not changed in more than 25 years.[43] There continues to be work to do. Intention is only the beginning of outcomes in creating the desired outcomes—diversity, equity, and inclusion. In academic settings, to mitigate the impact of bias in hiring, it has been suggested that search committees be composed of at least 35% women.[44] All qualifications being equal, this is the threshold at which men and women are equally likely to be hired.[45] It stands to reason that similar thresholds are necessary for equity in selection of those URiM. Faculty development programs that foster mentorship facilitate a successful academic career. Additional efforts in undergraduate and graduate medical education also should be considered.[33,34] Similarly, in meta-analyses, the composition of review committees also had a significant impact on performance evaluations. When raters were all male, men were rated significantly more favorably than women. When evaluators were a mixed group of men and women, this gender bias was eliminated or women were rated more highly.[46–55] Ideally, efforts at increasing representation in decision making are paired with systematic efforts to increase awareness of the negative impact of unconscious bias on the advancement of women and other underrepresented groups.[44,45] Addressing the disparities of DEI is the responsibility of the whole. Culture change begins with leadership and progresses when a critical mass of those URiM, women and others, bring new perspectives that reshape strategy. Interventions begin by reassessing the value placed on DEI, frank communication, and the development of recruitment and retention strategies. Without responsibility and accountability for DEI efforts, it will be hard to develop and maintain a strategy. Maintaining the DEI strategy requires focusing on outcomes rather than activities. The number of DEI activities is less valuable than defining metrics that meaningfully measure progress and accountability in the achievement of these goals. Finally, know that the conversation around DEI will be ongoing. We should incorporate the same diligence and results-driven orientation to DEI that normally are reserved for daily clinical operations, research productivity, and program development.

In conclusion, a diverse nation requires a culturally competent and diverse physician workforce. Otolaryngology historically has lagged behind other specialties with respect to DEI and remains one of the least diverse specialties, with women and racial/ethnic minorities significantly underrepresented. Without active discourse around DEI, there remains a barrier for URiM undergraduate and graduate students and URiM faculty development and achievement. Similar to a labyrinth, issues common for underrepresented groups in medicine are complex and multidimensional, requiring a variety of strategies to succeed. Strategies aimed at increasing DEI include programs designed to provide mentorship, coaching, and sponsorship. Pipeline efforts, inclusivity on committees, bidirectional communication, and equal pay are additional DEI inclusion efforts that have been successful in increasing URiM representation. Closing the diversity gap is a long-term process; although action should be taken daily and progress measured regularly, culture changes slowly. Focus on performance and promotion. Finally, accept feedback and use it to make refinements—opportunities exist to continually improve diversity, equity, and inclusion efforts.

DISCLOSURE

The authors have nothing to disclose.

REFERENCES

1. Steinecke A, Beaudreau J, Bletzinger RB, et al. Race-neutral admission approaches: Challenges and opportunities for medical schools. Acad Med 2007; 82(2):117–26.
2. Shay S, Shapiro NL, Bhattacharyya N. Pediatric otolaryngologic conditions: Racial and socioeconomic disparities in the United States. Laryngoscope 2017;127(3):746–52.
3. Smith DF, Boss EF. Racial/ethnic and socioeconomic disparities in the prevalence and treatment of otitis media in children in the United States. Laryngoscope 2010; 120(11):2306–12.
4. Ruthberg JS, Khan HA, Knusel KD, et al. Health disparities in the access and cost of health care for otolaryngologic conditions. Otolaryngol Head Neck Surg 2020; 162(4):479–88.
5. Nocon CC, Ajmani GS, Bhayani MK. A contemporary analysis of racial disparities in recommended and received treatment for head and neck cancer. Cancer 2020;126(2):381–9.
6. Suen JJ, Marrone N, Han H-R, et al. Translating public health practices: community-based approaches for addressing hearing health care disparities. Semin Hear 2019;40(1):37–48.
7. Ly CL, Chun MBJ. Welcome to cultural competency: surgery's efforts to acknowledge diversity in residency training. J Surg Educ 2013;70(2):284–90.
8. Metzl JM, Roberts DE. Structural competency meets structural racism: race, politics, and the structure of medical knowledge. Virtual Mentor 2014;16(9):674–90.
9. Metzl JM, Hansen H. Structural competency: theorizing a new medical engagement with stigma and inequality. Soc Sci Med 2014;103:126–33.
10. Simonsen KA, Shim RS. Embracing diversity and inclusion in psychiatry leadership. Psychiatr Clin North Am 2019;42(3):463–71.
11. Sullivan LW. Missing persons: minorities in the health professions, a report of the sullivan commission on diversity in the healthcare workforce. drum.lib.umd.edu. 2004. Available at: https://drum.lib.umd.edu/handle/1903/22267. Accessed April 13, 2020.

12. Ukatu CC, Welby Berra L, Wu Q, et al. The state of diversity based on race, ethnicity, and sex in otolaryngology in 2016. Laryngoscope 2019. https://doi.org/10.1002/lary.28447.

13. Weissman JS, Betancourt J, Campbell EG, et al. Resident physicians' preparedness to provide cross-cultural care. JAMA 2005;294(9):1058–67.

14. ABIM Foundation. American Board of Internal Medicine, ACP-ASIM Foundation. American College of Physicians-American Society of Internal Medicine, European Federation of Internal Medicine.. Medical professionalism in the new millennium: a physician charter. Ann Intern Med 2002;136(3):243–6.

15. Castilla EJ. Gender, race, and meritocracy in organizational careers. AJS 2008; 113(6):1479–526.

16. Castilla EJ, Benard S. The paradox of meritocracy in organizations. Adm Sci Q 2010;55(4):543–676.

17. Hallock VH. Perceptions of the professoriate: anticipatory socialization of undergraduate students from underrepresented groups 2003. Available at: https://surface.syr.edu/cfe_etd/21/. Accessed April 20, 2020.

18. Betancourt JR, Green AR. Commentary: linking cultural competence training to improved health outcomes: perspectives from the field. Acad Med 2010;85(4): 583–5.

19. Hayes D. Point: Introducing Diversity Into a Medical Group: How to Do It and Why. J Am Coll Radiol 2015;12(9):972–4.

20. Chapman EN, Kaatz A, Carnes M. Physicians and implicit bias: how doctors may unwittingly perpetuate health care disparities. J Gen Intern Med 2013;28(11): 1504–10.

21. Schwartz JS, Young M, Velly AM, et al. The evolution of racial, ethnic, and gender diversity in US otolaryngology residency programs. Otolaryngol Head Neck Surg 2013;149(1):71–6.

22. Fairmont I, Farrell N, Johnson AP, et al. Influence of gender and racial diversity on the otolaryngology residency match. Otolaryngol Head Neck Surg 2020;162(3): 290–5.

23. Bowe SN, Schmalbach CE, Laury AM. The state of the otolaryngology match: a review of applicant trends, "impossible" qualifications, and implications. Otolaryngol Head Neck Surg 2017;156(6):985–90.

24. Hafferty FW, Franks R. The hidden curriculum, ethics teaching, and the structure of medical education. Acad Med 1994;69(11):861–71.

25. Hafferty FW. Beyond curriculum reform: confronting medicine's hidden curriculum. Acad Med 1998;73(4):403–7.

26. Fan APC, Chen C-H, Su T-P, et al. The association between parental socioeconomic status (SES) and medical students' personal and professional development. Ann Acad Med Singapore 2007;36(9):735–42.

27. Le HH. The socioeconomic diversity gap in medical education. Acad Med 2017; 92(8):1071.

28. McGaghie WC, Downing SM, Kubilius R. What is the impact of commercial test preparation courses on medical examination performance? Teach Learn Med 2004;16(2):202–11.

29. Pingleton SK, Jones EVM, Rosolowski TA, et al. Silent bias: challenges, obstacles, and strategies for leadership development in academic medicine-lessons from oral histories of women professors at the University of Kansas. Acad Med 2016;91(8):1151–7.

30. Rodríguez JE, Campbell KM, Pololi LH. Addressing disparities in academic medicine: what of the minority tax? BMC Med Educ 2015;15:6.

31. Campbell KM, Rodríguez JE. Addressing the minority tax: perspectives from two diversity leaders on building minority faculty success in academic medicine. Acad Med 2019;94(12):1854–7.

32. Carson TL, Aguilera A, Brown SD, et al. A seat at the table: strategic engagement in service activities for early-career faculty from underrepresented groups in the academy. Acad Med 2019;94(8):1089–93.

33. Nivet MA. Minorities in academic medicine: review of the literature. J Vasc Surg 2010;51(4 Suppl):53S–8S.

34. Lin SY, Francis HW, Minor LB, et al. Faculty diversity and inclusion program outcomes at an academic otolaryngology department. Laryngoscope 2016;126(2): 352–6.

35. Cohen JJ. The consequences of premature abandonment of affirmative action in medical school admissions. JAMA 2003;289(9):1143–9.

36. Levine SR. Diversity confirmed to boost innovation and financial results. Forbes Magazine 2020. Available at: https://www.forbes.com/sites/forbesinsights/2020/01/15/diversity-confirmed-to-boost-innovation-and-financial-results/. Accessed April 13, 2020.

37. Phillips KW. How diversity makes us smarter. Sci Am 2014. https://doi.org/10.1038/scientificamerican1014-42.

38. Phillips KW, Northcraft GB, Neale MA. Surface-level diversity and decision-making in groups: when does deep-level similarity help? Group Process Intergroup Relat 2006;9(4):467–82.

39. Jones CM. The moral problem of health disparities. Am J Public Health 2010; 100(Suppl 1):S47–51.

40. Lovelace by R. Ruth Bader Ginsburg: "There will be enough women on the Supreme Court when there are nine." Washington Examiner. 2017. Available at: https://www.washingtonexaminer.com/ruth-bader-ginsburg-there-will-be-enough-women-on-the-supreme-court-when-there-are-nine. Accessed April 22, 2020.

41. NewsHour PBS. When will there be enough women on the Supreme Court? Justice Ginsburg answers that question. PBS NewsHour. 2015. Available at: https://www.pbs.org/newshour/show/justice-ginsburg-enough-women-supreme-court. Accessed April 22, 2020.

42. World Economic Forum. Global gender gap report 2020. 2019. Available at: http://www3.weforum.org/docs/WEF_GGGR_2020.pdf.

43. Quillian L, Pager D, Hexel O, et al. Meta-analysis of field experiments shows no change in racial discrimination in hiring over time. Proc Natl Acad Sci U S A 2017; 114(41):10870–5.

44. Carnes M, Bland C. Viewpoint: A challenge to academic health centers and the National Institutes of Health to prevent unintended gender bias in the selection of clinical and translational science award leaders. Acad Med 2007;82(2):202–6.

45. Yoder JD, Crumpton PL, Zipp JF. The power of numbers in influencing hiring decisions. Gend Soc 1989;3(2):269–76.

46. Bowen CC, Swim JK, Jacobs RR. Evaluating gender biases on actual job performance of real people: a meta-analysis1. J Appl Soc Psychol 2000;20(10): 2194–215.

47. Eagly AH, Karau SJ, Makhijani MG. Gender and the effectiveness of leaders: a meta-analysis. Psychol Bull 1995;117(1):125.

48. Bickel J, Wara D, Atkinson BF, et al. Increasing women's leadership in academic medicine: report of the AAMC Project Implementation Committee. Acad Med 2002;77(10):1043–61.

49. Brown FW, Moshavi D. Herding academic cats: faculty reactions to transformational and contingent reward leadership by department chairs. Journal of Leadership & Organizational Studies 2002;8(3):79–93.
50. Eagly AH, Johannesen-Schmidt MC, van Engen ML. Transformational, transactional, and laissez-faire leadership styles: a meta-analysis comparing women and men. Psychol Bull 2003;129(4):569–91.
51. Rosser VJ. Faculty and staff members' perceptions of effective leadership: are there differences between women and men leaders? Equity Excell Educ 2003; 36(1):71–81.
52. Eagly AH, Karau SJ. Role congruity theory of prejudice toward female leaders. Psychol Rev 2002;109(3):573–98.
53. Heilman ME, Wallen AS, Fuchs D, et al. Penalties for success: reactions to women who succeed at male gender-typed tasks. J Appl Psychol 2004;89(3):416–27.
54. Lowery BS, Hardin CD, Sinclair S. Social influence effects on automatic racial prejudice. J Pers Soc Psychol 2001;81(5):842–55.
55. Hassett JM, Zinnerstrom K, Nawotniak RH, et al. Utilization of standardized patients to evaluate clinical and interpersonal skills of surgical residents. Surgery 2006;140(4):633–8 [discussion: 638–9].

UNITED STATES POSTAL SERVICE®
Statement of Ownership, Management, and Circulation
(All Periodicals Publications Except Requester Publications)

1. Publication Title	2. Publication Number	3. Filing Date
OTOLARYNGOLOGIC CLINICS OF NORTH AMERICA	466 – 550	9/18/2020

4. Issue Frequency	5. Number of Issues Published Annually	6. Annual Subscription Price
FEB, APR, JUN, AUG, OCT, DEC	6	$424.00

7. Complete Mailing Address of Known Office of Publication (Not printer) (Street, city, county, state, and ZIP+4®)

ELSEVIER INC.
230 Park Avenue, Suite 800
New York, NY 10169

Contact Person
Malathi Samayan

Telephone (Include area code)
91-44-4299-4507

8. Complete Mailing Address of Headquarters or General Business Office of Publisher (Not printer)

ELSEVIER INC.
230 Park Avenue, Suite 800
New York, NY 10169

9. Full Names and Complete Mailing Addresses of Publisher, Editor, and Managing Editor (Do not leave blank)

Publisher (Name and complete mailing address)

TAYLOR BALL, ELSEVIER INC.
1600 JOHN F KENNEDY BLVD. SUITE 1800
PHILADELPHIA, PA 19103-2899

Editor (Name and complete mailing address)

STACY EASTMAN, ELSEVIER INC.
1600 JOHN F KENNEDY BLVD. SUITE 1800
PHILADELPHIA, PA 19103-2899

Managing Editor (Name and complete mailing address)

PATRICK MANLEY, ELSEVIER INC.
1600 JOHN F KENNEDY BLVD. SUITE 1800
PHILADELPHIA, PA 19103-2899

10. Owner (Do not leave blank. If the publication is owned by a corporation, give the name and address of the corporation immediately followed by the names and addresses of all stockholders owning or holding 1 percent or more of the total amount of stock. If not owned by a corporation, give the names and addresses of the individual owners. If owned by a partnership or other unincorporated firm, give its name and address as well as those of each individual owner. If the publication is published by a nonprofit organization, give its name and address.)

Full Name	Complete Mailing Address
WHOLLY OWNED SUBSIDIARY OF REED/ELSEVIER, US HOLDINGS	1600 JOHN F KENNEDY BLVD. SUITE 1800 PHILADELPHIA, PA 19103-2899

11. Known Bondholders, Mortgagees, and Other Security Holders Owning or Holding 1 Percent or More of Total Amount of Bonds, Mortgages, or Other Securities. If none, check box ➤ ☐ None

Full Name	Complete Mailing Address
N/A	

12. Tax Status (For completion by nonprofit organizations authorized to mail at nonprofit rates) (Check one)
The purpose, function, and nonprofit status of this organization and the exempt status for federal income tax purposes:
☒ Has Not Changed During Preceding 12 Months
☐ Has Changed During Preceding 12 Months (Publisher must submit explanation of change with this statement)

PS Form 3526, July 2014 [Page 1 of 4 (see instructions page 4)] PSN: 7530-01-000-9931 PRIVACY NOTICE: See our privacy policy on www.usps.com

---

13. Publication Title	14. Issue Date for Circulation Data Below
OTOLARYNGOLOGIC CLINICS OF NORTH AMERICA	JUNE 2020

15. Extent and Nature of Circulation			Average No. Copies Each Issue During Preceding 12 Months	No. Copies of Single Issue Published Nearest to Filing Date
a. Total Number of Copies (Net press run)			287	230
b. Paid Circulation (By Mail and Outside the Mail)	(1)	Mailed Outside-County Paid Subscriptions Stated on PS Form 3541 (Include paid distribution above nominal rate, advertiser's proof copies, and exchange copies)	144	113
	(2)	Mailed In-County Paid Subscriptions Stated on PS Form 3541 (Include paid distribution above nominal rate, advertiser's proof copies, and exchange copies)	0	0
	(3)	Paid Distribution Outside the Mails Including Sales Through Dealers and Carriers, Street Vendors, Counter Sales, and Other Paid Distribution Outside USPS®	101	69
	(4)	Paid Distribution by Other Classes of Mail Through the USPS (e.g. First-Class Mail®)	0	0
c. Total Paid Distribution (Sum of 15b (1), (2), (3), and (4))			245	182
d. Free or Nominal Rate Distribution (By Mail and Outside the Mail)	(1)	Free or Nominal Rate Outside-County Copies included on PS Form 3541	22	28
	(2)	Free or Nominal Rate In-County Copies Included on PS Form 3541	0	0
	(3)	Free or Nominal Rate Copies Mailed at Other Classes Through the USPS (e.g. First-Class Mail)	0	0
	(4)	Free or Nominal Rate Distribution Outside the Mail (Carriers or other means)	0	0
e. Total Free or Nominal Rate Distribution (Sum of 15d (1), (2), (3) and (4))			22	28
f. Total Distribution (Sum of 15c and 15e)			267	210
g. Copies not Distributed (See Instructions to Publishers #4 (page 3))			20	20
h. Total (Sum of 15f and g)			287	230
i. Percent Paid (15c divided by 15f times 100)			91.76%	86.66%

* If you are claiming electronic copies, go to line 16 on page 3. If you are not claiming electronic copies, skip to line 17 on page 3.

16. Electronic Copy Circulation	Average No. Copies Each Issue During Preceding 12 Months	No. Copies of Single Issue Published Nearest to Filing Date
a. Paid Electronic Copies ➤		
b. Total Paid Print Copies (Line 15c) + Paid Electronic Copies (Line 16a) ➤		
c. Total Print Distribution (Line 15f) + Paid Electronic Copies (Line 16a) ➤		
d. Percent Paid (Both Print & Electronic Copies) (16b divided by 16c × 100) ➤		

☒ I certify that 50% of all my distributed copies (electronic and print) are paid above a nominal price.

17. Publication of Statement of Ownership
☒ If the publication is a general publication, publication of this statement is required. Will be printed
in the October 2020 issue of this publication.
☐ Publication not required.

18. Signature and Title of Editor, Publisher, Business Manager, or Owner

Malathi Samayan

Malathi Samayan - Distribution Controller

Date 9/18/2020

I certify that all information furnished on this form is true and complete. I understand that anyone who furnishes false or misleading information on this form or who omits material or information requested on the form may be subject to criminal sanctions (including fines and imprisonment) and/or civil sanctions (including civil penalties).

PS Form 3526, July 2014 (Page 3 of 4) PRIVACY NOTICE: See our privacy policy on www.usps.com

Printed and bound by CPI Group (UK) Ltd, Croydon, CR0 4YY

13/10/2024

01773588-0001